WITHDRAWN

Specialist Training in
NEUROLOGY

This book is due for return on or before the last date shown below.

Commissioning Editor: Timothy Horne
Development Editor: Hannah Kenner
Project Manager: Elouise Ball
Design Direction: George Ajayi
Illustrator: Robert Britton
Illustration Manager: Bruce Hogarth

Specialist Training in
NEUROLOGY

R. Jon L. Walters BSc MBBS MD MRCP

Consultant Neurologist
Department of Neurology
Morriston Hospital
Swansea, Wales, UK

Adrian Wills BSc(Hons) MBBS MD FRCP MMed Sci

Consultant Neurologist
Queen's Medical Centre
Nottingham, UK

Philip Smith MD FRCP

Consultant Neurologist
University Hospital of Wales
Cardiff, Wales, UK

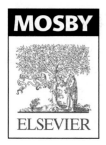

MOSBY
ELSEVIER

Edinburgh   London   New York   Oxford   Philadelphia   St Louis   Sydney   Toronto 2007

MOSBY
ELSEVIER

First published 2007

ISBN-13: 978-0-7234-3390-3
ISBN-10: 0-7234-3390-9

British Library Cataloguing in Publication Data
A catalogue record for this book is available from the British Library

Library of Congress Cataloging in Publication Data
A catalog record for this book is available from the Library of Congress

Notice
Knowledge and best practice in this field are constantly changing. As new research and experience broaden our knowledge, changes in practice, treatment and drug therapy may become necessary or appropriate. Readers are advised to check the most current information provided (i) on procedures featured or (ii) by the manufacturer of each product to be administered, to verify the recommended dose or formula, the method and duration of administration, and contraindications. It is the responsibility of the practitioner, relying on their own experience and knowledge of the patient, to make diagnoses, to determine dosages and the best treatment for each individual patient, and to take all appropriate safety precautions. To the fullest extent of the law, neither the Publisher nor the Authors assume any liability for any injury and/or damage to persons or property arising out or related to any use of the material contained in this book.

The Publisher

 your source for books,
journals and multimedia
in the health sciences

www.elsevierhealth.com

The
Publisher's
policy is to use
paper maufactured
from sustainable forests

Printed in China

Preface

Observe, record, tabulate, communicate. Use your five senses … Learn to see, learn to hear, learn to feel, learn to smell, and know that by practice alone you can become expert
William Osler

Specialist Training in Neurology is primarily intended for trainees in neurology and related specialities. The book is suited to either occasional browsing or reading end to end. We have emphasized clinical rather than theoretical neurology, and where possible used bullet points, text boxes and diagrams to clarify the text. Each chapter begins with an illustrative case history and ends with a list of key learning points. The book is lavishly illustrated and has been rigorously edited. A book of this size and weight can never be comprehensive; but it is an overall guide to clinical practice, and a stimulus for self-directed learning.

Clinical neurology demands intellectual rigour, attention to detail, good communication and history-taking skills and the capacity to reappraise all the evidence in the light of new information. This book emphasizes all these qualities as well as providing a wealth of clinically relevant information. The combining of these skills with compassion, intuition and experience distinguishes the great neurologist from the rest. These characteristics cannot be imbibed by reading any number of books. However, the authors have a wealth of clinical experience and have tried to convey their enthusiasm for the subject as well as highlighting many 'smart handles', previously only available to the cognoscenti!

We hope that you find reading this book as educational as we did writing it.

RJLW
AW
PS

Contents

The neurological consultation

1

The art of medicine remains the art of identifying the patient's problem – which is something more than merely diagnosing the disease

Sir Douglas Black, 1998

INTRODUCTION

The structure of an ideal consultation is outlined in Box 1.1. This is founded on several important principles:

- **Patient centredness.** The patient, not the clinician, should determine the content and pace of the consultation.
- **Active listening** is the clinician's main role in the consultation.
- **Patient perspective.** To understand the patient's illness involves more than knowing their symptoms. Remember that what is routine for you may be a major and frightening event for a patient; they might remember this day for the rest of their lives.
- **Clear and detailed documentation** is essential, especially in chronic conditions. Every page should have the patient's name and hospital number and each entry dated and signed.

HISTORY TAKING

Despite the emphasis upon physical examination in teaching and postgraduate examinations and notwithstanding the importance of neurological investigations, detailed and empathic history taking remains central to clinical neurology (Box 1.2). Targeting the history to specific conditions is emphasized in each chapter of this book.

Preparation

- **Reading notes.** Although it is good practice to read the referral letter and notes before the consultation, it is a mistake to assume the patient's presenting complaint. In review consultations, the patient's agenda may differ markedly from that inferred from previous notes.

Box 1.1: Consultation framework (adapted from the Calgary–Cambridge observation guide)

1. Opening
- Establish rapport:
  - Greet and obtain patient's name.
  - Introduce self and clarify role.
  - Demonstrate interest and respect, attend to patient's physical comfort.
- Identify reasons for the consultation:
  - Opening question, e.g. 'What would you like to discuss?'
  - Listen attentively to the patient's opening statement without interrupting or directing the patient's response.
  - Screen: check and confirm the problem list, e.g. 'So that's headaches and tiredness: is there anything else you would like to discuss?'

2. Information gathering
- Explore problems:
  - Patient's narrative: encourage patient to describe each problem in own words.
  - Question style: move appropriately from open to closed questions (coning in).
  - Listen attentively and allow patient to complete statements without interrupting and allow silences.
  - Facilitate responses using encouragement, silence, repetition, paraphrasing, interpretation.
  - Clarify, e.g. 'Could you explain what you mean by light-headed?'
  - Summarize periodically to verify own understanding: this invites patient's correct interpretation and provides further information.
- Understand the patient's perspective:
  - Beliefs, concerns, expectations, verbal and non-verbal cues.
- Provide structure to the consultation:
  - Summarize, signpost, sequence, keep interview on task.

3. Explaining and planning
- Provide the correct amount and type of information including 'chunking and checking'.
- Aid accurate recall and understanding, including organizing explanation into discrete sections, signposting, repetition and summarizing.
- Achieve a shared understanding: incorporating the patient's perspective and relating to previously elicited ideas, concerns and expectations.
- Planning: shared decision making, make suggestions rather than directives, negotiate and offer choices.

4. Closing
- Summarize the session briefly and clarify plan of care.
- Contract with patient re the next steps for patient and clinician.
- Safety netting: explain possible unexpected outcomes, what to do and where to seek help.
- Final check that patient agrees and is comfortable with the plan and ask if any corrections, questions or other items to discuss.

- **Optimize interaction.** Arrange the room for the patient's comfort and dignity. Try their chair beforehand to see their viewpoint. Right-handed clinicians prefer patients on the left side of the desk to allow writing while turned towards them.
- **Phone/bleep.** Within reason, you should not be available for phone, bleep or other interruptions during a consultation.
- **Focus.** Clear your head before the patient comes in. It is their time and you should not still be thinking about the last case.
- **Trainees** risk some patient disappointment that they are seeing the deputy and not the chief; rising to this challenge through a detailed and structured consultation is satisfying for both patient and clinician.
- **Greet** your patient, be welcoming and positive; shaking hands is not obligatory.

Box 1.2: Aids to neurology history taking

1. Facilitate the history by giving patients space and time to tell their story: resist shaping the story to fit preconceived ideas.
2. Minimize interruptions and value silences: let patients tell their story in their own way.
3. Use open questions: the answers are far more meaningful than those to closed questions.
4. Use the patient's own words when documenting the history: paraesthesiae is not the same as tingling.
5. Clarify non-specific terms such as dizziness (spinning vs light-headed) or numbness (loss of feeling vs weakness).
6. When giving an opinion on a patient, do not accept other clinicians' histories or diagnoses: hearing the story first hand is much more revealing.
7. Value seemingly throwaway lines: 'it's probably not important but …', or lines delivered with a laugh, denote history details of importance to the patient.
8. Do not blame the patient for an inadequate history: 'poor historian' often means impatient or hurried clinician.
9. 'What would you like to ask?' discloses more concerns than, 'Do you have any questions?'
10. Last words: important concerns may emerge after the discussion, e.g. fear of brain tumour or Alzheimer's disease.

Opening

The clinician's opening statement influences the whole consultation. Start with an open question ('What would you like to discuss?' or 'Please tell me about your symptoms'), not a closed one ('How long have you had headaches?'). Follow this by silence and (preferably non-verbal) encouragement to allow the patient to express their symptoms and concerns uninterrupted. Open questions with active listening and encouraged silences are less stressful for the patient (no barrage of questions) and for the clinician (not constantly having to think of the next question).

Exploring

After the patient's opening response, questions can become increasingly closed (coning in) to explore individual symptoms, e.g. 'Did you feel tired afterwards?' However, information provided spontaneously is far more valuable than the answers to closed questions. Silences are an important part of history taking, allowing the patient time to think, unpressured, and to voice concerns.

Understanding the patient's perspective, e.g. asking what they consider the cause of their symptoms, is often revealing and may give unexpected insights into their problem and agenda. An explanation and management plan taking account of the patient perspective is more likely to be accepted and followed.

Summarizing information obtained during the consultation is a useful technique, ensuring adequate understanding and often prompting disclosure of more information.

Past, family and social history

Any neurological symptom must be set into the context of the previous and family history and social background.

Handedness

Although traditionally asked at the start of a neurological consultation, this is a rather distracting first question for a patient anxious to tell their story. It needs to be asked, but later.

EXAMINATION

General points

- Most people think (wrongly) that neurologists reach diagnoses by detailed neurological examination. In fact, the history is their main focus and the examination is of more limited value (Box 1.3).
- Physical examination alone rarely provides the diagnosis, but can confirm hypotheses generated by the history. With no diagnosis after the history, it is likely that none will be reached following the examination.
- Neurological examinations are usually focussed; a 'full neurological examination' is almost never done on any one patient. To know what to include, trainee neurologists must acquire experience in examining every aspect in detail through repetition and supervision.
- Examination tools: Neurologists should possess a portable examination set, especially if visiting other units. This should include stethoscope, ophthalmoscope (with otoscope), pen-torch, tendon hammer, cotton wool, disposable sensory testing pins, a two-point discriminator, a red topped (blunted) pin for visual fields, a visual acuity chart, tuning forks (128 and 256 Hz), spare batteries and alcohol wipes for instruments.
- Full exposure of the relevant area is important. Remember that the upper limbs include the shoulders and scapulae and the lower limbs include buttocks and lower spine.
- You should consider the need for a chaperone for every consultation, particularly if examining an intimate area, and document this in the notes.
- Wash or wipe your hands after every examination and be seen to do so. In the intensive care unit (ICU) or barrier nursed cases, you should also use alcohol wipes on your instruments.
- Summarize physical signs using neurology shorthand, e.g. spastic paraparesis (or paraplegia if complete) with sensory level at T10; asymmetrical flaccid tetraparesis R > L; left spastic hemiparesis; flaccid monoparesis right arm.

Conscious level

In patients with disordered consciousness, it is essential to quantify the problem using the Glasgow Coma Scale (see Ch. 6).

Box 1.3: *Neurological examination: limitations*

1. The diagnosis usually comes from the history: regard the examination as the first and only essential investigation.
2. If you have no neurological diagnosis after the history, you are unlikely to reach it at all: consider continuing the history during the examination.
3. The diagnosis and management plan are usually clear from the history alone: however remember that patients are often more impressed by the examination and investigations.
4. Examination is easier to teach and to assess: postgraduate examinations therefore emphasize examination more than history.
5. Most patients attending a neurology clinic have a normal examination: this surprises non-neurologists who think neurologists deal mainly with abnormal neurological signs.
6. Neurological signs without corresponding symptoms are usually unimportant: this principle does not apply to other disciplines, e.g. cardiology, where signs without symptoms are common.
7. Non-organic signs are common in neurology: do not assume them to mean that the patient does not have an organic problem as well.
8. Undressing patients in preparation for the examination before the history is a self-defeating surgical trait: patients give better histories when comfortable, secure and fully dressed.
9. Reserve discussion of the diagnosis until after examination: although examination often adds little, the patient, who values the examination highly, might feel you are jumping to conclusions.
10. Neurological examination can be performed without a history: however you should reserve this for life-threatening situations such as the patient in coma or professional examinations.

Higher mental function

Arousal and attention

It is essential to assess arousal and attention in all patients before testing other domains. Useful tests include serial 7s, digit span forwards (normal 7 ± 2); months of the year forwards and backwards; orientation in time (normal is within 4 h for the time of day) and place. Loss of orientation in person implies a psychiatric problem. Slow speed of accomplishing these tasks suggests a subcortical process.

Note: Alzheimer patients may appear disorientated in time and place owing to memory difficulties.

Language

Spontaneous speech, e.g. describe a magazine page: is the speech fluent?

Comprehension: follow instructions, e.g. 'touch your nose'; the three-object test; understanding a simple sentence, e.g. is a hammer good for cutting wood?

Reading aloud and writing: this can identify surface dyslexia, e.g. pronouncing PINT to rhyme with MINT, suggesting a semantic dementia.

Repetition: e.g. repeat 'no ifs ands or buts' will identify dysphasia.

Other language abnormalities may be noted in the patient's speech, especially in frontotemporal dementias.

- Echolalia: repetition of other people's words.
- Echopraxia: copying examiner's movements.

- Palilalia: repetition of own words.
- Logoclonia: repetition of a final syllable.
- Speech stereotypies: e.g. repeating phrases, regularizing verbs, e.g. 'falled' instead of 'fell'.
- Paraphasias may be phonemic (similar sounding word substitute) or semantic (incorrect word).

Memory testing

Declarative memory (see Ch. 2):

- **Working (immediate) memory:** repeat and remember a list of objects:
  - With three objects, normal people register and repeat all three and recall all three after 5 min.
  - With 8–10 objects, normal people recall all objects after 3–5 attempts and repeats.
  - After 10–15 min, normal people recall two-thirds of the list.
- **Episodic memory** (autobiographical, time and place related). Ask for recall of past experiences, e.g. that holiday in Majorca.
- **Semantic memory** (for facts and word meaning unrelated to time or place). Ask for interpretation of a word, e.g. 'What is a river?'
- **Non-verbal memory:** test visual memory by recall of a diagram, e.g. the Rey–Osterrieth complex figure.

Non-declarative (skill or procedural) memory:

e.g. for playing sport. Problems here will be evident from the history.

Note: the term 'short-term memory' means different things to different people and is best avoided.

Calculation

Serial 7s. Subtract 7 from 100 and continue. This test result depends on educational background.

Frontal lobe cognitive function

Patients with suspected frontal lobe dementia (see Ch. 6) require more detailed frontal lobe function examination.

- **Initiation**
  - Category fluency: e.g. generating names of animals (normal 18 ± 6 in 1 min).
  - Phonemic fluency: e.g. generating words beginning with letters F, A and S (normal 15 ± 5 in 1 min).

Category fluency is normally easier than phenomic fluency. However, in semantic dementias, this is reversed.

- **Similarities and differences**, e.g. what is the similarity/difference between a child and a dwarf, or between a poem and a statue?
- **Abstraction**, e.g. proverb interpretation ('A rolling stone gathers no moss').
- **Cognitive estimates (judgement)**, e.g. how long is your spine? 'How fast do racehorses gallop?'

Frontal disinhibition reflexes

- **Visual rooting reflex:** ask the patient to look at a tendon hammer head brought towards the mouth. The mouth opens and the lips follow the hammer moved to the side.
- **Tactile rooting reflex:** draw the tendon hammer handle laterally across the upper or lower lip; the lips move and the mouth opens in that direction.
- **Palmomental reflex:** draw the tendon hammer handle medially across the palm and observe elevation of the ipsilateral lower lip.
- **Grasp reflex:** draw two fingers medially across the patient's palm: the patient grasps the fingers involuntarily without being asked to do so.

Note the **pout reflex** (myotactic stretch reflex) elicited by tapping the upper or lower lip and observing for lip protrusion is a sign of facial hyper-reflexia and not specifically of frontal dysfunction.

Non-dominant hemisphere testing

Disorders of the non-dominant hemisphere are very disabling, but may be difficult to appreciate because language and memory are usually normal. Right-sided parietal lobe damage typically presents with impaired visuospatial skills. Tests specific for non-dominant function should include the following:

- **Dyspraxia.** This is the inability to perform a task despite otherwise normal neurological function. For example, in upper limb dyspraxia, tone, strength, reflexes, sensation are normal, yet the patient cannot organize complex actions on command. Ideomotor dyspraxia tests include:
  - Transitive tasks (using tools), e.g. mime cutting bread, or using a hammer.
  - Intransitive tasks (gestural), e.g. wave goodbye, thumb a lift, or shadow box. Transitive tasks are usually affected before intransitive ones.
- **Agnosia.** 'Gnosis' is the organization of sensory information, allowing recognition of a shape, face or object. Agnosia (not knowing) often relates to bilateral temporal and occipital damage. Generally, memory about an object is preserved; touching or smelling it may enable patients to name it.
  - Astereognosis is the inability to recognize a shape or object placed in the hand, despite intact position sense, pinprick sensation and two-point discrimination.
  - Prosopagnosia, inability to recognize faces, is usually due to a right-sided lesion.
  - Agraphaesthesia is an inability to recognize a number or shape from the feeling of it being drawn on the hand with the eyes closed.
  - Anosognosia is a lack of insight into agnosia, i.e. they do not know that they do not know.
- **Inattention or neglect** may be identified during visual field testing. Does the head only look to the right, ignoring items and people to the left? It may be better quantified using cancellation testing (e.g. marking all the stars in a picture), drawing a clock face, naming objects around the room (are they all on one side?) and bisecting vertical and horizontal lines (this helps to distinguish hemianopia from neglect) (Fig. 1.1).

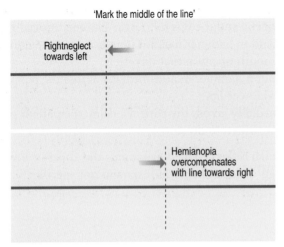

Figure 1.1
Neglect analysed by line bisection. Line bisection illustrating neglect vs hemianopia.

Brief assessment

A brief psychometric assessment, e.g. using the Mini-Mental State Examination (MMSE) (Box 1.4) is appropriate for outpatient clinics. More detailed cognitive function testing (psychometry) may be undertaken on selected patients, usually by a clinical psychologist.

Box 1.4: *The Mini-Mental State Examination (MMSE)*

1. **Orientation**
   - Time: day, month, season and year (**5 points**).
   - Place: building, ward, city, county and country (**5 points**).

2. **Attention and calculation together**
   - Serial 7s: subtract 7 from 100 and continue to subtract 7 from each answer. One point for each correct answer (**5 points**).

3. **Memory (verbal)**
   - Immediate recall (working memory): Repeat three named objects (dog, blackboard, lettuce) on first hearing them (**3 points**).
   - Delayed recall: Recall the three objects after 5 min (**3 points**).

4. **Dominant hemisphere (language)**
   - Naming: Name two objects (watch, pencil) (**2 points**).
   - Repetition: Repeat a short sentence ('No ifs ands or buts') (**1 point**).
   - Comprehension (spoken): three-stage command ('Pick up this paper, fold it and put it on the floor') (**3 points**).
   - Comprehension (written): Read and follow a written command ('Close your eyes') (**1 point**); write a simple sentence without help or prompting (**1 point**).

5. **Non-dominant hemisphere**
   - Construction: Copy a simple figure (intersecting pentagons) (**1 point**).

The MMSE can detect important higher mental function deficits sufficient to localize the cognitive lesion, establish the need for more detailed testing and help the patient and carers understand the problems. Clinicians must memorize a short series of questions and tasks and become familiar with the reasons why patients might be unable to complete them. The MMSE is easy to use and forms the basis for supplementary questions and tests but has several limitations:

- Verbal and memory skills are assessed well (excellent for detecting Alzheimer's disease); frontal function is not. Frontal lobe dementia patients may even score full marks on MMSE.
- Visuospatial problems from non-dominant parietal lesions may be very disabling, yet on MMSE give difficulty only with drawing (29/30).
- Adding MMSE scores together can give a deceptive impression of precisely quantifying a cognitive deficit (e.g. inferring that 20 out of 30 equals two-thirds intact). Yet it is no more meaningful to score physical examination by adding sensory loss, nystagmus and sluggish pupils. MMSE scores should therefore always be qualified (e.g. '29/30, missing one object on immediate recall').

Coverings

The main neurological examination begins by considering:

- **Scalp:** including scars, naevi, temporal arteries.
- **Skull:** shape, size, irregularity, bruit.
- **Spine and neck:** mobility, scars, shape, masses, neck hairline, lumbar hairy patch, tenderness and bruit.

Cranial nerves

Olfactory (1)

- 'Is your sense of smell normal?'
- Test using sample aromas (bottles or 'scratch and sniff') separately, beneath each nostril.

Optic (2), Oculomotor (3), Trochlear (4), Abducens (6)

Acuity

- 'Is your vision normal?'
- 'Do you wear glasses?' Acuity measurement is meaningless without optimal refraction (clean reading glasses or pinhole).
- Snellen chart at 6 m or standard reading chart assessed and recorded separately for each eye.

Fields

- Brief assessment if no abnormality suspected:
  - With both eyes open, hold up both hands towards patient.
  - 'Look at my eyes. Can you see both of my hands? Which finger am I moving?'
- Detailed assessment if abnormality suspected:
  - The room's light behind the patient, seated at same level.
  - Comparing your right visual field with the patient's left and vice versa (patient and doctor close/cover one eye); 'Look into my eye'.

- Bring a red-headed pin initially from behind the patient along the diagonal of each of four quadrants.
- Compare blind spots and red perception in the central fields.
- Document fields from the patient's viewpoint (the doctor's right and left view of the fields should be reversed).

Fundi

- 'Look at that object and try to keep looking at it even though I am in your way'.
- Right eye: hold the ophthalmoscope in the right hand, look with the right eye and examine from the right side and vice versa.
- First focus on the iris from 10–20 cm, looking for cataract etc.
- With lens initially on 0 (or corrected to your own vision), move as close as possible to the patient's eye.
- Examine the disc, vessels and macula.
- Fundoscopy offers the opportunity to see the only nerves and blood vessels directly visible.

Pupils

- **Light response:** using a bright pen-torch, not an ophthalmoscope, to assess direct and consensual response in each eye.
- **Accommodation:** this can be assessed during eye movements (convergence).

Eye movements

- **Pursuit**
  - With one hand on the patient's forehead, 'Follow my finger and tell me if you see double'.
  - Move finger in an 'H' shape to allow assessment of individual muscles, e.g. vertical movement with eyes left involves left eye superior and inferior recti and right eye inferior and superior oblique. Test convergence while watching for pupil constriction.
- **Saccades**
  - Ask the patient to look quickly to right and left, then up and down (opening and closing your outstretched hands as a target).

Trigeminal (5)

Sensory

- Light touch and pinprick perception in each of the three trigeminal dermatomes on each side.
- Corneal reflex:
  - 'Look up and away' and touch the cornea (over the iris) with cotton wool.
  - Note direct and consensual blink.
  - Take care with interpretation in contact lens wearers.

Motor

- Note bulk and symmetry of temporalis and masseter.
- 'Open your mouth and keep it open' (against resistance): the jaw opens to the side of weakness.

Facial (7)

Motor

- Observe facial symmetry.
- 'Close your eyes tightly', noting extent of lash burial; try to pull eyelids apart.
- 'Close your lips tightly'; try to pull them apart.

Taste

- The chorda tympani travels with the facial nerve, though is not actually part of it.
- Taste assessed on each side, without tongue movements, using three flavours (sweet, salt, sour).

Vestibulo-cochlear (8)

Acuity

- 'Repeat these numbers after me'.
- Whisper numbers at increasing amplitude into each ear while tapping a finger in the opposite ear.

Rinné test

- Vibrating tuning fork (256 Hz) on mastoid:
  - 'Tell me when the sound is gone', then move in front of the ear: 'Can you hear it now?'
  - or, 'Which is loudest, there (mastoid), or there (in front)?'
  - Note 'Rinné positive' is air conduction better than bone conduction.

Weber test

- Vibrating 128 Hz tuning fork on forehead:
  - 'In which ear is this loudest?'
  - Louder in deaf ear = conductive; louder in non-deaf ear = sensorineural.

Vestibular function

- Dix–Hallpike testing is described in Ch. 5.

Glossopharyngeal (9)

- This is sensory to the posterior tongue and pharyngeal wall.
- Say 'Ahh'. With the palate elevated, touch the posterior pharyngeal wall on each side with an orange stick, 'Does it feel the same on each side?'

Vagus (10)

- This is motor to the palate and larynx.
- Note quality and clarity of speech.

- Say, 'Ahh' and observe palate elevated in the midline (watch midline raphe not the uvula); the palate is pulled away from the weak side.

Accessory (11)

- Note bulk of sternomastoid and trapezius.
- Sternomastoids together: Place one hand on the patient's forehead and the other (as a precaution) behind the patient's head, 'Push forwards as hard as you can'.
- Sternomastoids individually: Lateral head rotation, 'Push your chin against my hand', noting that the left sternomastoid pushes the head to the right.
- Trapezii: 'Shrug your shoulders' against resistance.

Hypoglossal (12)

- Note bulk and fasciculation of resting tongue.
- 'Put your tongue out'. Note movement in the midline (moves towards weak side).
- 'Push your tongue into your cheek'. Assess tongue strength on each side by pushing it back.

Limbs

Posture, stance and gait

Arms: 'Close your eyes and hold your arms straight out with the palms upwards'. Watch for tremor, chorea, signs of pyramidal weakness (downward drift, elbow flexion and pronation) or for 'pseudoathetosis' of sensory ataxia (wandering movement of the fingers or arms from altered position sense).

Legs: Lower limb examination must include observation of stance and gait, including Romberg's test for sensory ataxia, tandem walking for cerebellar ataxia, observing posture and arm swing for parkinsonism and Trendelenburg test (stand on one leg and observe pelvic tilt) for proximal muscle weakness.

Inspection

Full inspection requires full limb exposure. The upper limbs include the neck, shoulders and scapulae (e.g. scapular winging); the lower limbs include the lower spine and buttocks.

Search for burns, scars, wasting (especially small hand muscles and extensor digitorum brevis in the foot), fasciculation, tremor, foot deformity and pressure sores (heels and buttocks).

Tone

- Spasticity (pyramidal) varies with speed and direction of passive movement and is best felt during forearm supination or knee flexion. Compare with opening a 'clasp knife' or penknife; initial movement is difficult and then it gives way and opens easily.
- Rigidity (extrapyramidal) is unchanged with speed and direction of passive movement. 'Lead pipe' or 'cogwheel' is best felt at the wrist and can be enhanced by active movement of the contralateral limb.

- Gegenhalten (holding against) is an involuntary active resistance to movement, suggesting frontal lobe dysfunction.

Strength

The principles of strength testing:

- The patient makes the movement; the examiner tries to overcome it.
- Assess one muscle group at a time, not two limbs together.
- Inherently weaker muscles are more likely to be helpful, e.g. extensors in the arms, flexors in the legs, finger abduction, toe dorsiflexion.
- Quantify strength either as MRC scale 1–5, or, more meaningfully, as normal, mild, moderate and severe.
- Patients may need encouragement to maximum effort: ask them to look at the limb as you exhort one big effort.

Selecting muscles

It is helpful to remember some routinely tested muscle groups and their nerve and root supplies (Table 1.1).

- Motor ulnar function is best tested using first dorsal interosseous because it is its most distally innervated muscle; an ulnar lesion is unlikely if it is spared. Abductor pollicis brevis is the best to assess motor median function (the thumb is lifted vertically from the palm against resistance over the proximal phalanx).
- Neck flexion strength (sternomastoids) can distinguish generalized weakness (motor neurone disease, polymyositis) from cervical myelopathy.

Patterns of weakness

- **Pyramidal** weakness (extensors in arms, flexors in legs) characterizes an upper motor neurone lesion.
- **Proximal** (symmetrical) weakness suggests myopathy (also myasthenia, Guillain–Barré syndrome).
- **Distal** (symmetrical) weakness suggests peripheral neuropathy (also myotonic dystrophy, inclusion body myositis).

Table 1.1: Muscle, nerve and nerve root for several selected muscles

Limb movement	Muscle	Nerve	Nerve root
Shoulder abduction (from 90°)	Deltoid	Axillary	C5
Elbow extension	Triceps	Radial	C7
Finger extension	Extensor digitorum	Posterior interosseous (radial)	C7
Index finger abduction	First dorsal interosseous	Ulnar	T1
Hip flexion	Iliopsoas	Femoral	L1, 2
Knee flexion	Hamstrings	Sciatic	S1
Ankle dorsiflexion	Peroneals	Common peroneal and sciatic	L4, 5
Great toe dorsiflexion	Extensor hallucis longus	Common peroneal	L5

Reflexes

Deep tendon reflexes

- Observe the muscle being tapped as well as its movement.
- Reinforce apparently absent reflexes using Jendrassik's manoeuvre (pull apart clasped hands) or teeth clenching.
- Elicit ankle jerks by tapping the Achilles or by tapping the hammer onto your hand over the metatarsal heads.
- Root innervation is easily remembered: S1, 2 (ankle), L3, 4 (knee), C5, 6 (biceps), C7, 8 (triceps).
- Hoffmann's reflex (thumb adduction on striking the palmar aspect of the fingers) is a sign of upper limb hyperreflexia; it is significant if asymmetrical, but rarely adds new information.

Superficial reflexes

- **Plantar response:** 'I am going to scratch your foot: try to keep your toes still'. Use an orange stick and observe the first movement of the big toe. Chaddock's manoeuvre involves scratching the foot's lateral border while observing the big toe.
- **Superficial abdominal reflexes** are reliable only in the young and the nulliparous. Stroke each abdominal quadrant with an orange stick, observing for local muscle contraction. They are lost early in multiple sclerosis, but may be preserved in hereditary spastic paraparesis and motor neurone disease.

Coordination

- **Gait** in cerebellar disease is broad-based and unsteady. 'Tandem gait' can exaggerate the difficulties, 'Look at your feet and walk on a tightrope'.
- **Intention tremor** is assessed in the arms by the finger to nose test and in the legs by the heel to shin test. Observe for tremor just before the finger touches the nose or as the heel touches the shin. The tremor is exaggerated by exaggerating the movement, e.g. stretching forward to your finger.
- **Dysdiadochokinesis** is assessed in the arms by rapidly tapping the thumb and index finger, or rapidly pronating and supinating the forearm.
- **Nystagmus and dysarthria** are additional features of cerebellar disorder (and with limb ataxia comprise Charcot's triad of MS).

Sensation

The patient shows you the area of sensory loss before testing.

Method

Pinprick. Use disposable pins only. Patients do not need to close their eyes. First, demonstrate normal pinprick sensation, remembering to press sufficiently hard to test pain sensation not light touch. Compare affected and unaffected areas asking, 'Does this feel sharp?' not, 'Can you feel this?'

Temperature perception is assessed to confirm spinothalamic loss. Use a tuning fork and ask, 'Does this feel cold?'

Light touch. Use cotton wool and ask, 'Does this feel normal?'

Position sense. Holding the finger or toe at its sides, demonstrate movements with the patient's eyes open. 'Close your eyes and tell me if it moves up or down', then make small (2–3 mm) movements. Romberg's sign can also indicate poor position sense.

Vibration. Using a 128 Hz tuning fork, demonstrate normal vibration feeling on the sternum. Test over bony prominences or the tips of fingers or toes asking, 'Do you feel this buzzing or just pressing?'

Two-point discrimination is used particularly if there are sensory symptoms but no other signs, e.g. in suspected MS. With the patient's eyes closed and testing over the finger tips or toes using two points each time, ask, 'Can you feel one or two points?'

Patterns of sensory loss

- **Stocking** (and later glove) implies peripheral neuropathy.
- **Sensory level** implies a spinal cord lesion (labelled from the lowest normal level).
- **Hemianaesthesia** suggests a contralateral cerebral lesion or, with no other signs, a non-organic disorder with hyperventilation.
- **Dissociated sensory loss** with lost spinothalamic but preserved dorsal column function suggests hemicord damage, e.g. anterior spinal artery syndrome, Brown–Séquard syndrome (usually MS), or syringomyelia. Sensory loss that is both dissociated and suspended (preserved sensation above and below, 'cape and balaclava'), characterizes syringomyelia.

Perineal examination

This is particularly important in patients with sphincter disturbance, potency changes, or perineal pain and numbness.

Inspection should include scars from previous surgery or trauma. Note that perianal skin breakdown is a consequence not a cause of incontinence.

Digital rectal examination should include:

- Exclusion of impaction or tumours in the lower rectum causing overflow incontinence.
- Assessment of anal sphincter tone and the patient's ability to augment it with voluntary squeeze effort.
- Identification of reduced perineal sensation and loss of anal wink as pointers towards neurogenic incontinence.

SCREENING EXAMINATION

Most neurology patients are examined without expecting to find abnormal physical signs. These patients require a 5–7 min screening examination.

General

Assume your history taking has not identified cognitive dysfunction.

Patient is undressed except underwear.

Inspect scalp, neck and spine.

Cranial nerves

- Ask about sense of smell.
- Measure visual acuity in each eye.
- With both eyes open, test fields by holding up both palms towards the patient: 'Look at my eyes; can you see both my hands? Touch the finger that moves' (right, left, both).
- Pupil light response, direct and consensual.
- Pursuit eye movements, including convergence pupil response.
- Examine the fundi.
- 'Do you hear this noise?' (examiner's fingers).
- Cotton wool sensation testing of the three trigeminal divisions bilaterally.
- 'Close your eyes tightly; put your lips hard together'; examiner tries to open them.
- 'Open your mouth and keep it open'; examiner tries to close it.
- 'Say "Ahh"', observing the palate.
- 'Put your tongue out', observing for deviation.
- 'Push your head forwards against my hand', testing sternomastoids together.

Arms

- Patient extends arms (palms upwards) with eyes closed.
- Inspect the arms and hands.
- Muscle tone.
- Strength of shoulder abduction, elbow extension, finger extension.
- Biceps, supinator and triceps reflexes.
- Finger nose test and dysdiadochokinesis.
- Pinprick testing of upper arm, forearm and hands.

Legs

- Inspect the legs and feet.
- Muscle tone.
- Strength of hip flexion, knee flexion, toe dorsiflexion.
- Knee, ankle and plantar reflexes.

- Heel shin test for coordination.
- Pinprick testing of upper leg, lower leg and feet.
- Observe gait and stance.

More detailed examination might then be needed if abnormal signs are found.

GIVING INFORMATION

Explaining and planning. Provide the appropriate amount and type of information. This may include using appropriate language, drawing diagrams, showing the patient their radiographs, etc. It also involves using 'chunking and checking' where a chunk of information is provided and the clinician checks understanding with the patient.

Aiding recall and understanding includes organizing the explanation into discrete sections, using signposting ('That's the cause of your headaches, I'm now going to move on to possible treatments'), repetition and summarizing.

Achieving a shared understanding involves incorporating the patient's perspective. For example, knowing that the patient expects a scan can be incorporated into the explanation 'With such clear symptoms of migraine I was not planning to arrange a scan at the moment'.

Planning involves shared decision making, making suggestions rather than directives, negotiating and offering choices.

CLOSING THE CONSULTATION

Summarizing. The consultation should ideally end with a brief summary, clarifying the plan of care, outlining the next steps, informing the patient what to expect during the treatment plan, where to seek help if needed (safety netting) and a final check that the patient is comfortable with the plan.

Final questions. 'What would you like to ask?' induces more response than 'Do you have any questions?' Doctors usually emphasize the diagnosis, investigation results and treatment, but patients often want to know the cause of the condition and its prognosis. Written information is important, including information sheets, details of websites and local support groups. Most powerful is a personalized letter summarizing the consultation and giving specific information. Copying the standard clinic letter is a useful alternative.

A word on reassurance. A doctor saying there is nothing to worry about without presenting the reasons is not necessarily reassuring for a patient and risks being seriously wrong. Patients need to derive their own reassurance from the evidence and explanation that you offer.

Expert patients. Patients with chronic conditions are experts in their individual condition since they constantly live with it. Providing individualized information and offering specialist nurse telephone contact are steps towards encouraging greater patient involvement in their long-term management.

CONSULTING WITH SPECIAL GROUPS

- **Emergency unit consultations** differ from outpatient practice. Patients may be confused, amnesic, uncooperative and unkempt. There is often limited availability of background information, case notes and out-of-hours investigations; tests may be needed before a full history (e.g. glucose in coma) and treatment may be needed before investigation (e.g. of airway in comatose patients). Witness (and ambulance personnel) accounts are important, e.g. medication bottles at the scene, previous health. Where rarer chronic conditions present acutely, be sensitive to the patient being better informed about the condition than you are: use this, rather than deny it. In emergency situations, the general and neurological examinations are equally important, e.g. signs of head injury, breath smell, coma score, neck stiffness, etc. Conditions presenting as emergencies include blackouts (seizure, syncope, psychogenic), status epilepticus (consider pseudostatus epilepticus), headache (meningitis, subarachnoid, migraine), stroke (infarction, haemorrhage, migraine), trauma (head or spinal cord but also consider internal bleeding), delirium and coma (toxic, stroke, meningitis, metabolic, psychiatric), paralysis (Guillain–Barré, cord compression) and visual loss (giant cell arteritis, glaucoma, optic neuritis).
- **ICUs** can be daunting for a neurology trainee. Approach the patient in the normal way, read all available notes and speak to clinicians who know the patient. Address apparently comatose patients as if they are awake, at least until it is confirmed that they are not locked in. Remember the risk of cross infection: not only should visiting clinicians wash hands, wear aprons and wipe medical instruments, they should be seen to do so.
- **Severe learning disability** can give very challenging consultations even in optimal circumstances. Again the history is crucial and so a carer who knows the patient well must accompany the patient. As far as practical, the conversation should be directed at the patient rather than the carers. Close liaison with the community learning disabilities team is essential.
- **Suspected dementia** patients should be seen initially with their carer. However, carers are often reluctant to disclose frank details in the patient's presence; a full history requires seeing the carer separately. Dementia consultations are often lengthy and include a full mental state examination.
- **Teenagers** should be treated as adults in the consultation, the parents literally taking a back seat. Teenagers are often reluctant to talk in front of parents and where possible the consultation should continue during a period alone. An opportunity arises during the physical examination which where possible should be done in a separate cubicle.
- **Other clinicians.** Consultations with doctors and nurses are often not optimal and colleagues risk receiving less good care than other patients. The preferred and safest approach is to treat clinicians exactly as you would any other patient. Importantly, do not assume a detailed knowledge and less need for explanation. Knowledgeable or medical patients might use technical terms such as 'paraesthesiae in L5' rather than 'tingling, pricking or fizzing in the leg'. The more technical description does not necessarily give the clearest possible symptom information and should be clarified.

KEY POINTS

- For most neurology outpatients, the history is more important than the examination; having no diagnosis after the history usually means there will still be no diagnosis after the examination.
- In general, direct the conversation to the patient rather than the parents or relatives. However, in dementia and learning disability, the patient and carer need to be seen independently. In teenagers, it is helpful to hear the teenager's viewpoint independently.
- Do not accept other people's diagnoses (e.g. of MS) without question, especially if no diagnostic test is available, e.g. blackouts.
- Fully expose patient for neurological examination.
- Err on the side of seeing urgent referrals yourself rather than relying on other people's accounts of history and examination.
- Never accept an invitation to 'just look at the fundi', or to do a mini-assessment of a clinical colleague 'while you're here': either you take responsibility for the patient or you do not.
- Carry your own examination tools (emergency units and non-neurology wards often do not have these available): a neurology registrar should never say 'Fundi: no ophthalmoscope available'.
- After every examination wash your hands (and be seen to wash them); in ITU and haematology wards, consider alcohol wiping your instruments.
- Update your ALS skills if you are dealing with emergencies.

Further Reading

Fuller GN. Neurological examination made easy, 3rd edn. Edinburgh: Churchill Livingstone; 2004.

Anatomy

Case history

A 70-year-old right-handed woman presented to casualty. Earlier that day she had noticed that she was unable to read. She could speak perfectly and understand spoken language. She was obviously alert. Her writing seemed to be normal but she was unable to read words aloud. The remaining neurological examination was normal apart from a right homonymous hemianopia.

FRONTAL LOBE

The frontal lobe generates novel strategies and has executive functions (motivating to put these in practice). It also enables self-criticism and 'trying again'. The prefrontal cortex connects extensively to other association cortices and to the basal ganglia, limbic cortex, thalamus and hippocampus.

- **The orbitofrontal cortex** tailors responses to primitive stimuli, e.g. hunger, thirst, sexual urges. Damage here causes disinhibited behaviour.
- **The dorsolateral prefrontal cortex** tailors responses to external situations, e.g. executing work responsibilities.
- **The cingulate gyrus and dorsomedial frontal lobe** (connected to the limbic system) govern motivation. Damage here causes abulia (lack of will), or even akinetic mutism with the patient mute and without motivation, although sometimes reacting to external cues (rather than internal), e.g. a telephone ringing.

The frontal lobes are very large. There are many and varied signs associated with frontal lobe dysfunction:

- **Personality dysfunction**, including abulia (cingulate gyrus), disinhibition (orbitofrontal area), or dysexecutive problems (dorsolateral frontal area).
- **Paraparesis** (often asymmetric) may accompany a parasagittal lesion, often with few other features of the upper motor neurone syndrome, e.g. tone may appear almost normal. Cerebral imaging is therefore important for paraparesis with normal cord imaging.
- **Paratonia** (*gegenhalten*: resistance to passive movement): the patient finds it hard to relax.
- **Grasp reflex** (see Ch. 1) is a form of motor disinhibition.
- **Frontal gait dysfunction** occurs with small vessel disease or, less commonly, hydrocephalus. On attempting to walk, the feet appear stuck to the floor (magnetic gait). This contrasts with a relatively normal examination on the couch and if pushed in a wheelchair with feet touching the ground, patients may move their feet normally.

- **Cortical hand.** The homunculus has disproportionate hand representation; a cortical lesion may cause only lost hand dexterity.
- **Seizures.** Simple partial seizures from motor strip involvement may manifest only as involuntary lateralized jerking. Classical frontal lobe epilepsy with seizures arising in the supplementary motor area, manifests as brief, lateralized motor seizures, often arising from sleep and with some retained awareness; the EEG may even remain normal during seizures.
- **Incontinence.** The timing and suitability of occasions to micturate may be disturbed.
- **Visual field deficit.** The anterior visual pathways (including chiasm) are beneath the frontal lobes.
- **Visual response disinhibition.** The patient keeps looking to target during visual field testing.
- **Expressive dysphasia.** Broca's area is in the dominant frontal lobe.
- **Anosmia.** Olfactory pathways lie beneath the frontal lobes.

TEMPORAL LOBE

Temporal lobe disease may cause several problems.

- **Memory dysfunction** (see below), particularly episodic memory relating to verbal (left side) and visual (right side) events. The adjacent diencephalic structures also have a major memory function.
- **Agnosia,** especially for visual and other sensory modalities.
- **Language disorder** (see below), especially receptive dysphasia (Wernicke's area, dominant hemisphere).
- **Visual field deficit.** Involvement of Meyer's loop causes a congruous upper homonymous quadrantanopia.
- **Auditory dysfunction.** Involvement of the auditory cortex (Heschl's gyrus and association cortices) may, for example, impair appreciation of music (non-dominant cortex). Because hearing is represented bilaterally, deafness is not a feature of cerebral (or brainstem) disease, unless the lesions are extensive and bilateral.
- **Limbic dysfunction,** with some features of Klüver–Bucy syndrome (see below) and disinhibition may occur through amygdala involvement.
- **Temporal lobe epilepsy.** See ch. 3

Limbic lobe

Broca described the cortex bordering the corpus callosum and diencephalon as the *limbus* (border; Latin). Papez, trying to locate the emotional brain, described the limbic system. The system now includes the *amygdala* (almond; Latin) rostral to the hippocampus and with extensive connections. Bard and Hess's animal experiments suggested emotional visceral and somatic reactions were generated in the hypothalamus. However, human emotions are not predictable or stereotyped and certainly more complicated than the sham rage from hypothalamic stimulation of experimental cats.

An 'emotional' pathway, separate from the pyramidal, innervates motor nuclei, e.g. causing dissociation between voluntary and emotional facial movements: following stroke, emotional smiling is preserved but voluntary smiling is asymmetric. The opposite rarely occurs, for example after a striatocapsular infarction voluntary smiling is symmetrical but emotional smiling is asymmetric.

Hypothalamic release (from the limbic system) phenomena were shown in classical animal experiments.

- **Klüver–Bucy syndrome.** Removing both medial temporal lobes of Rhesus monkeys caused visual agnosia, increased sexual activity and hyperorality.
- **Disinhibition.** Removing both amygdalae from Macaque monkeys caused breakdown of strict hierarchical behaviour, e.g. mating with the females of higher status males.
- **Aggression.** Removing the lateral septal nuclei created extreme aggression.

PARIETAL LOBE

- **Visual field deficit.** Involvement of the upper fibres of the optic radiation causes lower homonymous quadrantanopia.
- **Sensory dysfunction.** Impairment of accurate localization of touch, two-point discrimination, appreciation of shape, size, or texture of an object and for stereognosis.
- **Gerstmann's syndrome.** This suggests disease of the (dominant) angular gyrus, part of the inferior parietal lobe. There are four classical features:
  - **Dysgraphia.** Inability to write, often with inability to read (central alexia).
  - **Left–right disorientation.** 'Point to your right elbow, your left knee, etc'.
  - **Finger agnosia.** 'Show me your index finger, etc'.
  - **Acalculia.** Inability to do sums.
- Dyspraxia:
  - **Dominant parietal lobe.** This contains praxicons (see below) and hence damage leads to dyspraxia.
  - **Disconnection syndromes.** Damage to the dominant parietal lobe's projections (to the right-sided frontal premotor areas via the corpus callosum) also causes loss of praxis information; hence a left frontal infarction involving the corpus callosum may paradoxically cause left-sided limb dyspraxia.
  - **Non-dominant parietal lobe** damage characteristically causes dressing dyspraxia.
- **Inattention** suggests non-dominant angular gyrus involvement.
- **Denial** includes denial of any problem (anosognosia) or of existence of a body part (asomatognosia).

OCCIPITAL LOBE

Anatomy

- **The lateral geniculate nucleus** (projecting to the occipital lobes) has two portions:

- **Parvocellular portion** (receiving afferents from the parvocellular retinal ganglion cells) is responsible for size, shape and colour.
- **Magnocellular portion** conveys information about perception of quickly moving targets.
- **Streams of vision.** Two streams are anatomically distinct:
  - **Ventral** (mainly inferior temporal) is responsible for the 'what': high-resolution recognition of an object, colour recognition (area V4).
  - **Dorsal** (middle temporal and parietal) is responsible for the 'where': spatial aspects of vision and analysis of motion.
- The primary visual cortex connects to many extrastriatal areas in the temporal and parietal lobes.

Syndromes

- **Balint syndrome** relates to bilateral posterior occipito-parietal lobe damage. The triad comprises:
  - **Simultagnosia** is caused by a severely restricted visual field of attention, giving an inability to see the 'whole picture', e.g. a beach scene, but still able to identify parts of a scene.
  - **Optic ataxia** (visuomotor ataxia or visual disorientation). The person may be unable to grasp an object until a different cue is presented, e.g. when a bell is offered the patient cannot grasp it; when rung it may be located and reached.
  - **Optic apraxia** (psychic gaze paralysis) is the inability to look right or left voluntarily.
- **Alexia without agraphia.** Disruption to the corpus callosum (splenium) disconnects the intact right occipital cortex from the dominant language area; reading becomes impossible. Writing does not require this connection and so is unaffected.

LANGUAGE

Aphasia

Aphasia (or dysphasia) is an acquired disorder of language (distinct from speech) resulting from brain damage.

Language components

- Phoneme: smallest discrete unit (sound) of language.
- Grapheme: a phoneme written down.
- Lexicon: internal dictionary.
- Morphology: appropriate word endings (singular/plural, or verb tense).
- Semantics: word meanings.
- Syntax: word order.

Language anatomy

- **Heschl's gyrus**: in the superior temporal lobe (primary auditory cortex): sounds initially arrive here.
- **Wernicke's area** (Brodmann area 22) in the superior temporal gyrus: phonemes are decoded into recognizable words here. It is linked to association cortices, e.g. inferior frontal cortex (semantics), limbic lobe (feelings, e.g. emotional response to a word).
- **Broca's area** (Brodmann area 44 and 45), adjacent to the pre-motor cortex: here, words are converted into motor signals to the larynx, tongue, lips, etc.

Figure 2.1 describes a model of the anatomy of language. However, particular language functions are not confined to single cortical areas, e.g. Broca aphasics often show some comprehension difficulty. A working model, termed the 'Wernicke–Geschwind model', is used by many clinicians (Fig. 2.1). It has several shortcomings, for instance there is no space for the considerable role of the subcortex in language function, but it remains a useful working model. The model is outlined in Figure 2.1 for spoken words and the principles remain the same for written words.

Reading

Reading involves two processes: phonemic (word sounds) and semantic (word understanding).

- **Surface dyslexia** implies a problem with phonology (grapheme to phoneme conversion). Patients mispronounce irregularly spelt words, e.g. 'PINT' to rhyme with 'MINT' (left posterior temporo-parietal cortex in semantic dementia).
- **Deep dyslexia** patients cannot say non-words (those without semantic representation) and substitute words with related meanings, e.g. 'boy' for 'man' (left perisylvian region in Broca's dysphasia).

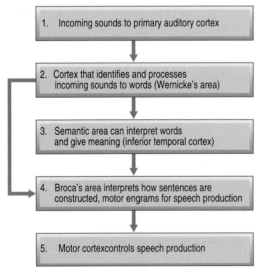

Figure 2.1
Wernicke–Geschwind model.

Pure alexia without agraphia

The visual cortex is disconnected from the word decoding apparatus (Fig. 2.2).

- Patients cannot read words, but can say them if they are spelt aloud (because the auditory cortex is 'wired up to' the semantic and motor phoneme parts).
- Patients can match colours but not name them.

Alexia with agraphia

This is caused by a lesion in the decoding apparatus itself (usually the angular gyrus). It may be part of Gerstmann's syndrome or occur with Wernicke's aphasia (area 22 is nearby).

Aphasic alexia

Aphasia is often accompanied by some alexia (grapheme and phoneme representations are very close).

Examination

Examination of language focuses on seven aspects.

1. **Comprehension** is either intact (e.g. Broca's) or affected (e.g. Wernicke's).
2. **Spontaneous speech** is either fluent (posterior, e.g. Wernicke's) or non-fluent (anterior, e.g. Broca's).
3. **Repetition** of something said to a patient is impaired in Broca's and Wernicke's aphasia. When a Wernicke's patient attempts to whisper, this may prompt attempted repetition. In *transcortical* aphasia, the perisylvian cortex is intact and so repetition is possible, despite adjacent association cortex damage; transcortical motor or sensory aphasias are similar to Broca's or Wernicke's aphasias apart from preserved repetition.
4. **Naming difficulty** (anomia) in isolation is non-localizing, e.g. accompanying visual agnosia or aphasia (anomic aphasia). Naming errors include neologisms (nonsense

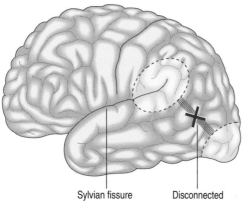

Sylvian fissure   Disconnected

Figure 2.2
Alexia without agraphia. Disconnection of visual cortex from word decoding apparatus.

words), phonemic paraphasias (phonologically similar words, e.g. 'claw' for 'door'), or semantic paraphasias (words meaningfully related, e.g. 'pencil' for 'Biro').
5. **Written words.**
6. **Reading** (silently and aloud). In conduction aphasia, reading comprehension is normal (the grapheme to semantic base is intact) but reading aloud is difficult because the patient cannot translate the words into a motor programme.
7. **Associated signs**, e.g. right hemiparesis.

Broca aphasia

- **Non-fluent speech.** Patients may still say well-rehearsed things, e.g. days of the week.
- **Good comprehension**, except with difficult sentences, e.g. 'The girl who the boy is chasing is tall; who is tall?'
- **Impaired naming**, although often the sounds are slightly wrong (phonemic errors). With frequent phonemic errors, especially with successive attempts to self-correct (*conduit d'approche*), consider conduction aphasia.
- **Impaired reading and writing** is common.
- **Impaired repetition.**
- **Associated signs** include right hemiparesis, orofacial dyspraxia (for premotor programmes: ask the patient to lick the lips or cough) and left arm dyspraxia.

Aphemia

This is pure speech apraxia: written and auditory comprehension is completely normal.

Wernicke aphasia

- Fluent speech: to a non-native speaker, it sounds normal.
- Impaired comprehension.
- Impaired naming, often with bizarre results.
- Impaired repetition: prompt by asking the patient to whisper.
- Impaired reading and writing (not invariable).
- Associated signs: usually no weakness but may have homonymous hemianopia.

Conduction aphasia

- Fairly fluent speech.
- Good comprehension.
- Impaired repetition (cannot say 'no ifs, ands or buts').

MEMORY

Memory is either declarative or non-declarative.

Declarative

- **Semantic memory** is information memory, unrelated to time, e.g. reading a book.
- **Episodic memory** is autobiographical, e.g. remembering when or where you read it.
- **Remote memories** are stored in association cortices; new declarative memory requires the hippocampal system.
- **Recent** (or working) **memory**, e.g. memorizing a telephone number, is stored in the auditory association cortex. Activity increases within a specialized group of cells in a certain pattern, without activity in other cells; these memories are therefore fleeting.

Non-declarative

- **Procedural** (or skilled) **memory**, e.g. playing golf or learning to mirror-write, is stored in the motor and pre-motor cortex, cerebellum and basal ganglia.

Physiology of memory

Physical representation of a memory is termed an engram. Hebb hypothesized that the internal representation of objects comprised an assembly of cortical cells: if these cells were stimulated, the rest would fire. Learning results from changing the strength of neuronal interconnections: 'cells firing together will wire together', hence allowing long-term potentiation.

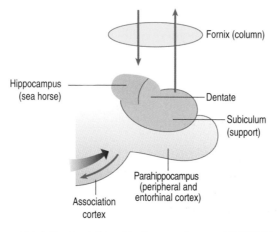

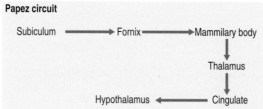

Figure 2.3
Functional anatomy of memory. Two important regions: medial temporal lobe and medial diencephalic area. Input from association cortex to entorhinal cortex, output to association cortex, fornix, mamillary bodies and thalamus. Papez circuit: subiculum → fornix → mamillary body → thalamus → cingulate hypothalamus.

The hippocampal system allows acquisition and consolidation of memories (Fig. 2.3). Declarative memory depends upon the hippocampal system and the strength of its neuronal connections, e.g. cortex to parahippocampus to hippocampus (subiculum) to parahippocampus and back to cortex.

MOTOR SYSTEM

Extrafusal muscles (myofibres) are individual muscle fibres innervated by α-motor neurones. During muscle contraction, small α-motor neurones fire first; later, with greater force, larger α-motor neurones are recruited (Fig. 2.4a).

Intrafusal fibres are contained within muscles and feed back to the spinal cord (Fig. 2.4b).

- **Group 1A afferents** detect rate of change of muscle length: this is the afferent path for myotactic reflexes.
- **Group 2 afferents** detect muscle length.
- **Group 1B afferents** relay information from Golgi tendon organs, informing about muscle tension and regulating contraction force by inhibiting synergists and exciting antagonists.

Hughlings Jackson's 'hierarchy of influences', where higher centres constrain lower ones, helps to understand 'disinhibition'.

- **Decerebrate posturing**. Disinhibition of postural stability pathways, e.g. vestibulospinal tracts, affects extensors more than flexors.
- **Decorticate state**. Lesions at or above the midbrain disinhibit the tracts flexing the arms and extending the legs (e.g. causing pronator drift).
- **Nociceptive flexion reflex**. Nociceptive (pain) fibres (C, δ) generally excite flexors and inhibit extensors. Lesions that affect the descending inhibitory influence of the reticulospinal tract disinhibit the nociceptive flexion reflex, clinically manifesting as a Babinski response.

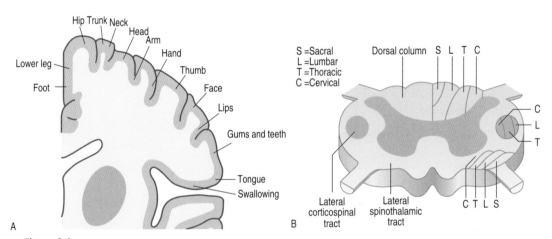

Figure 2.4
The motor system. (a) Motor homonculus (coronal section). (b) Spinal cord cross-section showing motor and sensory lamination. S, sacral; L, lumbar; T, thoracic; C, cervical.

- **Tetanus and strychnine poisoning** cause loss of Renshaw cell inhibitory influence (glycine-mediated), manifesting as muscle spasms Renshaw cells. These (interneurones) receive collateral afferents from α-motor neurones; these in turn synapse with the same α-motor neurones (and their synergists), so preventing the motor system running away with itself.

Several descending tracts influence the anterior horn cells, either directly (corticospinal tract) or through interneurones.

- **The corticospinal tract** arises from Brodmann area 4. Signals travel directly to the anterior horn cells, particularly those destined for the hands and feet, enabling performance of precision movements.
- **The tectospinal tract** originates in the superior colliculus and so deals with orientating head movements, e.g. looking towards a noise.
- **The vestibulospinal tract** innervates the ventromedial (axial) musculature, so allowing corrective movements in maintaining the upright posture. Parkinson's disease may affect this tract, occasionally with marked postural instability.
- **The medullary and pontine reticulospinal tracts** maintain proximal limb posture, e.g. providing a steady base for finer hands movements.

HIGHER CORTICAL MOTOR FUNCTION

The higher cortical centres tell the motor system (pyramidal, extrapyramidal and cerebellar) when and how to move. Movements may reflect internal wishes (endo-evoked) or external stimuli (exo-evoked), e.g. fire alarms.

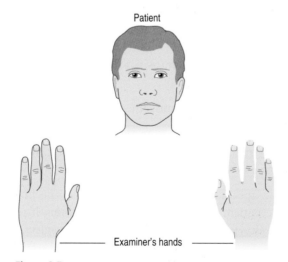

Patient

Examiner's hands

Figure 2.5
Crossed response task. 'Look towards the hand if it goes up but look away if it goes down'. If the patient fails to look at the hand when raised this may imply sensory neglect but failing to look away when the contralateral hand is lowered implies directional akinesia.

When to move

The following deficits follow bilateral cortical lesions, although sometimes isolated right hemisphere lesions.

- **Akinesia** is failure to move, despite normal comprehension and attention, and intact upper or lower motor neurones. It is assessed using the crossed response task (Fig. 2.5).
- **Motor impersistence** is tested by failure to maintain a posture for 20 sec (e.g. protrusion of the tongue or arm), or to look right or left for 20 sec.
- **Defective response inhibition**, e.g. the wrong hand moves when testing the crossed response task, or the patient looks the wrong way on the crossed response eye test. The patient cannot suppress the urge to look at fingers when testing one hemifield but not the other.
- **Perseveration** is becoming stuck repeating the same thing, e.g. clapping more than three times (*signe d'applause*), or copying loops.

How to move (praxis)

Praxicons (motor representations of tasks) are impaired in dominant parietal lobe lesions. This lobe is linked to the left premotor and motor cortex directly and (via the corpus callosum) to the right motor cortex. The impairment may therefore reflect disease in the parietal lobes, the frontal lobes (premotor/supplementary motor area), or the corpus callosum.

- Ask the patient to perform transitive (using tools, e.g. hammer) and intransitive tasks (gestures, e.g. wave goodbye, salute, shadow box). Transitive tasks usually show more deficits. Test orofacial praxis by asking the patient to cough, blow a kiss and smack their lips. Understanding these tasks clearly involves language (left hemisphere), which must first be assessed carefully. Note Broca patients often have left limb dyspraxia, so ensure a good understanding before testing praxis.
- Ask the patient what you are doing, e.g. cutting bread. Recognizing the task indicates the posterior praxicons are intact.
- Copy what you do: this is easier than asking for a transitive task but more difficult if there is a conduction dyspraxia.

Assess the timing, trajectory of movements and joint movements strictly.

- **Ideomotor apraxia** is most people's idea of dyspraxia (as above).
- **Ideational apraxia** implies difficulty in performing a task in sequence, e.g. write this letter, put it in the envelope, put on a stamp and address it.

Brodmann area 7 lesions can mimic apraxia due to difficulty relating the internal body image to the external world, e.g. the patient sits but cannot orientate himself properly; he looks as though he might miss the chair, yet has full visual fields and no neglect, etc.

Neglect

Attention may be intentional or reactive.

- **Intentional** attention is a deliberate 'willed' act (frontal cortex).
- **Reactive** attention is a reflex full attention to a significant stimulus, e.g. fire alarm (thalamus and brainstem). At a cortical level, many background stimuli (e.g. constant sensory information) are normally ignored.

Neglect is common (up to two-thirds of right hemisphere strokes) and reflects attention or spatial representation deficits. It may be sensory or motor (motor akinesia: see above). Right-sided lesions more commonly cause neglect, classically with an inferior parietal lobe or right angular gyrus lesion.

Test for neglect by asking the patient to name ten objects around the room, to bisect a line, or to perform a cancellation task.

Distinguish neglect from hemianopia using two tests:

1. Retest for neglect (as above) with eyes turned away from the neglected side.
2. Analyse line bisection (see Fig. 1.1): left-sided neglect causes bisection to the right of the midline; left-sided hemianopia without neglect causes bisection of the line to the left.

BASAL GANGLIA

The basal ganglia are large subcortical nuclear masses comprising the caudate, putamen, pallidum, nucleus accumbens and (usually included) the amygdala.

- **Input** is mainly from the striatum (caudate and putamen).
- **Output** is mainly to the medial globus pallidus, the pars reticulata of the substantia nigra, the motor thalamus and pedunculopontine nucleus.

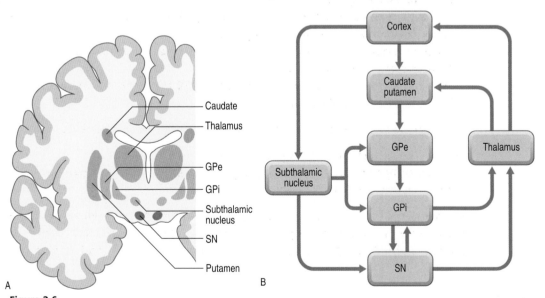

Figure 2.6
Functional anatomy of the basal ganglia. (a) Basal ganglia. (b) Connections of the basal ganglia (schematic). GPi, globus pallidus (internal); GPe, globus pallidus (external); SN, substantia nigra.

Motor function

Basal ganglia motor function is well established (Fig. 2.6a,b) in both health and in disease, e.g. Parkinson's disease. This model acts as a template for the other circuits mentioned below. Large cortical areas are funnelled to a restricted part of the basal ganglia and then relayed back to a circumscribed area of cortex (usually prefrontal) (Fig. 2.7).

In Parkinson's disease, there is loss of dopaminergic neurones from the substantia nigra (pars compacta). Dopamine loss causes overactivity of the subthalamic nucleus and globus pallidus (medial), inhibiting the thalamus (with loss of cortical excitation) and the prepontine nucleus (important for ambulation).

The direct pathway neuromodulators are substance P and opioid peptides (derived from preproenkephalin-B (PPE-B), e.g. dynorphin).

The indirect pathway neuromodulators are derived from PPE-A.

Psychomotor function

The basal ganglia are surprisingly important for behaviour and cognition, especially the 'ventral striatum' (those parts of the basal ganglia linked to the limbic lobe). Cognitive and behavioural dysfunctions are common in basal ganglia conditions, e.g. Parkinson's disease.

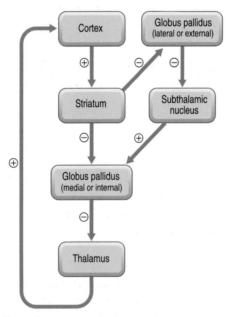

Figure 2.7
Model of basal ganglia pathways.

CEREBELLUM

Anatomy

The cerebellum has three anatomical divisions.

- **Vestibulocerebellum** governs posture, equilibrium and eye movements. The flocculonodular node receives afferents from the vestibular apparatus and sends efferents to the fastigial and vestibular nuclei.
- **Cerebrocerebellum** (connected to the dentate nucleus) receives afferents from area 4, 6 and association cortices and sends efferents to the ventrolateral thalamus and red nucleus and hence to motor and premotor cortex. The 'thinking part' (feed-forward) aspects of the cerebellum are important in movement initiation, planning and timing. There is also a cognitive and behavioural aspect to cerebellar function – the cerebellar cognitive affective syndrome includes disrupted executive function, spatial cognition, language and emotional regulation of behaviour.
- **Spinocerebellum** includes the midline vermis (connected to the fastigial nucleus) and is involved with limb movements. It receives afferents from the spinocerebellar and vestibular apparatus and sends efferents to the ventromedial spinal cord, influencing posture. Alcohol impairs its function, hence causing predominantly gait difficulty with a few eye movement problems or upper limb ataxia.

Coordination

The cerebellum is principally a comparator, adjusting motor outputs according to afferent signals and allowing coordinated skilled movements. It influences all motor tone, posture and gait.

- **Impaired feedback.** Most cerebellar clinical signs reflect impaired correction of movement errors, e.g. intention tremor.
- **Impaired 'feed-forward'.** Accurate planning of the direction, force and timing of multi-jointed movements, relies on predicting previously learned movements.

Figure 2.8 shows the basic cerebellar circuit.

Motor learning

The cerebellum is important in motor learning. For example, if the lateral rectus tendon is cut and the intact eye patched, the saccade will be hypometric. The cerebellum then changes the gain on saccadic eye movements, regaining their accuracy; if the intact eye is now unpatched, the saccades become temporarily hypermetric.

A simplified explanation of the mechanism is as follows:

- The inferior olive receives information from muscle proprioceptors and sends information (climbing fibres) to Purkinje cells of an aspect of the movement that failed.
- Mossy fibres from pontine nuclei that are connected to cortical areas synapse with granular cells, which send parallel fibres that synapse with many Purkinje cells.

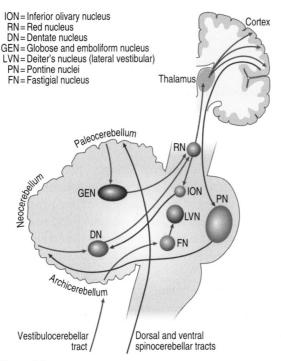

ION = Inferior olivary nucleus
RN = Red nucleus
DN = Dentate nucleus
GEN = Globose and emboliform nucleus
LVN = Deiter's nucleus (lateral vestibular)
PN = Pontine nuclei
FN = Fastigial nucleus

Figure 2.8
Cerebellar connections. ION, inferior olivary nucleus; RN, red nucleus; DN, dentate nucleus. INPUTS: (1) Cortex → pons → middle cerebellar peduncle; (2) Spinal cord – via dorsal spinocerebellar (legs) and cuneocerebellar (arms) systems; (3) Sensory, e.g. vestibular. OUTPUTS: (1) Lateral system → ION/RN/DN; (2) Intermediate system → medial motor → rubro and tectospinal tracts; (3) Medial system → vermis → flocculonodular system.

- Pairing signals from climbing fibres and mossy fibres result in smaller Purkinje post-synaptic responses (long-term depression), hence plasticity and motor learning.

CRANIAL NERVES AND BRAINSTEM

Motor tracts

The motor pathways are anterior and decussate at the medullary pyramid, with the leg fibres below the arm fibres.

Sensory tracts

The sensory pathways in the brainstem and cord are easily disrupted by inflammation (e.g. in multiple sclerosis) but are generally more resistant to tumours (and also to central pontine myelinolysis).

In the medulla, the spinothalamic tracts (pain and temperature) are separate from the medial lemnisci (extensions of the dorsal column) and run close to the sympathetic chain. A brainstem Horner's syndrome is therefore often associated with contralateral pain and temperature loss.

Brainstem stroke syndromes

Brainstem anatomy is complicated and best illustrated by recognizable stroke patterns (Fig. 2.9a–c).

Midbrain

The classical midbrain infarction syndromes illustrate the anatomy.

- **Basal (anterior) midbrain infarction** disrupts the corticospinal tracts and the emerging 3rd nerve, causing *Weber syndrome*:
  - Contralateral hemiparesis.
  - Ipsilateral 3rd nerve palsy.
- **Paramedian midbrain** (red nucleus) **infarction** causes *Benedikt syndrome:*
  - Contralateral cerebellar dysfunction.
  - Partial ipsilateral 3rd nerve palsy.
- **Dorsolateral midbrain infarction** damages the spinothalamic tracts and medial lemniscus (running closely together), the sympathetic pathway, 3rd nerve nucleus and the superior cerebellar peduncle. This causes *Nothnagel syndrome:*
  - Complete loss of sensation (contralateral).
  - Horner's syndrome (ipsilateral).
  - 3rd nerve palsy (ipsilateral).
  - Cerebellar signs (ipsilateral).

Pons

Basal

Limited basal pontine lesions often affect the 6th and 7th nerve nuclei together, e.g. *Millard-Gubler syndrome* comprising:

- Contralateral hemiparesis.
- Ipsilateral 6th and 7th nerve palsies.

More extensive basal pontine lesions also cause:

- Vertigo (involving the vestibular nucleus, Fig. 2.10).
- Contralateral facial spinothalamic loss (5th nucleus).
- Horner's syndrome.
- Deafness.

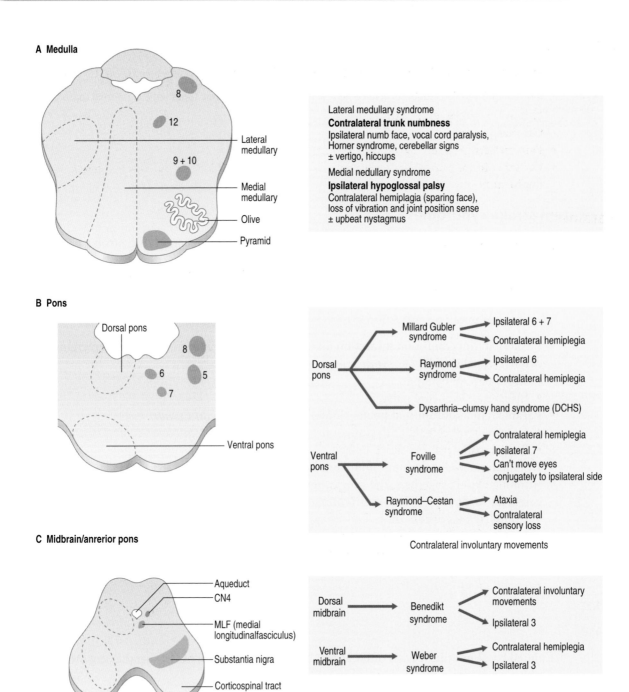

A Medulla

Lateral medullary
Medial medullary
Olive
Pyramid

Lateral medullary syndrome
Contralateral trunk numbness
Ipsilateral numb face, vocal cord paralysis,
Horner syndrome, cerebellar signs
± vertigo, hiccups

Medial nedullary syndrome
Ipsilateral hypoglossal palsy
Contralateral hemiplagia (sparing face),
loss of vibration and joint position sense
± upbeat nystagmus

B Pons

Dorsal pons
Ventral pons

Dorsal pons → Millard Gubler syndrome → Ipsilateral 6 + 7
→ Contralateral hemiplegia
→ Raymond syndrome → Ipsilateral 6
→ Contralateral hemiplegia
→ Dysarthria–clumsy hand syndrome (DCHS)

Ventral pons → Foville syndrome → Contralateral hemiplegia
→ Ipsilateral 7
→ Can't move eyes conjugately to ipsilateral side
→ Raymond–Cestan syndrome → Ataxia
→ Contralateral sensory loss

Contralateral involuntary movements

C Midbrain/anrerior pons

Aqueduct
CN4
MLF (medial longitudinalfasciculus)
Substantia nigra
Corticospinal tract

Dorsal midbrain → Benedikt syndrome → Contralateral involuntary movements
→ Ipsilateral 3

Ventral midbrain → Weber syndrome → Contralateral hemiplegia
→ Ipsilateral 3

Figure 2.9
Brainstem stroke syndromes. Stroke patterns in the brainstem. (a) Lateral medullary stroke: Ipsilateral – numb face, vocal cord paralysis, Horner syndrome, cerebellar signs ± vertigo and hiccups. Contralateral – trunk numbness. Medial medullary stroke: Ipsilateral – hypoglossal palsy. Contralateral – hemiplegia (Sparing face), loss of vibration and joint position sense ± upbeat nystagmus; (b) pons and (c) midbrain.

Dorsolateral

Dorsolateral pontine lesions disrupt the spinothalamic tract, sympathetic chain and the cerebellar pathways causing:

- Horner's syndrome (ipsilateral).
- Cerebellar signs.
- Pain and temperature loss (contralateral).
- Dorsal column function is preserved (the medial lemnisci lie deep and medial and so are unaffected).

Paramedian

Paramedian pontine lesions cause:

- Ipsilateral light touch and position sense loss (medial lemniscus disrupted).
- 6th or 7th nerve palsy, or conjugate gaze palsy.

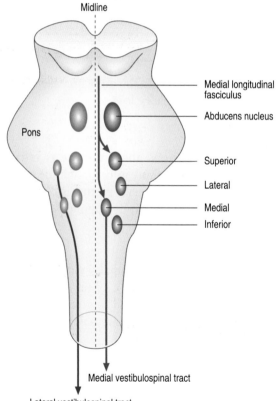

Figure 2.10
Vestibular pathways (posture, tone and eye movements). Lateral vestibulospinal tract: increases extensor tone and activates extensor muscles, especially axial. Medial vestibulospinal tract: coordinates movements of eyes, head and neck with vestibular input.

Medulla

Dorsolateral

A dorsolateral lesion causes the celebrated *Wallenberg syndrome*, comprising:

- Vertigo (vestibular nucleus), often the most prominent first symptom.
- Ataxia (inferior cerebellar peduncle).
- Disruption of 9th and 10th nerve nuclei (swallowing).
- Altered facial sensation.
- Contralateral spinothalamic loss.
- Horner's syndrome.

Sometimes the spinal cord is affected (the anterior spinal artery is derived from the vertebral arteries). *Opalski syndrome* is ipsilateral hemiparesis with *Wallenberg syndrome*.

Paramedian

This causes disruption to the 12th nerve, the medial lemniscus and the motor pathways (causing locked-in syndrome if bilateral).

Upper cranial nerve nuclei

Trigeminal

The trigeminal nucleus is very extensive: a dorsolateral lesion anywhere between C2 and the mid-pons may cause crossed facial spinothalamic sensory loss.

Oculomotor

The 3rd nerve anatomy (Fig. 2.11) allows predictions about nuclear vs infranuclear 3rd nerve palsies. The three 'inferior' muscles (inferior rectus, inferior oblique and medial rectus) are ipsilaterally supplied; the 'superior' muscle (superior rectus) is contralaterally supplied and the 'supra' muscle (orbicularis oculi) is bilaterally supplied (the central caudal nucleus (CCN) is in the midline). Thus:

- **Nuclear 3rd nerve palsy**
  - The classical presentation is ipsilateral partial 3rd nerve palsy with contralateral superior rectus palsy.
  - A midline nuclear 3rd nerve lesion involves the CCN and so gives bilateral ptosis.
  - A ventral lesion, sparing the CCN, gives bilateral 3rd nerve palsy without ptosis.
- **Not nuclear 3rd nerve palsy**
  - A unilateral dilated pupil must be a fascicular 3rd nerve palsy, because the Edinger–Westphal nucleus is in the midline.
  - Contralateral superior rectus sparing in a 3rd nerve palsy is unlikely to be nuclear.

Eye movements

Saccades

These are rapid eye movements (800°/sec).

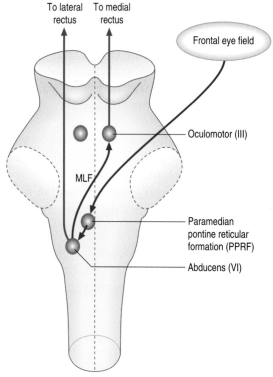

Figure 2.11
Control of eye movements. 6, Abducens nucleus; PPRF, paramedian pontine reticular formation; 3, oculomotor nucleus; MLF, medial longitudinal fasciculus.

Physiology of saccades

Saccades may be triggered externally (to noise or new visual stimulus) or internally.

- **Burst neurones** are tonically inhibited by pause neurones in the nucleus raphe interpositus. In a rapid eye movement, a high frequency pulse (phasic discharge) is needed to overcome the viscous orbital forces. Disruption of burst neurones cause *slow saccades* (the examiner can see the eyeball move): the patient is usually unaware of the problem.
- **Pause neurones** can be disinhibited by the cortex or the superior colliculus.
- **The neural integrator** (medial vestibular nucleus and nucleus prepositus hypoglossi) generates a pulse (velocity command) and hence a 'step' discharge (a position command), which facilitates the 'step change' in innervation, required to maintain the new eye position.

Anatomy of saccades

Saccades involve several brain structures. Horizontal and vertical saccade systems are anatomically distinct but work on the same principles.

- **The parietal lobes** stimulate reflexive saccades.
- **The frontal lobes** stimulate 'higher order' voluntary saccades.

- The **prepontine reticular formation** (PPRF), rostral to the 6th nerve nucleus, contains burst neurones that generate rapid horizontal eye movements. A PPRF lesion disrupts horizontal saccades, but spares vestibulo-ocular movements.
- The **6th nerve nucleus** contains motor neurones for the lateral rectus, but also contains interneurones to the contralateral 3rd nerve nucleus via the medial longitudinal fasciculus (MLF). A fascicular 6th nerve palsy causes a lateral rectus palsy alone, whereas a nuclear 6th nerve palsy also disrupts horizontal gaze (saccadic and pursuit).
- The **cerebellum and PPRF** maintain the output of the neural integrator by controlling gain. The gain is the ratio of output to input; a faulty gain will lead to a drift off the target and a corrective saccade: gaze evoked nystagmus.
- The **basal ganglia** are also involved in saccades. There is output from the frontal lobe to the caudate nucleus and then to the superior colliculus via the basal ganglia output – the substantia nigra pars reticularis.

Figure 2.12a,b illustrates the lesions causing internuclear ophthalmoplegia (INO) and lateral one-and-a-half syndrome. The posterior INO of Lutz causes restricted volitional abduction but reflex manoeuvres (cold calorics) are unaffected; it is usually caused by a lesion in the rostral pons.

Pursuit

These are eye movements (70° per sec), which track a target.

Motion detection depends upon the afferent pathway. The geniculostriatal cortex projects to the middle temporal and medial superior temporal cortex, which in turn project to the dorsolateral pontine nuclei.

- **Impaired pursuit** leaves the eyes unable to keep up with a target; hence the fovea 'slips', producing corrective saccades (broken pursuit movements). Bi-directional broken pursuit movements are non-specific (e.g. anxiety, stress, tiredness, medication, older age). However, unilateral broken pursuit is a localizing sign.
- **Convergence** of the eyes allows binocular fixation to be maintained with close vision, allowing single vision and depth perception; it can be considered as a dysconjugate eye movement in the horizontal plane.

Supranuclear eye movement disorders

Saccades are affected first in supranuclear lesions: examining saccades (rather than just pursuit) is therefore important in cerebral disorders.

Supranuclear gaze dysfunction implies an interruption to the 'voluntary' motor pathways projecting to the eye movement generators in the midbrain or PPRF. The lesion spares the final common pathway (nuclear and infranuclear) and hence preserves reflexive eye movements such as Bell's phenomenon, vestibular and caloric reflexes.

Vestibular (otolith) tone disruption influences the vertical eye position, causing:

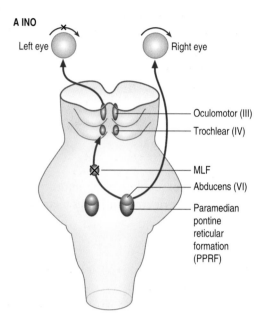

A INO

Left eye   Right eye

Oculomotor (III)

Trochlear (IV)

MLF

Abducens (VI)

Paramedian
pontine
reticular
formation
(PPRF)

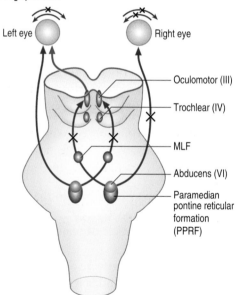

B 1¹/₂ syndrome

Left eye   Right eye

Oculomotor (III)

Trochlear (IV)

MLF

Abducens (VI)

Paramedian
pontine reticular
formation
(PPRF)

Figure 2.12
(a,b) (a) Internuclear ophthalmoplegia (INO). 6, Abducens nucleus; PPRF, paramedian pontine reticular formation; MLF, medial longitudinal fasciculus; 4, trochlear nucleus; 3, oculomotor nucleus. (b) One and a half syndrome. X, lesion.

- A dysconjugate movement: skew deviation, often with associated head tilt.
- A conjugate movement: torsion, documented with fundal photographs. With the head erect, the optic disc and macula should be level; when there is torsion, the relative positions change so the disc is either above or below the macula (globe intorted or extorted, respectively).

Cerebellum and eye movements

Cerebellar disease affects several aspects of eye movements:

- **Loss of smooth pursuit**: this involves the flocculus.
- **'Leakiness' of the neural integrator**, leading to gaze evoked nystagmus.
- **Inaccuracy of saccades**, leading to dysmetric (hypermetric and hypometric) saccades: this involves the fastigial nucleus.

Lower cranial nerves

Glossopharyngeal

- **Sensory.** The 9th nerve is practically entirely sensory, providing taste to the posterior tongue and somatic sensation to the pharynx and Eustachian tube; these fibres terminate in the tractus solitarius. The somatic sensation of the area of skin behind the ear ends in the nucleus and tract of the trigeminal nerve.
- **Motor function** is limited to the stylopharyngeus (nucleus ambiguus).
- **Autonomic function.** The 9th nerve is secretomotor to the parotid gland (inferior salivatory nucleus). The carotid nerve conveys chemoception information from the carotid body (respiratory reflex) and stretch information from the carotid sinus (circulation reflex).

Vagus

- **Dorsal motor nucleus** gives preganglionic parasympathetic fibres to the abdominal viscera (bronchi, gastrointestinal tract and heart).
- **Nucleus ambiguus** gives motor fibres to the striated muscle of pharynx, larynx and soft palate.
- **Tractus solitarius** receives afferents from the abdominal viscera and some taste fibres from the epiglottis. Somatic afferents from the pharynx and larynx go to the spinal nucleus of the 5th cranial nerve.

A vagus nerve lesion gives weakness of two laryngeal muscle groups (Fig. 2.13).

- Tensors (superior laryngeal nerve).
- Adductors and abductors (recurrent laryngeal nerve).

Accessory

The accessory nerve gives motor innervation to the sternocleidomastoid and trapezius.

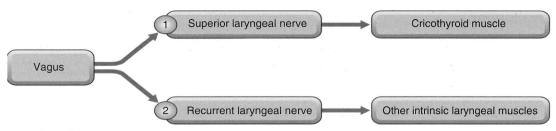

Figure 2.13
Vocal cord palsies. Lesions of (1), mild weakness of phonation; complete lesion of (2), mild weakness of phonation. Ipsilateral cord takes up neutral position; incomplete lesion of (2), abductors affected more than adductors (Semon's Law). Affected cord adopts adducted position, stridor; bilateral complete lesion of (2), aphonia and stridor.

Nucleus

The accessory nerve nucleus has two components:

- The lowest part of the nucleus ambiguus.
- The ventral grey matter of the upper five cervical segments.

Fibres from each join before exiting the skull through the jugular foramen.

Supranuclear

Supranuclear innervation is ipsilateral to sternocleidomastoid, but contralateral to trapezius. Thus in a cerebral infarction the head turns towards the side of the lesion.

Hypoglossal

The 12th nerve is motor to the tongue. The proximity of the last four cranial nerves (particularly beneath the skull) makes them often affected together.

- The 9th, 10th and 11th nerves exit through the adjacent jugular foramen.
- The 12th nerve exits through the hypoglossal canal.
- The sympathetic chain is close by as it courses up the carotid artery.

This anatomy leads to three classical syndromes.

- **Jugular foramen (Vernet's) syndrome.** A jugular foramen lesion inside the skull affects 9th, 10th and 11th cranial nerves. A meningioma or cholesteatoma causing this combination often gives additional 5th and 7th cranial nerve damage, as well as long tract signs.
- **Intercondylar space (Collet–Sicard) syndrome.** A jugular foramen lesion just outside the skull affects 9th, 10th, 11th and 12th cranial nerves, but spares the sympathetic chain.
- **Retropharyngeal space (Villaret's) syndrome.** A jugular foramen lesion outside the skull (9th, 10th, 11th and 12th cranial nerve palsies), but also involving the retropharyngeal space (Horner's syndrome).

The latter two patterns also occur if a meningioma (or neurofibroma) extends out through the jugular foramen.

Swallowing

Reflex swallowing involves the coordinated activity of many structures.

- **The larynx is pulled upwards and forwards** by the muscular sling (suprahyoid muscula-ture) suspending the larynx and hyoid bone. This comprises the myohyoid and anterior belly of digastric (5th nerve and C1-3) anteriorly and stylohyoid and posterior belly of digastric (7th cranial nerve) posteriorly.
- **The anterior upper oesophageal sphincter (cricopharynx) is pulled open** as the larynx moves, since it is attached to its posterior wall. The opening oesophagus pulls the bolus into it and peristalsis starts. The base of the tongue and posterior pharyngeal wall ensure the bolus is cleared.
- **The larynx closes as it moves forwards**: the true cords, false cords, arytenoids and epiglottis (10th cranial nerve).

A neurogenic cause of dysphagia is suggested by abnormalities of:

- **Voice** (phonation, articulation).
- **Tongue and palate** movements.
- **Cough.**

An ear, nose and throat opinion is usually advisable as malignancies can mimic these neuro-logical diseases. Malignancy is often painful, whereas neurogenic dysphagia seldom is.

Case history outcome

The patient had alexia without dysgraphia due to an infarction involving the posterior corpus callosum (see above). The symptoms improved slowly over several weeks.

KEY POINTS

- Single limb involvement suggests a cortical lesion; arm, leg and face involved together suggests capsule or brainstem involvement.
- Parasagittal lesions may present with paraparesis: cerebral imaging is essential in patients with paraparesis with normal cord imaging.
- Saccades are affected earlier than pursuit movements in cerebellar disease: do not rely upon pursuit movements only.
- Bilateral broken pursuit movements are non-specific: unilateral broken pursuit is a local-izing sign.
- Anatomy may be learnt 'stroke by stroke' - so reflect on patterns seen in patients (and texts).
- Anatomy is potentially complicated and confusing. Concentrate upon the pattern of sensory and motor deficits you find. Mastering and recognizing these patterns will often mean you are more than half way there.

- Observe and record your findings. Try to make sense of them anatomically. Do not decide where the lesion is first and then try and fit signs to confirm your hypothesis.
- Think where a lesion is and then what process may be causing it.

Further Reading

Chusid JG. Correlative neuroanatomy and functional neurology, 16th edn. California: Lange Medical Publishers; 1976.

Blackouts and sleep disorders

3

Case history

A 30-year-old woman with a previous diagnosis of epilepsy had been treated for 10 years with sodium valproate. She continued to experience occasional events. She had lost her job since the diagnosis and had been ineligible to drive for 10 years. On re-taking the history, she reported the episodes occurred only in the upright posture. Each would begin with blurring of vision, feeling hot and light-headed, followed by loss of consciousness and brief asymmetric limb shaking with no tongue biting or incontinence and rapid recovery afterwards. The EEG had shown non-specific sharpened theta over one hemisphere; CT brain scan had been normal.

INTRODUCTION

Diagnosing blackouts requires a detailed history including a witness account; investigations are less important than the history. The common causes of blackouts are seizures, syncope and psychogenic attacks. Epilepsy has a broad clinical spectrum with many possible underlying causes; furthermore, many other conditions can present in a similar way. Diagnosing episodic altered consciousness therefore requires a general medical perspective, an understanding of the differential diagnosis and knowledge of seizure and epilepsy classification. Where there is doubt (this is common), re-taking the history is more helpful than repeating tests. Table 3.1 lists the common causes of blackouts other than seizures and Table 3.2 gives the characteristics helpful in distinguishing the three most common causes of blackouts: syncope, seizures and psychogenic episodes.

EPILEPSY

Epidemiology

The prevalence of epilepsy is 750 per 100 000. Most patients become seizure-free on medication and can live normal lives, but 30% have continued seizures and/or significant medication side-effects; these require regular specialist review.

The incidence of epilepsy is 50 per 100 000 people per year. However, for each person diagnosed with epilepsy, 4–5 people with blackouts must be assessed; thus 250 per 100 000 people per year require specialist assessment.

Seizure classification

Seizures are either generalized or focal.

Table 3.1: Differential diagnosis of epileptic seizures

Neurally-mediated syncope	Vasovagal syncope
	Carotid sinus syncope
	Cough and micturition syncope
Orthostatic syncope	Autonomic failure
	Age related autonomic dysfunction
	Medications, esp. vasodilators
Cardiogenic syncope	Tachyarrhythmia
	Bradyarrhythmia
	Structural cardiac disease
Cerebral syncope	Ictal bradycardic syncope (seizure causing bradycardia)
	Migraine (especially hemiplegic and basilar artery migraine)
	Chiari malformation, colloid cyst
Psychogenic	Panic disorder
	Dissociative non epileptic attack disorder ('pseudoseizures')
Sleep disorders	Parasomnia
Acute vertigo	Acute labyrinthitis, Ménière's disease
Paroxysmal movement disorders	Familial kinesigenic dystonia
Endocrine, metabolic, toxic	Hypoglycaemia, hypocalcaemia, poisoning (including date rape drugs)
Transient ischaemic attack (TIA)	'Shaking TIA' (critical carotid stenosis with hypotension)
	Brainstem TIA (with vertigo and diplopia)

Table 3.2: Distinguishing syncope, seizures and psychogenic episodes

	Vasovagal syncope	Cardiac syncope	Seizure	Psychogenic episode
Trigger	Common (upright, bathroom, blood, needles)	Uncommon (exertion)	Rare (flashing lights, hyperventilation)	Common (anger, panic)
Prodrome	Almost always	Uncommon	Common (aura)	Uncommon (anxiety symptoms)
Onset	Gradual	Sudden	Usually sudden	Often gradual
Duration	1–30 sec	1–30 sec	1–3 min	Often prolonged (occasionally hours)
Colour	Very pale	Very pale	Cyanosed	Usually normal
Convulsions	None or brief	None or brief	Common (prolonged)	Atypical (fighting, pelvic thrusting, erratic movements)
Eyes open	Often	Often	Usual	Rare (resists eye opening and eye contact)
Incontinence	Uncommon	Uncommon	Common	Uncommon
Lateral tongue bite	Rare	Rare	Common	Very rare (may bite front of tongue or cheek)
Breathing	Quiet	Quiet	Apnoea (expiration)	Hyperventilation or apnoea (inspiration)
Post-ictal confusion	Rare	Rare	Common	Rare
Recovery	Rapid (wakes on floor)	Very rapid	Slow (wakes in ambulance)	Variable, repeated episodes, may be tearful
Fatigue	Minutes to hours	None	Minutes to hours	May report fatigue
Injury	Rare	Common	Common	Uncommon (carpet burn, wrist from fall on to arm)

- **Primarily generalized seizures** include typical absences (abrupt onset and offset, 3 Hz spike-and-wave on EEG, usually normal intellect), atypical absences (less abrupt onset and offset and lasting longer, with 2–4 Hz spike-and-wave and often learning disability), myoclonic jerks and generalized tonic-clonic seizures.
- **Focal (partial-onset) seizures** include *déjà vu* or epigastric aura of medial temporal lobe epilepsy, head and eye turning (adversive seizure) of frontal lobe epilepsy, or visual aura of occipital epilepsy. Generalized tonic-clonic seizures in adults are usually secondarily generalized.

Epilepsy classification

Epilepsies are classified as generalized or focal (localization-related) according to the predominant seizure type, but also with reference to the underlying cause:

- **Idiopathic epilepsies** typically have an age-specific onset (child or adolescent), favourable response to antiepileptic drugs (AEDs), normal cerebral imaging and a presumed genetic aetiology. Idiopathic generalized epilepsies (e.g. juvenile myoclonic epilepsy) comprise 30% of epilepsies and present with combinations of generalized seizures.
- **Symptomatic epilepsies** have a known underlying cause (usually structural), such as mesial temporal sclerosis (Fig. 3.1), tumour or cortical dysplasia. They mainly have focal seizures resistant to medication.
- **Cryptogenic epilepsies** are probable symptomatic epilepsies, but a definite explanation cannot be found (normal imaging).

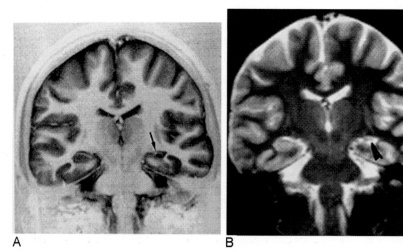

A   B

Figure 3.1
Brain section illustrating mesial temporal sclerosis. (a) T1 weighted MRI, (b) T2 weighted MRI. Arrows show hippocampal sclerosis. Note the hippocampus, temporal lobe/cortex and fornix are smaller on the left than the right. (Courtesy of M O'Donoghue, Queen's Medical Centre, Nottingham).

Provoked or unprovoked?

Provoked (acute symptomatic) seizures occur with transient cerebral insults, e.g. alcohol withdrawal, drug intoxication, meningitis/encephalitis, head injury and intracerebral haemorrhage. Long-term antiepileptic medication is usually not indicated.

Single seizure or epilepsy?

Most people with epilepsy are diagnosed following a first major seizure, but often have had preceding minor events. People may not consider myoclonic jerks, absence seizures, simple or even complex partial seizures to have been epileptic events and they often go unreported.

Acute seizures

- **Emergency resuscitation.** 'ABC' is rarely required following a first seizure since patients are usually already recovering on arrival.
- **Acute seizure control.** Lorazepam is preferable to diazepam for rapid seizure control (less lipophilic, smaller volume of distribution, better clearance, less accumulation and hypoventilation). Seizures persisting beyond 5–10 min should be treated as status epilepticus (see below).
- **Treat underlying cause.** If there is an obvious precipitating factor (Table 3.1), then investigation and treatment of the underlying condition is appropriate.
- **Investigations.** Emergency management takes priority over investigations in acute situations. The exception is blood glucose, essential in all patients presenting with altered consciousness: ambulance personnel will often already have done this.

Emergency history

The diagnosis depends upon an accurate and detailed history, preferably with witness account, taken by an appropriately experienced clinician. Certain details influence acute management (previous seizures, medications, alcohol, illicit drugs), yet emergency unit histories are necessarily limited for several reasons:

- **Patients** may be amnesic for the event, confused post-ictally, or drowsy following lorazepam.
- **Witnesses** may be frightened and unreliable. Also, many episodes are unwitnessed, especially in elderly people.
- **Previous notes** are rarely immediately available.

Emergency unit clinicians must therefore maximize the available history.

- **Clinicians** in the emergency unit often will witness further seizures themselves.
- **Paramedic crews** may describe seizures at the scene or in transit, or have spoken to witnesses.
- **Telephoning** a relative or friend, especially with confused patients, is recommended.

Emergency examination

Physical examination infrequently reveals the cause of a seizure.

- **Emergency assessment.** Assessing conscious level and airway protection is essential for safe clinical management.
- **Cardiovascular examination** (lying and standing blood pressure, heart auscultation) is important since syncope is more common than epilepsy, especially in the elderly.
- **Neurological examination** includes searching for head injury, tongue biting, meningism, papilloedema and focal signs including visual field defects. Upgoing plantars are common post-ictally.
- **General examination.** Epilepsy specialists also habitually examine for skin stigmata (neurofibromata, tuberous sclerosis), dysmorphic features, body size asymmetry (e.g. nail size) and cerebral bruits.

Investigating a first seizure

'Everyone is allowed one seizure' is nonsense and potentially dangerous; all first seizures must be investigated and explained.

- **Blood tests** other than glucose are rarely necessary following an isolated seizure. With pre-existing epilepsy, serum antiepileptic drug level measurement may help in confirming poor compliance. Blood alcohol levels, liver function tests and calcium levels may be relevant. Serum prolactin (often normal following a non-epileptic seizure) is not sufficiently reliable or available out of hours to be useful.
- **Electrocardiogram** is indicated following all blackouts and first seizures. This is particularly relevant if first seizures or syncope occur in the elderly or on exertion. Although significantly abnormal in only about 5% of patients with syncope, emergency unit clinicians must recognize potentially fatal conditions diagnosable on electrocardiogram that commonly present as blackouts, e.g. long QT syndrome.
- **Electroencephalography** (EEG) is especially useful in children and young adults following a first seizure. EEGs show 'epileptiform' changes in about 35% of people following a first seizure, increasing to 50% on EEGs performed within 24 h. The EEG should therefore, if considered necessary, be performed as soon as practicable after a first seizure. It must be interpreted in the light of the history and can support (but never exclude) a diagnosis of epilepsy, can help with classification and exclude photosensitivity. Over-interpreting minor EEG anomalies encourages a misdiagnosis of epilepsy.
- **Imaging.** Computed tomography (CT) scanning is the most practical emergency cerebral imaging method, being readily available and allowing close monitoring if necessary. However, most patients presenting with a spontaneous seizure will require magnetic resonance (MR) brain scanning at some stage. Only MR imaging can identify many of the major causes of focal epilepsy, such as mesial temporal sclerosis or cortical dysplasia. It is therefore indicated following a spontaneous seizure, unless idiopathic generalized epilepsy is confidently diagnosed and responsive to the first antiepileptic medication.
- **Cardiovascular tests.** Echocardiogram, tilt table and exercise tests may be useful to investigate syncope, along standard consensus guidelines.

Examples of cards for patients and carers following an epileptic seizure are shown in Boxes 3.1 and 3.2.

Box 3.1: Patient

You have had an epileptic fit.
- The doctor has examined you. You do not require admission to hospital.
- It is necessary that a responsible adult observes you for 24 h.
- Please rest, take your usual medication and do not drink alcohol.
- Arrange to see your family doctor as soon as convenient and give him/her the letter describing what has happened to you.
- Do not drive until you have discussed the fit with your doctor.

Box 3.2: Carer

Please bring the patient back to the hospital if he or she:
- Becomes increasingly sleepy.
- Has another fit.

What to do if another fit occurs:
- Lie the patient down on one side (the recovery position).
- Try to ensure that he/she can breathe easily. This means that their airway must be clear.
- Do not insert objects or fingers into the mouth.
Usually the fit will subside in a few minutes. Stay with the patient. If the attack lasts for many minutes or you feel unable to cope, then seek urgent medical help or dial 999 and ask for an ambulance. The ambulance personnel will know what to do.

Subsequent management

Following suspected spontaneous seizures, patients need rapid specialist access, for confirmation of diagnosis, relevant investigations, consideration of treatment, informed lifestyle advice and appropriate follow-up. Ideally, emergency units should make fast-track links to local epilepsy specialist services, thereby often avoiding the need for hospital admission.

History taking in suspected epilepsy

Presenting complaint

The clinician should take time to listen and document carefully the symptoms of the patient's episodes. Time at this stage saves much uncertainty later. Important pointers to seizure (rather than syncope or psychogenic event) are a stereotyped warning (e.g. epigastric aura or *déjà vu* in temporal lobe epilepsy, head turning in frontal lobe epilepsy), stereotyped automatisms (lip smacking, hand movements, vocalizations), lateral tongue biting, post-event confusion (patients following a seizure typically wake in the ambulance or emergency unit; following syncope they wake on the floor) and post-ictal muscle aching.

Previous blackout events must be explored in detail and patients asked specifically for any history of absences, myoclonus or photosensitivity.

Medication history

- Current and previous AEDs, including dose, formulation, dates, benefit and adverse effects.
- Potentially epileptogenic medications, e.g. ciprofloxacin, tramadol, antimalarials.
- Drugs with important AED interactions, e.g. warfarin, digoxin, oral contraceptive.

Previous history

The history should include potential cerebral insults, e.g. premature and/or traumatic birth, febrile seizures, meningitis/encephalitis and head injury. Heart disease (congenital or acquired) may suggest syncope. Depression and anxiety commonly accompany epilepsy, but a significant psychiatric history (including abuse and illicit drug dependence) might favour psychogenic events.

Family history

The family history should include epilepsy, febrile seizures, syncope and sudden or young deaths. Family histories are notoriously unreliable, often incomplete, sometimes deliberately concealed and may require repeated enquiry or even direct assessment of affected individuals.

Social history

This includes education, employment, driving status, family planning, home situation, sporting interests, use of alcohol and illicit drugs.

Examination

Physical examination often contributes little to blackout diagnosis.

- **Epilepsy:** Examination includes a search for skin stigmata (neurofibromatosis, tuberous sclerosis), dysmorphic features, body size asymmetry (e.g. nail size) and cerebral bruits. Long-term AEDs may result in tremor, hair loss, weight gain (e.g. sodium valproate, gabapentin), gum hypertrophy, hirsutism, acne, ataxia or absent reflexes (e.g. phenytoin). Patients with focal-onset seizures require examination for visual field defects or long tract signs. Field defects from vigabatrin therapy or temporal lobe epilepsy surgery may have implications for driving, even when seizure-free.
- **Probable syncope:** Cardiovascular examination is essential, particularly in the elderly. The pulse rate, rhythm and blood pressure (BP) require particular attention. The supine and standing BP and heart rate is usually unhelpful because in those with suspected vasovagal syncope it remains unchanged or even rises a little on first standing; its main value is in patients (usually elderly) with possible orthostatic hypotension. BP in each arm may help to diagnose brainstem transient ischaemic attacks due to subclavian steal syndrome. Cardiac auscultation is important to identify structural, particularly valvular, heart disease. Carotid sinus massage should not usually be undertaken in a neurology clinic without special arrangements.
- **Psychogenic episodes:** If hyperventilation is suspected as a cause of blackouts, it can be helpful (to patient and clinician) to provoke the physical symptoms in the clinic by deep breathing for 3 min. Hyperventilation may also induce typical absences in children.

Investigations

All first seizures must be explained and usually investigated. Electroencephalogram (EEG) and MR brain scanning may help to identify the causes and classification of epilepsy, but alone rarely provide the diagnosis. Note that normal EEG and brain scans do not exclude epilepsy.

Electroencephalogram

EEG can help to distinguish generalized from focal epilepsies (Fig. 3.2), support an epilepsy syndrome diagnosis and localize the focus of partial seizures. However, the EEG is normal in about 60% of people following a single spontaneous seizure and in about 40% with epilepsy. EEGs are most useful soon after the seizure and before AEDs are prescribed (it is worth finding the patient's first EEG). Prolonged video-EEG is helpful in patients with frequent events in distinguishing epileptic from non-epileptic attacks.

Brain imaging

This is indicated for spontaneous seizures either of presumed focal onset (aura, focal signs or EEG focus) or refractory to medical treatment. Spontaneous seizures arising in adults are mostly focal and so all should be considered for cerebral imaging. MR is the imaging of choice because computed tomography (CT) scanning often misses epilepsy causes such as mesial temporal sclerosis (Fig. 3.1), cortical dysplasia, cavernoma and benign temporal lobe tumours, e.g. ganglioglioma, dysembryoplastic neuroepithelial tumour.

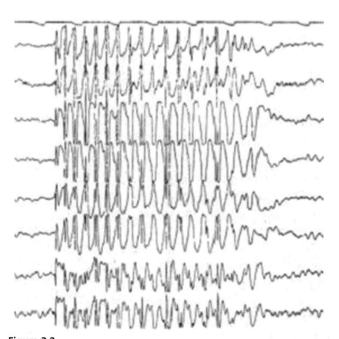

Figure 3.2
EEG showing generalized 3/sec spike and wave. Right-sided leads: upper four tracings; left-handed leads: lower four tracings.

Electrocardiogram (ECG)

A 12-lead ECG is indicated following all undiagnosed blackouts, especially suspected syncope and in the elderly (Fig. 3.3). Rare cardiac causes of syncope (long QT, Brugada syndrome) may mimic epilepsy (seizures in sleep) and can induce sudden death.

Epilepsy management

Starting medication

Antiepileptic drugs are considered usually following more than one spontaneous epileptic seizure. Long-term medication is usually withheld following a single seizure. However, highly epileptogenic causes such as glioma, or subclinical epileptiform EEG changes may justify medication after a single event. Antiepileptic medication is usually long term, requiring informed discussion with an epilepsy specialist. Short-term trials are rarely justified. The patient must balance the seizure morbidity, including the small risk of sudden unexpected death (SUDEP) against the consequences, inconvenience and the adverse effects for that individual (including potential teratogenicity).

Choosing medication

Initial treatment is usually with either carbamazepine (focal seizures) or sodium valproate (generalized or focal seizures). Women of childbearing potential (including girls requiring medication into their childbearing years) should probably not be prescribed valproate as first-line owing to

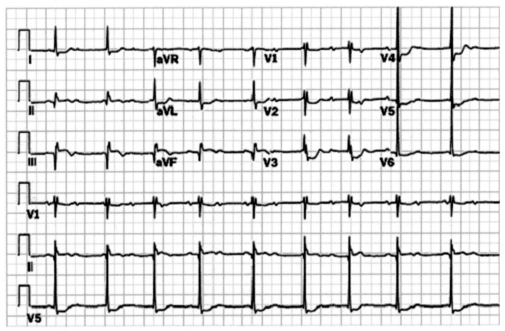

Figure 3.3
EEG showing complete heart block presenting as syncope.

teratogenicity. Alternative monotherapy should be tried before considering polytherapy. Vigabatrin is no longer started (except in babies with West syndrome) because of problems with permanent visual field constriction. The role of other newer drugs (gabapentin, levetiracetam, oxcarbazepine, pregabalin, tiagabine, topiramate, zonisamide) will become clearer with their more widespread use and with the results of comparative pragmatic clinical trials.

Antiepileptic medications

The following are brief prescribing summaries for each of the commonly used antiepileptic medications.

Carbamazepine

- First-line treatment for partial seizures and generalized tonic-clonic seizures; may worsen absences or myoclonic seizures.
- Start low and build to a maintenance (twice daily) dose (600–1800 mg daily).
- Use slow release preparation where possible, especially for higher doses.
- Blood levels not essential.
- Warn about rash, tiredness.
- Warn of the interaction with other medications, including the need for a higher dose contraceptive pill and the need for additional contraception.
- Restrict alcohol use.
- Hyponatraemia is uncommon but in elderly patients on diuretics check electrolytes before prescribing (and in the first few weeks of treatment).
- Warn about potential teratogenicity (malformations in 2.5%) and prescribe folate 5 mg in women of childbearing potential who are not taking definite contraceptive measures.
- If given with lamotrigine, toxic symptoms may be due to an increase in carbamazepine metabolites, despite a therapeutic carbamazepine level.

Gabapentin

- A second-line add-on treatment for partial seizures.
- Build the dose up quickly (three times daily) to maintenance (900–2700 mg daily) over 1–2 weeks.
- Side-effects are unlikely.
- No significant interactions.
- Blood levels are unnecessary.
- Teratogenicity potential appears favourable. Folate 5 mg daily is advised for women of childbearing potential who are not taking definite contraceptive measures.

Lamotrigine

- A first or second line treatment for partial onset and generalized seizures.
- Build up the dose (once or twice daily) slowly.
- The dose prescribed depends on other medications taken:
  - Maintenance 150–300 mg daily as monotherapy.
  - Halve the dose and speed of introduction when prescribed with valproate.

- Bigger doses are needed if prescribed with an enzyme inducer, with the contraceptive pill and in pregnancy.
- Warn about possible rash.
- Blood levels are unnecessary.
- Teratogenicity potential appears favourable at low dose. Folate 5 mg daily is advised for women of childbearing potential who are not taking definite contraceptive measures.

Levetiracetam

- A second line treatment for partial and generalized tonic-clonic seizures, myoclonus and possibly generalized absences.
- Build up the (twice daily) dose over 4–6 weeks to maintenance of 2000–3000 mg daily.
- Warn of the likely dose-related sedative side-effects.
- No significant interactions.
- Blood levels are unnecessary.
- The teratogenic potential in humans is unknown.

Oxcarbazepine

- A first line treatment for partial seizures and generalized tonic-clonic seizures; avoid for absences or myoclonic seizures.
- Build quickly to the maintenance (twice daily) dose 600–2400 mg daily.
- Warn of need for a higher dose contraceptive pill and of the need for additional contraception.
- Give with folate 5 mg in women of childbearing potential who are not taking definite contraception measures.
- The teratogenic potential in humans is unknown.

Phenytoin

- Use for partial and generalized tonic-clonic seizures but not for absences or myoclonic seizures.
- Particularly useful in the acute situation, e.g. status epilepticus.
- Blood levels are important for monitoring phenytoin dosing.
- Give an initial loading dose and then the (once daily) maintenance dose (around 300 mg daily).
- Make only small (e.g. 25 mg) changes when raising or lowering the maintenance dose.
- Warn about toxic unsteadiness and long-term cosmetic effects.
- Warn of need for a higher dose contraceptive pill and of the need for additional contraception.
- Care with interactions when used with other medications.
- Restrict alcohol use.
- Warn of potential teratogenicity.
- Give with folate 5 mg to women of childbearing potential not taking definite contraception measures.

- In elderly patients, phenytoin treatment may justify vitamin D supplements and mineral bone density assessment.

Pregabalin

- A second line treatment for adults with partial and generalized tonic-clonic seizures.
- Build the dose up quickly to maintenance (600 mg daily) over 1–2 weeks as a twice-daily dose.
- Warn of the possible sedative dose-related side-effects.
- There are no significant interactions; no effect on the oral contraceptive pill.
- Blood levels are unnecessary.
- The teratogenic potential in humans is unknown.

Tiagabine

- Use as an add-on agent for patients with partial seizures.
- Start with 15 mg twice daily (adults); 20 mg three times daily if combined with enzyme inducers, e.g. carbamazepine or phenytoin.
- Warn about dizziness, sedation and headache.
- It does not affect the oral contraceptive pill.
- The teratogenic potential in humans is unknown.

Topiramate

- Use as a second line treatment of partial and generalized tonic-clonic seizures and possibly for generalized absences and myoclonus.
- Build up the (once or twice daily) dose only slowly to maintenance of 100–600 mg daily.
- Warn of the likely sedative and ataxic dose-related side-effects and of potential weight loss. Warn about blurred vision (glaucoma).
- Avoid if there is a history of renal calculi; take care if there is a previous psychiatric history.
- Few interactions but a higher dosed oral contraceptive pill is needed with topiramate doses above 100 mg daily.
- Blood levels are unnecessary.
- The teratogenic potential in humans is unknown.

Valproate

- Suitable for all epilepsy types but remains first choice treatment for generalized seizures.
- Build dose (once or twice daily) to maintenance (600–3000 mg daily) over 2–8 weeks.
- Take care when combining with lamotrigine.
- Blood levels are unnecessary.
- Warn about weight gain, tremor, hair loss and polycystic ovaries.
- Warn that alcohol will appear more potent and sedative.
- Warn about potential for teratogenicity, including spina bifida. Women planning a pregnancy may wish to consider alternative antiepileptic drugs prior to conception.
- Give with folate 5 mg in women of childbearing potential who are not taking definite contraception measures.

Vigabatrin

- Vigabatrin (add on for partial and generalized tonic-clonic seizures) is now rarely used except in babies with West syndrome.
- Avoid in myoclonic or absence epilepsy.
- Build dose up slowly, over 4–6 weeks once or twice daily (maintenance 1000–3000 mg daily) in adults and over 7–10 days in infants.
- Warn of potential visual field impairment, sedation, or depression; monitor visual fields annually in patients taking vigabatrin and withdraw (slowly) on suspicion of field loss.
- Blood levels are unnecessary.
- No significant interactions.
- Teratogenicity potential unknown.

Zonisamide

- A second line add-on treatment for adults with partial and generalized tonic-clonic seizures.
- Build up the (once or twice daily) dose slowly over 4–6 weeks to maintenance of 300–400 mg daily.
- Warn of possible rash; avoid if there is a history of renal calculi.
- Carbamazepine or phenytoin increase metabolism of zonisamide; this may necessitate a higher dose.
- Blood levels are unnecessary.
- Teratogenicity potential in humans is unknown.

Stopping medication

Seizure-free patients require detailed discussion before stopping antiepileptic medications. In children, it is usual to try after 2 years seizure-free. In adults, continued seizure freedom for driving and employment often justifies the inconvenience of continued medication; many adults therefore remain on medication while seizure-free for years. Women wishing to conceive naturally wish to stop medication (see below) and often do so without consulting their doctor. Overall, 40% of adults seizure-free for 2 years will relapse. The risk is highest with previous tonic-clonic or myoclonic seizures, seizures after starting medication, needing more than one medication and in those with abnormal EEGs.

Epilepsy surgery

Symptomatic epilepsies, e.g. from mesial temporal sclerosis, are commonly resistant to antiepileptic medication and justify consideration of surgery. The detailed preparation for surgery (prolonged and sometimes invasive video EEG monitoring, sodium amytal testing) is available in only a few centres. Potentially curative procedures include removal of proven epileptogenic lesions, e.g. temporal lobectomy for mesial temporal sclerosis; palliative procedures include multiple subpial transection, corpus callosotomy and hemispherectomy in patients with severe symptomatic epilepsies. Vagus nerve stimulation is an option for adults and children with resistant epilepsy.

Special situations

Status epilepticus

Status epilepticus may be the first presentation of epilepsy. Generalized tonic-clonic status epilepticus is a medical emergency requiring immediate intervention. Traditionally, it is defined as seizures continuing for 30 min; in practice, however, status epilepticus treatment should begin if seizures persist for longer than 5–10 min. Perhaps half of apparent status episodes are psychogenic (pseudoseizures) and an ictal EEG may be very helpful. For those with frequent status needing out of hospital benzodiazepines (usually rectal diazepam), consider buccal midazolam administered at home as a more dignified and easier treatment.

Look for a cause: ask about drug compliance in pre-existing epilepsy, blood tests including glucose and if appropriate consider brain imaging and lumbar puncture. Outcome depends upon the aetiology, age and duration. The mortality is 10–30%; less is known about morbidity. The first 30 min are associated with profound compensatory changes including increased blood pressure and consumption of glucose and oxygen. However, after 30 min this decompensates with hypotension, hypoglycaemia and pulmonary oedema. Early treatment is therefore essential to avoid permanent damage (time is brain).

A treatment protocol agreed with your emergency unit and ITU is essential (Fig. 3.4). This involves resuscitation, drug treatment progressing from lorazepam (0.1 mg/kg bolus,

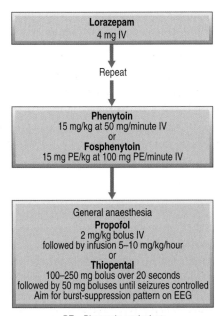

PE = Phenytoin equivalent

Figure 3.4
Emergency treatment of status epilepticus. PE, phenytoin equivalent.

repeated if necessary after 2 min) to phenytoin (20 mg/kg infusion at 50 mg/min), to phenobarbitone (20 mg/kg infusion at 100 mg/min) and if necessary anaesthetizing and ventilating preferably with continuous electroencephalography monitoring. Do not 'try another drug' before admission to ITU. Clinicians often give inadequate amounts of drugs, so give the full dose. Valproate may have a role for patients unresponsive to phenytoin or phenobarbitone.

If the seizures persist, remember again that non-epileptic attack disorder commonly mimics status epilepticus.

Refractory epilepsy

Refractory focal epilepsy demands a detailed search for structural pathology. Not all MR scans are equal in their quality of data acquisition or reporting (ideally brain MRI should include high definition, thin sliced images, with FLAIR sequences and reported by a neuroradiologist); repeat imaging may be necessary. Poor treatment compliance may cause apparently refractory epilepsy. Furthermore, 15% of patients with 'refractory epilepsy' have psychogenic seizures. Patients who have not responded to two first-line antiepileptic medications therefore require careful diagnostic review. The epilepsy classification must also be reviewed since certain medications indicated for focal epilepsies (e.g. carbamazepine, gabapentin) may be ineffective and even worsen absences, myoclonus and photosensitivity.

Learning disability

One-third of patients with severe learning disability have epilepsy. Such consultations can be very challenging. Again, the history is crucial and so a carer who knows the patient well must accompany the patient. As far as practical, the conversation should be directed at the patient rather than carers. Close liaison with the community learning disabilities team is essential.

Children and teenagers

Epilepsy in children is a major sub-speciality, not covered by this review. Teenagers with epilepsy can benefit from combined consultations with adult and paediatric specialists to address their complex medical and social problems.

Elderly

Blackouts management in the elderly is complicated for several reasons. Patients often live alone (no witness account), may have poor recall of events and other medical problems with pre-existing polypharmacy. Most importantly, both epilepsy and syncope are commoner in the elderly, but syncope presenting in old age requires urgent cardiological evaluation. Cerebrovascular disease is closely linked to elderly-onset epilepsy; such patients require consideration of antiplatelet and statin therapy, as well as antiepileptic medication.

Pregnancy

Young women need clear information about teratogenicity (see below) upon which to base treatment and lifestyle decisions. However, for women already pregnant, teratogenicity advice comes too late. Epilepsy nurse input into antenatal clinics help management of epilepsy in pregnancy (0.5% of all pregnancies). Combined neurologist and obstetrician clinics are useful for complicated cases.

Lifestyle implications

People with epilepsy should be encouraged to live normal lives, within sensible limits.

Driving

Loss of driving privileges contributes significantly to the social predicament of epilepsy. Many people are told that they cannot drive until seeing the specialist and eagerly await your advice. The driving regulations vary between countries, but it is usual to have some disqualification from driving in people with active epilepsy. This law usually applies even to minor seizures including epileptic myoclonic jerks. Provoked seizures, e.g. within 1 week of head injury, do not necessarily lead to a driving ban. Heavy goods and public service licences usually have different and stricter rules.

General advice

Sports and leisure: The seizure frequency and type influence advice for specific circumstances such as swimming, cycling on busy roads and isolation sports (e.g. horse riding, hill walking, etc).

Alcohol may provoke seizures through sleep loss, AED interaction (chronic alcohol intake induces liver enzymes), forgetting medication or inducing misplaced confidence that AEDs can be omitted. Pragmatic advice is that patients with epilepsy should limit alcohol consumption to four units in 24 h.

Sleep deprivation is an avoidable cause of lowered seizure threshold, especially in idiopathic generalized epilepsies.

Flashing lights: True photosensitivity is uncommon in adults especially on medication, but many people with epilepsy unnecessarily avoid computers, TVs and discos.

Teratogenicity

Women contemplating pregnancy require balanced and reliable information about the teratogenic potential of their medication. Unfortunately, such data are currently lacking and advice is based to an extent upon opinion and conjecture. Nevertheless, prospective observational data suggest valproate is associated with major congenital malformations more than carbamazepine. The risks are higher with bigger doses and with polytherapy. Furthermore, there are suggestions, awaiting prospective evaluation, of increased neuro-developmental delay among children exposed to antiepileptic medications *in utero*. Unfortunately, valproate is the medication of first choice for idiopathic generalized epilepsies and so changing drugs to protect unborn children risks compromising seizure control. Also, switching from valproate to lamotrigine is complicated, taking several months. Despite lack of conclusive proof and the inherent difficulties in researching this area, young women, particularly on valproate, require specialist review to inform decisions about long-term treatment.

Written information

Patients need opportunities to ask questions. Early follow-up after the initial diagnosis provides the opportunity to discuss concerns after a period of reflection. Patients with chronic conditions are expert in their individual condition since they constantly live with it.

Providing individualized verbal and written information and offering specialist nurse telephone contact encourage greater patient involvement in their long-term management. Most powerful is a personalized letter summarizing the consultation and giving specific information. Copying the standard clinic letter is a useful alternative. Recommended websites for patient and carer information are Epilepsy Action (www.epilepsy.org.uk) and the National Society for Epilepsy (www.epilepsynse.org.uk).

Follow-up

Epilepsy, more than many chronic disorders, justifies long-term follow-up. The diagnosis is history-based and too often is made incorrectly, particularly in non-specialist hands. The choice and need for prescribed medications may be inappropriate and patients may too easily accept medication side-effects and unnecessary lifestyle restrictions. Good practice would suggest annual review, including 'nurse-led' epilepsy specialist clinics, be offered to all patients with epilepsy. Proactive specialist review of those currently managed in the community may also be justified to check diagnoses, optimise clinical management and to provide information.

SLEEP DISORDERS

Sleep can be sub-divided. Rapid eye movement sleep (REM) occupies about 25% sleeping time and is associated with dreaming. In REM sleep, skeletal muscles become atonic with the exception of the eyes and diaphragm. Non-REM sleep is subdivided into four phases – with progressively slower waveforms on EEG. Normally, we spend 80% or more time asleep in bed (sleep efficiency); normal subjects will fall asleep after about 10 min with the first burst of REM sleep after 1 h or so.

What to do with the sleepy patient

This referral has many potential implications – notably with regard to safety when driving – the driving authorities will often need to be notified by the patient. There are sleepiness scales including the Epworth scale.

The age of the patient is a useful clue to aetiology: If young (<25 years), consider narcolepsy, drugs and sleep apnoea.

Narcolepsy – needs A and B to be present.

A. Irresistible urges to fall asleep for 15–30 min; patient awakes refreshed. Sleep at night is often disrupted.
B. Cataplexy: that is a loss of posture (head droops, eyelids droop or falling to floor) provoked by an emotional response, e.g. laughter.
C. Sleep paralysis: awakes not able to move – this can be a normal phenomenon.
D. Hallucinations just before dropping off to sleep.
E. Fugue-like states with automatic obedience – almost a waking prolonged absent-minded daydream state.

Pathophysiologically, narcolepsy appears to be a dysregulation of REM sleep, e.g. the REM atonia spilling into wakefulness with the cataplexy or sleep paralysis. Acetylcholine promotes REM sleep: aminergic transmissions inhibit it. Narcolepsy is diagnosed clinically and with the multiple sleep latency test – abnormal if a non-sleep deprived subject sleeps before 8 min (8–10 borderline) and REM onset. Treatment is modafinil/amphetamine for sleep disorder and tricyclic or SSRI for cataplexy.

Sleep apnoea is common: patients feel unrefreshed waking from sleep, have morning headaches and often snore. Sleep recordings reveal arousals from sleep (5–20/h mild, 20–40 moderate, >40 severe). A trial of continuous positive airway pressure (CPAP) may be necessary. The final answer, irrespective of the sleep study, is whether it is 'CPAP responsive'.

Idiopathic hypersomnolence: this condition is under-recognized and may affect the young. Urges to sleep occur and last for 1–2 h (longer than narcolepsy) and are unrefreshing. These patients do not have cataplexy. Treatment: modafinil.

Parasomnias

REM parasomnia (acting out dreams) often seen in α-synucleinopathies (e.g. MSA). The partner says the subject kicks and punches in his sleep. Waking is associated with dream content. Treat with benzodiazepine.

Non-REM parasomnia occurs in the first half of sleep and includes sleep walking and night terrors. Sleep walkers need to consider their safety: lock windows and inform family members.

Nocturnal frontal lobe seizures are brief stereotyped episodes of less than 2 min, often more than once per night that originally were thought to be forms of dystonia and now known to be epileptic.

SYNCOPE

There are two components to syncope: loss of consciousness (abrupt and transient) and loss of postural tone. It follows a sudden fall in cerebral perfusion. Syncope is far more common than epilepsy (syncope prevalence 20%; epilepsy prevalence 0.75%) and accounts for 3% of emergency department visits and 1% of hospital admissions. Syncope is often misdiagnosed and erroneously treated as epilepsy.

History taking in suspected syncope

The history should focus on each component of syncope:

- **Situations and triggers**: Hot, crowded, stressful or painful situations may provoke vasovagal syncope. Presyncope often leads patients to visit bathrooms, where syncope occurs. Micturition or vigorous coughing may prompt syncope in susceptible individuals; collapse from standing suggests either vasovagal or orthostatic syncope and collapse during exertion suggests cardiac syncope.
- **Prodrome**: Prodromal blacking of vision is a strong pointer towards syncope and prodromal nausea strongly suggests the syncope was vasovagal. Syncope without warning or with palpitations suggests cardiac (arrhythmogenic) syncope.
- **Event**: Syncope results in loss of consciousness for usually 15–45 sec. Patients appear pale, with pupils dilated and eyes elevated and may stiffen with minor convulsions (convulsive syncope) and sometimes incontinence and injury, but rarely lateral tongue biting (Table 3.1). Collapse in a confined space (e.g. toilet) may increase its severity by enforcing an upright posture (anoxic seizures).
- **Recovery**: Patients typically recover promptly from syncope. Patients with vasovagal syncope are quickly orientated but are typically fatigued for minutes to hours afterwards; by contrast, patients with cardiac syncope recover completely almost immediately on regaining consciousness. This is important because those patients who feel perfectly well afterwards and send away the ambulance are in fact at much higher risk of sudden death than those who feel unwell afterwards.

Vasovagal syncope

This is common, generally benign and is the usual explanation for fainting in otherwise healthy individuals of all ages, especially young adults. A patient's vasovagal tendency also influences the likelihood and severity of syncope developing from seemingly unrelated causes, e.g. aortic stenosis and hypertrophic cardiomyopathy. In vasovagal syncope, the blood pressure and heart rate are typically maintained until a sudden haemodynamic collapse.

- **Situations and triggers**: Vasovagal syncope episodes typically occur in bathrooms, hot restaurants, or crowded aeroplanes; specific triggers include prolonged standing, hot, crowded environments, emotional trauma and pain. In susceptible individuals, coughing, swallowing or micturition may provoke episodes. Exercise-induced vasovagal syncope must be investigated in detail to distinguish it from cardiac syncope.
- **Prodrome**: Developing over 1–5 min are light-headedness, nausea, sweating, greying or blacking of vision, muffled hearing and feeling distant and anxious.
- **Event**: A witness may describe pallor, sweating, cold skin and brief convulsive jerks. Incontinence and injury are uncommon and lateral tongue biting rare.
- **Recovery**: Any post-event confusion is typically brief, usually a few seconds, unless there had been associated head trauma.

Vasovagal syncope with specific triggers

Cough syncope, micturition syncope, swallow syncope, etc. are variants of vasovagal syncope where certain specific situations act as powerful triggers to vagus-mediated haemodynamic collapse.

Cardiac syncope

Cardiac syncope results from disorders of either cardiac rhythm or cardiac structure. Cardiac syncope can occur from any posture, usually with little warning and rapid recovery. The history must include a search for pointers towards structural heart disease (previous myocardial infarction or congestive heart failure) and a family history of sudden death before the age of 40 years. A detailed drug history must identify drugs associated with bradyarrhythmias (e.g. amiodarone, beta-blockers, calcium channel blockers) or acquired long QT syndrome (e.g. antipsychotics, erythromycin and antihistamines).

Arrhythmias can result in a sudden fall in cardiac output resulting in loss of consciousness, with little warning. Tachyarrhythmic syncope often occurs without perception of palpitations. Patients with significant structural heart disease (e.g. history of prior myocardial infarction) and scar-related ventricular tachycardia are at high risk of sudden cardiac death due to a cardiac arrest (10–20% annual risk). Patients with genetic disorders such as congenital long QT syndrome or Brugada syndrome can present with syncope and apparently normal hearts and be at risk of sudden and unexpected death. At the other end of the spectrum are patients with structurally normal hearts and regular forms of supraventricular tachycardia who may present with syncope rather than palpitations. Bradyarrhythmias occur mainly in the elderly due to fibrosis in the sinus node or the specialized conducting tissue. Evidence of conduction system disease such as complete left bundle branch block, trifascicular heart block or evidence of sinus node dysfunction such as pauses alternating with atrial tachyarrhythmias (tachy-brady syndrome) increase the possibility that syncope is due to a bradyarrhythmia.

Structural causes: Less commonly, syncope results from mechanical obstruction to either left ventricular outflow (hypertrophic cardiomyopathy, aortic stenosis) or left ventricular inflow (mitral stenosis, atrial myxoma). In patients with previous myocardial infarction, heart failure, or a family history of sudden, unexpected death below age 40 years, any unexplained syncope should be considered life threatening (ventricular tachyarrhythmia) requiring urgent cardiological assessment. Exertional syncope requires exclusion of mechanical obstruction; however, most aortic stenosis or hypertrophic cardiomyopathy patients experience syncope either at rest or at minimal exertion.

Orthostatic syncope

Orthostatic hypotension is where autonomic dysfunction impairs the normal vasoconstriction responses to a postural BP fall, allowing a systolic postural fall exceeding 20 mmHg soon after standing. Orthostatic syncope usually occurs in the elderly, but may accompany any autonomic peripheral neuropathy (diabetes, alcohol, amyloidosis) or complex autonomic failure (e.g. multiple system atrophy). Associated dysautonomic symptoms include impotence, urinary incontinence, nocturnal diarrhoea and constipation. Certain medications may exacerbate the problem, especially antihypertensives, diuretics, tricyclic antidepressants and anti-Parkinsonian treatment. Orthostatic syncope occurs within seconds or minutes of becoming upright, typically on rising and after meals. Unlike in vasovagal syncope, the skin stays warm, the heart rate is unchanged despite the BP fall and sweating is absent. BP and heart rate measured lying and standing usually confirm the diagnosis.

Carotid sinus syncope

Patients with carotid sinus syndrome have exaggerated baroreceptor-mediated reflexes, leading to symptomatic bradycardia and hypotension. It is rare below 50 years of age, but is an important yet frequently overlooked cause of syncope in the elderly. If specifically sought, carotid sinus syndrome is diagnosed in about 15% of elderly patients presenting with suspected presyncope or syncope. However, carotid sinus hypersensitivity (carotid sinus massage resulting in >3 sec asystole) is common in the elderly and so more malignant causes of syncope (e.g. scar-related ventricular tachycardia) should be considered before a diagnosis of carotid sinus syndrome is made.

Carotid sinus syndrome presents, usually in the elderly, with dizziness, syncope or falls, often with injury. Important precipitating factors include head movements (especially with tight neckwear or neck pathology), prolonged standing, heavy meals, or straining on micturition, defecation and coughing.

Central nervous system syncope

These are rare causes of syncope.

- **Seizure-induced arrhythmogenic syncope** results from heart rate and rhythm changes during seizures. Tachycardias commonly accompany seizures, though rarely lead to symptoms. Bradyarrhythmias are rarer, usually associated with left-sided partial seizure onset and lead to loss of consciousness which is syncopal rather than primarily due to the seizure. Such cases are often initially diagnosed as cardiac arrhythmogenic syncope, but partial seizures continue without collapse following cardiac pacing.
- **Intermittent obstructive hydrocephalus**, e.g. Chiari malformation, typically present as occipital 'pressure' headaches building over seconds before loss of consciousness. Third ventricular colloid cysts may present as 'drop attacks' (without loss of consciousness) owing to stretching of the corticospinal fibres supplying the lower limbs. Intermittent elevation of intracranial pressure is a potential cause of sudden death.
- **Transient ischaemic attacks** rarely lead to loss of consciousness, except with posterior circulation involvement with associated vertigo, ataxia, diplopia and paraesthesiae. 'Vertebrobasilar insufficiency' from cervical spondylosis is commonly diagnosed but exceedingly rare.
- **Migraine syncope** is typically associated with familial hemiplegic migraine and usually manifests as a gradual onset loss of consciousness in the context of other migraine symptoms. Basilar artery migraine presents with syncope (commonly prolonged), typically preceded by visual blackening, vertigo, or diplopia. There is overlap between basilar migraine and occipital epilepsy ('migralepsy').

Metabolic syncope

Syncope sometimes results from metabolic disturbances. Hypoglycaemia, easily diagnosed and readily reversed, should be considered in all patients with undiagnosed altered consciousness. Insulin treated diabetes mellitus is the obvious cause. Insulinoma is rare and frequently missed. Other metabolic disorders, e.g. hypocalcaemia, may present as pre-syncope and rarely syncope. Hypoglycaemic syncope presents as recurrent blackouts, often with behaviour disturbance, confusion and convulsions. Insulinoma-related neuroglycopenia occurs especially in sleep and in the early morning and is associated with weight gain from consumption of frequent sweet drinks. Hypocalcaemia (e.g. from hypoparathyroidism) may present as recurrent episodes of tingling, carpopedal spasm and syncope.

Investigations

Investigation of suspected syncope follows standard guidelines and includes electrocardiogram, echocardiogram, exercise testing, head-up tilt table testing and 24-h ECG. Suspected cardiogenic syncope requires urgent cardiology referral.

Electrocardiogram

A 12-lead ECG is indicated following all unexplained syncope, especially in the elderly. Important findings include ischaemic changes, varying degrees of heart block (Fig. 3.3), re-entry tachycardia markers and long QT syndrome.

Echocardiogram

Echocardiography is indicated in all patients with unexplained syncope, especially if a cardiac cause is suspected from certain clinical features:

- **Structural heart disease**, e.g. abnormal cardiovascular examination, abnormal ECG, exercise-induced symptoms, or major cardiac risk factors including age >60 years, smoker, diabetic, hypertensive, hyperlipidaemic patients.
- **Cardiac syncope**, e.g. brief syncope with onset from seated or lying posture, absence of prodrome and rapid recovery. Also, cardiac syncope should be considered in older patients or in those with associated history of palpitation.

Exercise tolerance test

An exercise test is indicated in patients with syncope where:

- The symptoms are associated with exertion or
- There is suspected coronary disease.

An echocardiogram is essential before exercise testing for exertional syncope.

Carotid sinus massage

Carotid sinus massage is indicated in elderly patients with recurrent unexplained syncope or falls ('drop attacks'), especially if the symptoms suggest carotid sinus syndrome. It is usually performed during tilt table testing.

Tilt table testing

Head-up tilt table testing is indicated in patients with recurrent unexplained syncope (likely to be vasovagal) where structural heart disease is either not suspected or has been excluded as the cause. It is indicated after a single episode only if syncope occurred in a high-risk setting, e.g. while driving, or causing significant injury. Anecdotally, a positive tilt table test helps the patient to understand the symptoms and can lead to improvement in syncope frequency.

Prolonged ECG monitoring

Cardiac arrhythmias causing syncope are rare in structurally normal hearts. Thus, ambulatory ECG monitoring (including longer-term ambulatory loop monitoring) is only indicated where:

- Syncope occurs with suspected structural heart disease, e.g. abnormal ECG or age over 60 years.
- In suspected arrhythmogenic syncope (brief loss of consciousness, palpitation with syncope, absence of prodrome, prompt recovery).
- Syncope in individuals with a family history of premature sudden unexpected death.

Management

Syncope management clearly depends upon its cause. Patients with vasovagal syncope are helped by an accurate diagnosis and by advice to prevent presyncopal symptoms from developing into faints (head down, or lying flat with feet elevated). Avoiding provoking situations and correctable causative factors (e.g. certain medications) are clearly important. Medication is rarely needed, but beta-blockers and SSRIs have been shown to be helpful for recurrent vasovagal syncope. Fludrocortisone, high salt content diet and support tights may help to prevent orthostatic syncope. The main priority is to identify or exclude potentially serious cardiac causes and close working with a cardiologist is essential for their safe management.

PSYCHOGENIC NON-EPILEPTIC ATTACK DISORDER

This important cause of blackouts is considered in detail in the 'non-organic neurology' chapter.

Case history outcome

The patient's symptoms were typical of vasovagal syncope, but previously misdiagnosed as epilepsy. The valproate was withdrawn and the episodes managed as faints. Sadly, at the time of the revised diagnosis, she already had a child with learning disability and spina bifida, almost certainly from valproate exposure during pregnancy.

KEY POINTS

- A detailed history with an eyewitness account is essential for blackout diagnosis.
- Epilepsy diagnosis is clinical; a normal EEG does not exclude epilepsy.
- All patients with undiagnosed blackouts should be asked about a family history of sudden explained death.
- The examination of patients with blackouts should include a detailed cardiovascular examination.
- An electrocardiogram (ECG) should be obtained in all patients with syncope.
- An MRI brain should be considered for all new onset spontaneous seizures in adults, unless definitely of generalized onset.
- All patients with unexplained blackouts or epilepsy must inform the relevant driving authorities.
- Females of childbearing potential must understand the potential teratogenicity of their antiepileptic medication.
- Misdiagnosis of epilepsy is common; perhaps 20% of people on medication for epilepsy have other causes for their blackouts.
- In difficult cases, retaking history (patient and eye witness) is more valuable than repeating tests.

Further Reading

Hadjikoutis S, O'Callaghan P, Smith PE. The investigation of syncope. Seizure 2004; 13: 537–548.

Wills AJ, Stevens DL. The management of epilepsy in the accident and emergency department. Br J Hosp Med 1994; 52(1): 42–45.

Headache

4

Case history

A 46-year-old man presented with sudden onset of severe occipital headache with neck stiffness but no pho-tophobia. On examination, he appeared marfanoid. Kernig's sign was positive. The neurological examination (including fundoscopy) was normal. CT brain scan and CSF analysis were normal, with no xanthochromia. CSF opening pressure was 2 cm water.

INTRODUCTION

Headache is the most common neurological referral, with a broad spectrum of presentations and causes.

- Tension type headache.
- Migraine and migraine variants.
- Mixed headache.
- Analgesic induced (chronic daily) headache.
- Raised pressure headache.
- Low-pressure headache.
- Trigeminovascular headache (cluster headache and its variants).
- Giant cell arteritis.
- Subarachnoid haemorrhage.

The main question in headache diagnosis is: 'Is this a primary headache (migraine, tension headache) or a secondary headache (a structural cause)?'

TENSION TYPE HEADACHE

Clinical features

This is the most common headache. It is distinguished from migraine by its continuous 'tight band' quality, generalized discomfort and its lack of systemic upset, photophobia or aura. Often the headache occurs daily, sometimes with a feeling of pressure at the vertex. The headache worsens towards the end of the day and with anxiety, noise or glare. It is closely associated with musculoskeletal problems, particularly neck muscle tension and neck trauma, e.g. whiplash. One-third of patients with tension type headache have accompanying depressive symptoms. Physical examination is normal, though there may be inappropriate muscle contraction over the forehead and neck.

Investigation and management

Imaging is not necessary if the history is typical. Management includes explanation of the symptoms, addressing specific exacerbating factors such as poorly fitting dentures, teeth grinding in sleep and refractive error. A programme of relaxation exercises is often helpful and reinforces to the patient the notion of neck muscle tension causing the headache. Medications must be used with caution, as they are often poorly effective if used in isolation. A non-steroidal preparation is best for pain relief, combined with amitriptyline 10–25 mg nocte, helping both the pain and the return of a normal sleeping pattern.

MIGRAINE

Migraine is common: £1.5 billion of working days are lost annually in the UK through migraine. The diagnosis is made clinically (Box 4.1). Typically it is episodic (lasting 4 h to 3 days) and the headaches are unilateral, throbbing, exacerbated by exertion or movement and associated with systemic upset including nausea, vomiting, phonophobia, photophobia, fatigue, hyperaesthesia and autonomic dysfunction. There are no diagnostic tests.

Box 4.1: *Clinical diagnostic criteria*

Core features (need both):
• Five attacks or more.
• Photophobia, phonophobia and/or nausea.

Additional features (need two or more):
• Moderate to severe headache.
• Unilateral.
• Throbbing.
• Worse on movement.

Migraine with aura

Some 30% of migraine patients have had an aura, either visual, dysphasic, or positive sensory, e.g. pins and needles.

Migraine management

Lifestyle and explanation

• Explain and discuss the diagnosis.
• Encourage regular meals (especially breakfast with high roughage), regular sleep and sensible exercise.
• Cut caffeine consumption (coffee, tea, cola).
• Avoid specific triggers (patients often discover these themselves).

Acute treatment

Start at step 1 and move to the next after three or more failures:

1. Soluble aspirin 600–1200 mg (in water or fizzy drink), with rectal or oral domperidone (anti-emetic and prokinetic, to encourage absorption).
2. Parenteral analgesics, e.g. diclofenac, with domperidone.
3. Triptans: take at headache onset, but not before. The newer triptans generally have fewer side-effects and longer action than sumatriptan. Note that a half dose should be used in patients taking propranolol.
4. Combinations of the above.
5. Intramuscular diclofenac or chlorpromazine.

Note: Ergotamine is relatively contraindicated in patients who have migraine with aura or migraine with additional vascular risk factors.

Prophylaxis

This is appropriate if migraine symptoms significantly interfere with lifestyle, or occur more than once a month.

- Atenolol 25–100 mg b.d.
- Amitriptyline 10–100 mg nocte.
- Sodium valproate 300–1000 mg b.d.
- Topiramate 25–50 mg b.d.
- Combinations of the above.
- Others: pizotifen, verapamil, methysergide, SSRIs.

Hormonal influences

Migraine can be hormonally sensitive.

- Menstrual migraine (exclusively) is rare: a headache diary over three cycles is helpful. Box 4.2 gives the management approach to menstrual migraine.
- Pregnancy often improves migraine.

Migraine in systemic disease

Several systemic conditions may give migraine-type symptoms (see Ch. 7).

Box 4.2: *Management of menstrual migraine*

- NSAIDs, e.g. mefenamic acid or naproxen.
- Oestrogen skin patches, 100 µg 3 days before and 7 days after period onset; reduce to 50 µg oestrogen (or use oestrogen gel) if effective but poorly tolerated.
- Hormone replacement therapy may improve or exacerbate migraine. If the symptoms worsen, reduce the dose or switch to a non-oral preparation. There is no definite evidence that it increases or decreases stroke risk.
- Migraine with aura is a relative contraindication to the combined oral contraceptive pill.

- Lupus anticoagulant syndrome.
- Mitochondrial cytopathy.
- Cerebral autosomal dominant arteriopathy with subcortical infarcts and leucoencephalopathy (CADASIL).
- Urea cycle disorders (children).

Migraine sine headache

Migraine aura with little or no headache poses a diagnostic problem.

- **'Migraine equivalent'** may cause transient monocular blindness and has important differential diagnoses (see below).
- **Retinal migraine.** More than six episodes of visual disturbance 'like ink spots', involving one or both eyes and lasting for minutes.

Sodium valproate, calcium-channel blockers or aspirin are usually effective; β-blockers may worsen vasoconstriction and are best avoided.

The differential diagnosis of migraine sine headache includes transient ischaemic attacks (symptoms appearing abruptly rather than spreading with time and negative rather than positive), glaucoma ('rainbows' around objects), focal brain lesions (often with positive motor symptoms) and occipital epilepsy (Box 4.3).

Box 4.3: Occipital epilepsy: distinction from migraine with aura

- **Duration of visual symptoms**. Migraine: >4 min; epilepsy: <4 min.
- **Aura characteristics**. Migraine: black and white linear aura (especially zigzags); epilepsy: coloured lights and shapes.
- **Frequency**. Migraine episodes are infrequent; epilepsy episodes are frequent (even daily).

MEDICATION OVERUSE HEADACHE

This common problem in neurological practice often complicates a chronic headache tendency. These patients take analgesia for headache (especially opiates and caffeine containing preparations) more than twice weekly. Often patients buy these 'over the counter' and carry pills with them, so ask to see them. Overcoming analgesic dependence is difficult, especially as preventative measures often are ineffective until analgesic overuse is stopped.

- Stop the analgesia, gradually or overnight (the latter is easier).
- Replace with a combination of amitriptyline 10–25 mg nocte and a non-steroidal such as naproxen 500 mg b.d. or mefenamic acid.
- Warn patients of a transient worsening but emphasize 'light at the end of the tunnel'.
- For more severe symptoms, consider hospital admission, adequate hydration, chlorpromazine (especially at night), intravenous aspirin 1 g with rectal domperidone, or even intravenous dihydroergotamine.
- A brief course of oral steroids for 5-10 days may also be useful.

MIXED (TENSION VASCULAR) HEADACHE

This is the most common headache referral to neurology. It is a combination of chronic migraine, with either tension headache or with medication overuse headache. Typically, there is continuous headache with episodes between of typical migraine. Management depends upon which is the predominant component, but usually focuses mainly on analgesic dependence and of chronic tension-type headache.

CHRONIC DAILY HEADACHE

In practice, patients referred for a neurological opinion about their headache initially carry a diagnosis of chronic daily headache. Patients have headaches on 15+ days per month: they almost have forgotten what it is like not to have pain. The important distinction is between primary daily headache (benign) and secondary daily headache (more sinister).

Primary daily headache

Many patients have combinations of all three main types (mixed headache, see above).

- Chronic migraine (frequent migraine episodes).
- Chronic tension-type headache.
- Medication overuse headache (analgesic dependent).

Secondary daily headache

New onset chronic daily headache should be considered initially as secondary, particularly from raised or lowered intracranial pressure.

Raised intracranial pressure

- History may include headache exacerbation in the mornings, on lying flat and by coughing or sneezing. Patients may wake at night with headache or report visual obscurations (blurred or lost vision) on standing. Ask about personality change and sense of smell, since large prefrontal cortex lesions may present with raised pressure without traditional sensory or motor signs.
- Examination should include a thorough general and neurological check. In particular, fundoscopy may show swollen optic discs (usually bilateral with haemorrhages). Examine the visual fields and blind spots (Fig. 4.1).

Idiopathic (benign) intracranial hypertension characteristically affects obese young women. Remember to ask about drugs and dietary habits (vitamin A toxicity). It is mandatory to exclude venous sinus thrombosis. CSF constituents are normal but the pressure is elevated (usually >25 cm water). Record the patient's weight; assess vision fully including colour vision and fields. Treat with acetazolamide or furosemide (if tolerated), sequential lumbar punctures and refer to dietician to assist with weight loss. If headaches persist or vision is

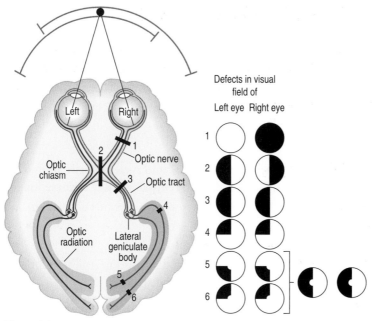

Figure 4.1
The visual fields.

deteriorating, consider neurosurgical (shunt procedure) or ophthalmological referral (optic nerve fenestration). Changes in visual fields are more important than symptoms in determining the management.

Low-pressure headache (or low volume CSF headache)

- **Clinical features:** The cardinal feature is a headache worsening on sitting up or standing, but relieved by lying flat. It may complicate trauma but many are spontaneous: Marfan's syndrome predisposes to low-pressure headache. Examination is normal apart from occasional 6th nerve palsy. In chronic cases postural features may be lost – so consider in a new onset chronic daily headache.
- **Investigations:** MR brain scan may show tonsillar herniation (Chiari malformation) and meningeal contrast enhancement reflecting increased venous perfusion with lower pressure (this also follows lumbar puncture). CSF shows low pressure (<6 cm water) and may contain lymphocytes. The pressure may be so low that air appears on subsequent CT brain images. Interestingly the older literature notes a low CSF pressure to indicate subdural collections (a recognized potentially serious complication of low-pressure headache). Radioisotope cisternography may show abnormal isotope accumulation at site of CSF leak and early tracer excretion.
- **Management:** General measures include bed rest, analgesia and caffeine, orally or intravenously (500 mg in 500 ml normal saline over 2 h, repeated after 2 weeks if necessary). Blood patching (30 ml autologous blood) is often highly effective, given either blindly or targeted within one interspace of any identified leak.

TRIGEMINAL AUTONOMIC CEPHALGIA

These syndromes typically give trigeminal distribution pain, usually ophthalmic, lasting <4h, with autonomic dysautonomia, e.g. lacrimation and Horner's syndrome. The spectrum includes cluster headache, paroxysmal hemicrania, hemicrania continua and SUNCT syndrome (see below).

Cluster headache

The prevalence is about 1:1000, mostly males (5:1) and onset usually in middle age. Most patients have a lifelong cluster tendency, although remissions may become longer. There are major and minor clinical diagnostic criteria.

Major

- **Unilateral headache**, often severe, in a trigeminal distribution (eye or temple).
- **Periodicity** (circadian and circannual), which can be striking.
- **Autonomic features**: One or more of the following symptoms (ipsilateral to the headache): Horner's syndrome (sympathetic underactivity), conjunctival injection, lacrimation, rhinorrhoea (parasympathetic overactivity). Horner's syndrome sometimes persists.

Minor

- **Headache duration**: Episodes usually last 45–90 min, but almost always <4h.
- **Cluster duration** is typically >1 week, with remissions for >2 weeks. 10–20% experience a more chronic cluster, without remission.
- **Restlessness** and pacing during episodes is characteristic (whereas migraine patients lie still).
- **Photophobia**, phonophobia and nausea occasionally occur.
- **Alcohol** precipitates headache within an hour (whereas alcohol provokes migraine after several hours). Alcohol does not provoke attacks during remission.

Differential diagnosis

- **Symptomatic cluster headache**, e.g. from pituitary lesions.
- **Other trigeminal autonomic cephalgias.** Paroxysmal hemicrania and SUNCT (see below).
- **Hypnic headache.** This is painful, without autonomic features, with headache lasting 5–180 min and awaking the patient at night. Caffeine, indomethacin or lithium help the symptoms.
- **Giant cell arteritis.** Always consider in those aged >55 years. The steroid responsiveness of cluster headache sometimes causes diagnostic confusion.
- **Trigeminal neuralgia** (see below).

Management

General measures: Provide information about cluster headache including the 'OUCH' website. Avoid alcohol and daytime naps during clusters.

Acute measures:

- **Triptan,** either subcutaneously or nasally (e.g. sumatriptan 6 mg up to twice daily).
- **100% oxygen** (7–12 L/min): an appropriate delivery device is essential, with high flow rate regulator (BOC Medical Gases; Multiflow regulator code 888842) and non-rebreathing face mask (code 888845).

Short-term prophylaxis:

- **Corticosteroids.** Use with other preventative measures, tapering the dose as the relapse resolves (60 mg for 5 days, reducing by 10 mg every 3–5 days).
- **Ergotamine** is useful given rectally before retiring to bed. Note that sumatriptan cannot be used with ergotamine.
- **Methysergide.** Consider if the cluster is usually short-lived (4–5 months). Start 1 mg daily, increase by 1 mg every 3 days (TDS regimen); at 5 mg daily, increase by 1 mg every 5 days (ceiling 12 mg). The concern about retroperitoneal fibrosis limits its use to 6 months. Repeated courses are acceptable after a break.

Long-term prophylaxis:

- **Verapamil.** Large doses are needed. After a baseline ECG, start verapamil 80 mg twice daily, increased by 80 mg weekly aiming for 240–960 mg daily. Repeat ECG before each dose increment.
- **Lithium.** Beware of the need for blood levels and the potential interactions with non-steroidal medications and diuretics.

Paroxysmal hemicrania

Characteristics

The headaches are brief (15–30 min) and much more frequent than in cluster headache: 1–40 attacks can occur per day and without a nocturnal emphasis. The pain is severe and usually ocular or temporal. Some patients pace around, others sit still.

Triggers

Head movement or pressure can provoke episodes, but alcohol rarely does.

Management

Indomethacin trial. Sensitivity to indomethacin is crucial to the diagnosis and management. Indomethacin is to certain headaches what levodopa is to movement disorders. Clinicians should have a low threshold for using indomethacin in suspected paroxysmal hemicrania, hemicrania continua, or idiopathic stabbing headache (see below).

- Indomethacin 25 mg t.d.s. for 2 weeks, with a proton pump inhibitor.
- If no benefit, try 50 mg t.d.s. (2 weeks) and eventually 75 mg t.d.s.
- If the highest dose gives no benefit at 2 weeks, the trial has failed.

Hemicrania continua

This is a chronic unilateral headache without autonomic features, which is responsive to indomethacin.

SUNCT syndrome

SUNCT (short-lasting unilateral neuralgiform headache with conjunctival injection and tearing) is a very brief, painful headache (duration seconds to minutes) in an ophthalmic distribution and with dysautonomia (particularly lacrimation). The attack frequency varies from two to hundreds per day.

Triggers

Attacks can be triggered by touch or by neck movement.

Treatments

SUNCT is usually fairly treatment-resistant. Some patients respond to topiramate (25–50 mg b.d.), lamotrigine or gabapentin.

Differential diagnosis

Conditions with similar pain but without the autonomic features include:

- **Idiopathic stabbing headache.** The pain is usually unilateral, ophthalmic and responds to indomethacin.
- **Trigeminal neuralgia (TN).** Box 4.4 gives the main features distinguishing TN from SUNCT.

Surgery

Surgery to interrupt the trigeminal sensory or autonomic pathways can be done for TN and sometimes for other trigeminal autonomic cephalgias.

- **Microvascular decompression.** Pledgets of shredded Teflon felt are used to separate the nerve from an aberrant vessel (usually superior cerebellar artery) in TN. Although avoiding nerve destruction, it still requires a craniotomy.
- **Glycerol rhizolysis** is useful in medically frail patients. Patients can go home the same day and avoid craniotomy. A needle is passed through the cheek into the foramen ovale; the trigeminal cistern is outlined with Iohexol dye and then glycerol (neurotoxic) is injected. This gives relief within hours. Complications may include CSF leak, carotid artery damage (fistula), corneal anaesthesia and anaesthesia dolorosa (numbness with severe dysaesthesia).
- **Other options** include radio frequency rhizotomy, balloon compression and radiosurgery.

OUTPATIENT HEADACHE CONSULTATIONS

As well as a full history and examination, there are additional points to include.

Box 4.4: Distinguishing TN from SUNCT

- **Pain**. TN: very brief lighting pain (1–2 sec); SUNCT: seconds to minutes.
- **Distribution**. TN: 1st and 2nd trigeminal dermatomes, or 2nd and 3rd; SUNCT: 1st division.
- **Autonomic features**. Absent in TN; prominent in SUNCT.
- **Responsiveness**. TN responds well to carbamazepine (also baclofen or phenytoin); SUNCT is generally unresponsive, although topiramate may help.
- **Remissions**. TN: typically persists for a few weeks, remits, but returns months later. SUNCT is less likely to remit.

TN and SUNCT both have no neurological signs (including normal corneal reflex).

History

- 'Tell me about the worst headaches you have' often prompts migrainous stories and helps to start the therapeutic discussion.
- Behaviour: what do patients do when the headache is at its worst, e.g. lie down, or pace around, switch the light off?
- Accompanying symptoms (photophobia, phonophobia, nausea, characteristics of headache, autonomic features).
- Triggers, coffee, tea, meals, alcohol, sleep pattern.
- Preceding factors (neck injury, medications).

Examination

- Note if there is frowning and dark glasses.
- Include examination of temporo-mandibular joints, temporal arteries, neck movements, palpable muscle tension and cranial bruit.

Investigations

- Consider ESR in anyone with headache aged >55 years.
- Imaging is often what patients are expecting will happen; if a scan is not indicated, this must be explained to the patient and not left unsaid.

EMERGENCY HEADACHE CONSULTATIONS

Headache is a common presentation to emergency units; 30% of those presenting acutely have serious pathology.

History taking

The emergency clinician should ask five questions:

1. **Is this the first or worst headache?** This suggests subarachnoid haemorrhage or other thunderclap headache (see below).
2. **Is there fever?** Headache with fever suggests infective causes, e.g. meningitis, encephalitis or abscess (see Ch. 13). If subarachnoid haemorrhage (SAH) is suspected, do not undertake lumbar puncture without a scan (SAH or meningitis can cause hydrocephalus). In suspected meningococcal meningitis, start antibiotics before investigation.
3. **Is there raised intracranial pressure?** Symptoms include visual obscuration, night time and morning headache, worse on coughing, sneezing and lying flat. These patients need urgent CT brain scanning to exclude a space-occupying lesion.
4. **Is it giant cell arteritis?** Criteria include new headache, age >50 years (usually 70+), high ESR or CRP (do both) and tender temporal arteries (palpate). Look for scalp or tongue ulceration (careful not to diagnose zoster). If in doubt, start prednisolone, possibly with an intravenous methylprednisolone loading dose. Temporal artery biopsy helps long-term management and should be done even if the patient has taken steroids for several days.
5. **Is it a primary headache syndrome?** Diagnose this only by exclusion. Patients with migraine can also have serious causes for headache.

Headache presenting to the emergency unit will broadly divide into acute onset (thunderclap) headache and other severe headache presenting subacutely.

Acute (thunderclap) headache

Thunderclap headache has an acute (explosive) onset, reaching peak intensity within 30 sec (like a clap of thunder) and lasting for >1 h. There are many important conditions to consider.

- Subarachnoid haemorrhage (SAH): new onset of thunderclap headache must be regarded as due to SAH until proven otherwise.
- Meningitis.
- Extracranial artery dissection.
- Spontaneous CSF leak with low-pressure headache.
- Idiopathic thunderclap headache (including benign sex headache).
- Cerebral venous thrombosis.
- Pituitary apoplexy.

Clinical note. Painful stroke implies bleeding, dissection, vasculitis and venous thrombosis.

Other emergency unit headache

Other headaches presenting acutely or subacutely include the following:

- Atypical or non-infective meningitis (e.g. fungal, malignancy, sarcoidosis): 25% of cryptococcal meningitis cases have a normal CSF, so test for the cryptococcal antigen.
- Cervical radiculopathy may cause surprising confusion with SAH.
- Idiopathic (benign) intracranial hypertension.

- Drugs causing raised intracranial pressure, e.g. corticosteroids, vitamin A, danazol.
- Malignant hypertension (rare, but always measure blood pressure in acute headache).
- Hypercapnia (consider measuring $PaCO_2$ for headache with obesity and/or COPD).
- Carbon monoxide poisoning (check the carboxyhaemoglobin level and look for polycythaemia, particularly if other household members are affected).
- Some systemic diseases, e.g. SLE.
- Some endocrine disorders, e.g. Cushing's disease.

Subarachnoid haemorrhage

Headaches presenting to emergency units must be taken seriously. One-quarter of sudden onset severe headaches are SAH (Fig. 4.2). If the headache is either the 'first or worst', treat as a SAH until proven otherwise. Some 12% of SAH present with headache only: these patients have the best prognosis: even though they may look well and their headache has settled, investigation and management must be prompt and appropriate.

Clinical features

- **Timing**: One-third develop SAH during normal daily activity, one-third during sleep and one-third during vigorous exercise or lifting (Valsalva manoeuvre).
- **Severity**: Poor initial grade has many potential causes, e.g. significant parenchymal damage or hydrocephalus. Note that hydrocephalus is potentially reversible so remain open-minded about those with a poor Glasgow coma score.

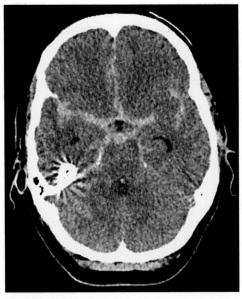

Figure 4.2
CT brain showing diffuse subarachnoid blood.

- **Photophobia** occurs with optic nerve irritation from blood within the CSF, so remember SAH as a differential for meningitis.
- **Collapse.** Some patients with SAH present with syncope because cerebral perfusion is impaired by raised intracranial pressure from an arterial bleed.
- **Meningism** and mild fever are common in SAH.
- **Sub-hyaloid haemorrhages** appear next to the disc as distinct well demarcated bright red lesions.

Causes

Berry aneurysm rupture causes 85% of SAH. Perimesencephalic haemorrhages (10%) have no detectable aneurysm and have a good prognosis. Other causes of SAH include arteriovenous malformations, pituitary apoplexy, dissection (see below), drug abuse (amphetamines/cocaine), vasculopathies, clotting abnormalities (including platelet abnormalities sometimes with a normal total platelet count).

Investigations

- **CT scanning.** This is essential in all suspected SAH, the earlier the better. It is almost 100% sensitive at 12 h and 60% at 5 days; the amount of blood can be graded (Fisher grade): more blood gives a greater risk of vasospasm. A CT sometimes shows the aneurysm.
- **Lumbar puncture.** With a positive CT, this is unnecessary; with a negative CT, CSF analysis is always required. Remember to measure the CSF pressure since venous thrombosis may be missed on CT and the only clue may be high CSF pressure.
  - Xanthochromia was first used to describe the yellow discolouration accompanying pneumococcal meningitis (in 1902) and later in the 1920s following a SAH as red cells haemolyse. This may take up to 12 h to appear and lasts for 2 weeks (therefore wait 12 h after onset before doing LP); jaundice will interfere with result. Visual inspection misses 50% of xanthochromia; spectrophotometry can demonstrate xanthochromia between 12 h and 2 weeks following bleeding in all cases but sometimes lacks specificity.
  - Traumatic tap. Inexperienced lumbar puncture operators may cause a traumatic tap. This is a big problem because repeating the LP will not help in diagnosis after blood has been introduced. Examination for blood in three consecutive CSF tubes may not definitely distinguish a bloody tap from SAH.
- **Digital subtraction angiography.** Neurological complications occur in 0.5% (permanent) and 1% (transient); note this is higher with spasm and in migraineurs. Diagnostic conventional angiography will become less utilized as MRI/CT techniques evolve.
- **Non-invasive angiography** is an option if CT and CSF are negative, yet the index of suspicion high: MR angiography has 95% sensitivity for aneurysms >6mm; CT angiography has similar sensitivity. The imaging choice depends upon local radiological preference and expertise.

Management

- **General measures:** These include resuscitation, hydration (3 L normal saline over 24 h), pain relief (codeine) and prevention of complications by medical, surgical and radiological interventions.

- **Cerebral vasospasm** can be prevented by nimodipine (60 mg orally q.d.s. or 1–2 mg/h i.v.). A young stroke occasionally presents 1–2 weeks after SAH, so ask about preceding headache in seemingly straightforward ischaemic stroke.
- **Definitive measures:** Aneurysm re-bleeding causes 30% of SAH deaths, so early definitive treatment impacts on mortality. Interventional radiological coiling is generally used following superiority demonstrated in the ISAT (International Subarachnoid Treatment) trial, which recruited >2000 patients and compared surgery with endovascular coiling; 76% of coiled patients were independent at 1 year compared with 69% of surgery patients.
- **Prognosis** overall is fairly poor: 25% die before or soon after reaching hospital, a further 25% die in hospital and 50% of the survivors remain disabled. The prognosis correlates with the Glasgow coma score at presentation and the patient's age.

Differential diagnosis

- **Cerebral venous thrombosis.** Up to 10% present with thunderclap headache. Some 25% of venous thromboses are overlooked on CT and so a venogram (CT or MRI) is needed.
- **Pituitary apoplexy** presents with severe headache, meningism, photophobia, field/visual loss, diplopia and hypotension leading to coma (Addisonian crisis). These patients need intravenous fluids, intravenous hydrocortisone, urgent imaging and neurosurgical advice.
- **Spontaneous CSF leaking** causes a low-pressure headache. Note that the meninges enhance on MRI and there may also be tonsillar herniation and even subdural collections.
- **Idiopathic.** This includes coital headache (see below) but also spontaneous idiopathic headaches (also called benign angiopathy or crash migraine). This diagnosis remains one of exclusion after other potential causes have been excluded. The condition often recurs, 30% having further episodes over subsequent months. Angiography may demonstrate vasospasm. The pathophysiology is unclear but excessive sympathetic activity may be involved since phaeochromocytomas and hypertensive crisis also cause angiospasm.
- **Arterial dissection.** The Lausanne study highlighted that headache is common in stroke (20%) with a higher incidence in those with extracranial arterial pathology (but not embolism), particularly dissection and posterior fossa stroke. Look for a Horner's syndrome (may accompany either carotid or vertebral dissections). Subarachnoid haemorrhage sometimes follows a subadventitial (as opposed to sub-intimal) vertebral dissection.
- **Viral meningitis** may rarely present as thunderclap headache.

Warning leaks

Some SAH patients report a preceding (warning or sentinel) headache in the weeks beforehand. However, this is less common than previously thought, the higher previous prevalence probably reflecting recall bias. Reports of unruptured aneurysms presenting as a thunderclap headache may represent sudden aneurysm expansion, but are probably coincidental.

Angiography is therefore probably not required in patients with negative CT brain and CSF examination.

Unruptured aneurysms

The prevalence of unruptured aneurysms is about 1%; approximately 0.05% of those <10 mm diameter rupture annually, increased to 0.5% if >10 mm diameter or with a history of previous aneurysm rupture. Other features increasing the rupture risk include high blood pressure, aneurysm site (higher in posterior circulation), aneurysm shape, female sex and a positive family history (e.g. polycystic kidneys). Some paradoxes include the fact that most ruptured aneurysms are <10 mm diameter, whereas during follow-up larger aneurysms are more likely to rupture. One possible explanation is that the risk of rupture is higher soon after aneurysm formation and then the lesion stabilizes. Giant aneurysms (>25 mm diameter) are dangerous and require a careful multidisciplinary approach.

Benign exertional headaches

Generalized headache immediately following coughing, exertion or sexual orgasm is well recognized and may cause great concern and limitation of activity. They are presumed to be migraine variants but no specific treatment is consistently helpful.

Giant cell arteritis

In individuals aged >55 years (but usually older), ask about systemic symptoms, local temporal artery tenderness and jaw claudication. Examine for skin necrosis (or tongue necrosis): do not be fooled into thinking it is herpes zoster. Diagnostic criteria are given elsewhere (see Ch. 7). Check the ESR and CRP, but note that the ESR is normal in 15%. Treatment is usually with hospital admission for intravenous methylprednisolone or high dose oral steroids.

Post-traumatic headache

The trauma may refer to intracranial infection or physical head trauma (sometimes mild). A substantial minority relate to cervical muscle tension following associated neck trauma. The issue of outstanding compensation following trauma involves complex factors. The same sort of medications are used as for tension-type headache, including amitriptyline and gabapentin.

Carbon monoxide poisoning

Environmental headache (better on holiday) associated with flu-like symptoms, cherry-red lips, generalized malaise, nausea and confusion. There may be associated parkinsonism. Check the carboxy-haemoglobin levels (>25%) and consider hyperbaric oxygen.

Case history outcome

The patient subsequently had a brain MRI with contrast, demonstrating diffuse meningeal enhancement and tonsillar herniation; this was sufficient without lumbar puncture to confirm the clinical diagnosis of intracranial hypotension. Subsequent radionuclide cisternography demonstrated the site of CSF leakage, which was repaired by an ENT surgeon.

KEY POINTS

- The history is much more important than examination or any test in headache.
- Red flags for headache are night pain (waking from sleep), morning vomiting and orthostatic headache.
- Brain tumour is rarely the explanation for isolated headache.
- Fundi: the earliest sign of raised pressure is loss of venous pulsation.
- Migraine is commonly provoked by missing meals and missing sleep; it is rarely provoked by chocolate and cheese.
- Caffeine is a useful acute treatment for migraine: excess caffeine consumption may worsen migraine owing to caffeine withdrawal.
- Migraine patients lie still; cluster patients move about.
- Cluster headache can be confused with giant cell arteritis because both respond to steroids.
- CSF examination is essential if the history suggests subarachnoid haemorrhage, but the CT scan is normal.
- The management of idiopathic intracranial hypertension depends upon the visual fields.

Further Reading

Silberstein SD. Migraine. Lancet 2004; 363: 381–391.

Dizziness

5

Case history

A 73-year-old man developed dizziness following cardiac surgery. He had undergone prosthetic aortic valve replacement, complicated by valve infection and required further surgery during a month in the intensive care unit. He was on warfarin and had a pacemaker. He had marked gait unsteadiness and could no longer walk to the toilet. His vision would jump (but not spin) when moving in his wheelchair, but not when stationary. Examination of eye movements, including pursuit and saccades, was normal.

INTRODUCTION

The vestibular system detects angular (semicircular canals) and linear (otolith organs) accelerations. Normally, the two sides are balanced: unbalanced 'pull' or 'push' to one side gives the illusion of rotation.

- **'Pull'**, from reduced function, e.g. vestibular neuritis.
- **'Push'**, from excess stimulation, e.g. Ménière's disease.

Dizziness and disequilibrium ('off-balance') are common. However, 'dizzy' can mean many things: you must first establish what the patient means (see below).

What is 'dizzy'?

- Spinning: true vertigo.
- Light-headedness from presyncope, e.g. vasovagal (including carotid sinus hypersensitivity), cardiogenic and orthostatic.
- Light-headedness from hyperventilation: anxiety provoked by situations, e.g. shops, fluorescent lights. Note this may follow or accompany true vestibular symptoms.
- 'Travel sickness': Mismatch between the visual and vestibular systems provoking dizziness, e.g. car journeys, ironing stripy shirts, or using computer screens (strobing).
- De-personalization (self is unreal) and de-realization (world is unreal) present usually as psychological problems.
- Unsteadiness ('off-balance' or disequilibrium): may be a manifestation of several important conditions (Box 5.1).

Box 5.1: Causes of non-specific unsteadiness ('off-balance')

- **Without obvious signs.** Some patients report persisting symptoms without an identified cause. Although many remain undiagnosed, several important conditions may present in this way:
  - Recovering from vestibular disease (often accompanied by anxiety).
  - Bilateral vestibulopathy. These patients do not have vertigo, but feel dizzy, fall and have oscillopsia (failure of vestibulo-ocular reflex (VOR); do a VOR head thrust and test visual acuity having rotated the head. Causes include drugs (e.g. aminoglycosides – there is no safe non-vestibulotoxic dose), aspirin, cisplatin, furosemide, erythromycin) and spinocerebellar ataxias.
  - Communicating (normal pressure) hydrocephalus.
- **With focal signs**
  - Early cerebellar disease.
  - Posterior fossa tumour. Note that CT scanning may miss this due to skull base artefact (Fig. 5.1).
  - Sensory ataxia, e.g. demyelinating peripheral neuropathy.
  - Lambert–Eaton myasthenic syndrome.
  - Orthostatic tremor. Patients are steady when walking but develop unsteadiness on standing still (see Ch. 9).

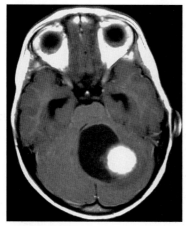

Figure 5.1
MRI showing cerebellar pilocytic astrocytoma.

VERTIGO

The clinician has the following questions:

- Is there *true vertigo*, i.e. spinning?
- Is it a *first and spontaneous* episode? The diagnosis of acute spontaneous vertigo depends whether it is peripheral (vestibulopathy) or central (cerebellar or brainstem) (Box 5.2).
- Is it *recurrent and positional*?
  - Common: Benign positional vertigo (see below).
  - Rare: multiple sclerosis, cerebellar disease and Chiari malformation.
- Is it *recurrent and spontaneous?* The likely cause then depends upon the presence of focal symptoms and/or hearing loss.
- With other focal symptoms:
  - Migraine.

> **Box 5.2:** *Acute spontaneous vertigo: Central vs peripheral features*
>
> - Causes:
>   - **Peripheral**, e.g. vestibular neuritis, labyrinthine infarction, autoimmune inner ear disease.
>   - **Central**, e.g. cerebellar or brainstem infarction, multiple sclerosis.
> - Symptoms:
>   - **Hearing loss and tinnitus** suggest a peripheral lesion.
>   - **Oscillopsia** suggests a central lesion.
>   - **Diplopia, weakness, or altered consciousness** suggest central pathology.
> - Signs:
>   - **Focal signs** (other than hearing loss) suggest a central cause.
>   - **Saccades, pursuit and vestibulo-ocular reflex (VOR) suppression** are normal with peripheral lesions, but abnormal with central lesions.
>   - **Abnormal head thrust test** suggests a peripheral cause (Fig. 5.1).
>   - **The Dix–Hallpike manoeuvre** demonstrates important differences (Fig. 5.2 and Table 5.1).
>   - **Nystagmus worsening with visual suppression** suggests a peripheral cause. Consider using Freznel spectacles during Dix–Hallpike testing.
> - Investigations:
>   - **Nystagmography** may highlight differences, e.g. a rectilinear waveform (peripheral cause) versus an exponential waveform (central cause).
>   - **MR imaging** helps to distinguish peripheral from central causes.

- Multiple sclerosis.
- Vertebrobasilar transient ischaemic attack (rare, must have other symptoms, not isolated vertigo).
- With hearing loss:
  - Ménière's syndrome.
  - Perilymph fistula.
  - Vestibular paroxysmia.
  - Syphilis.

Acute unilateral vestibulopathy

The otolith and vertical semicircular canals project to the 3rd, 4th and 6th cranial nerve nuclei and their supranuclear centres, allowing vestibulo-ocular reflex (VOR) movements. The intact side pushes the eyes towards the damaged side from where there is no output; corrective saccades then flick the eyes back towards the undamaged side (fast phase of nystagmus is away from the lesion). Vision is suppressed during this, so there is an illusion of rotation away from the damaged side.

Acute vestibular neuritis

This is relatively common and the classical cause of peripheral vestibulopathy, usually presenting in the sixth decade.

Symptoms

- **Prolonged severe vertigo.** The world appears to spin away from the damaged vestibular apparatus. The vertigo is severe, intermittent and provoked by head movement. Patients prefer to lie with the affected ear downwards. It is disabling at first but improves over a few days.

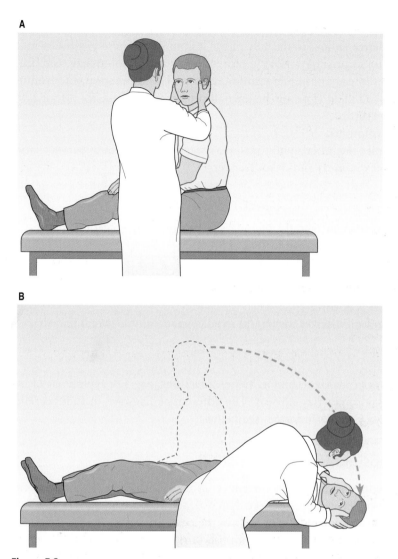

Figure 5.2
Dix–Hallpike manoeuvre. (a) Patient sitting up, head turned to left. (b) Head is rotated with respect to gravity in the plane of affected posterior canal.

Table 5.1: Dix–Hallpike manoeuvre: peripheral or central cause?

Lesion type	Nystagmus onset	Habituation	Nystagmus characteristics	Accompanying symptoms
Peripheral	Delayed	Yes	Horizontal or rotatory (torsion)	Prominent vertigo even with minimal nystagmus
Central	Immediate	No	Any direction (often with other eye movement abnormalities)	Vertigo not invariable, despite nystagmus

- **Unpleasant autonomic symptoms**, e.g. nausea and vomiting.
- **Postural imbalance**, falling to the side of the lesion. At the onset, standing and walking are difficult. Surprisingly, moving more quickly and running may stabilize the gait. Vision becomes important in maintaining balance: loss of fixation, e.g. from face washing, can provoke falling. The 'off-balance' feeling may continue for a time after the main symptoms have settled.
- **No auditory symptoms.**
- **Fear** accompanies the initial symptoms; persistent anxiety with hyperventilation can provoke further dizziness and delay recovery.

Signs

Eye movement assessment should include smooth pursuit, saccades, the vestibulo-ocular reflex (VOR) and VOR suppression (Fig. 5.3).

- **Nystagmus** with the fast phase away from the affected side.
- **Normal eye movements** and no diplopia, weakness etc.
- **Head thrust test** is positive.
- **Caloric testing** demonstrates ipsilateral hypo-responsiveness (canal paresis).

Aetiology

A viral infection is probably to blame. Other infections, e.g. TB, syphilis or *H. zoster* oticus (Ramsay Hunt syndrome) may cause it. The differential diagnosis includes cerebellar stroke, hyperviscosity and Cogan syndrome (see below).

Benign paroxysmal positioning vertigo (BPPV)

This is the most common cause of recurrent positional vertigo: one-third of patients >70 years have had BPPV. Females are affected more than males (2:1). It is explained by debris (canalolithiasis) within the canal endolymph, especially in the posterior vertical canal. The debris is denser than endolymph and acts as a plunger with head movements, inducing bidirectional (push or pull) forces on the cupula, triggering BPPV attacks. Unterberger's 'step' test can be useful in various labyrinthine disorders: the patient is asked to march on the spot with the eyes closed. A positive test is indicated by rotational movement of the patient towards the side of the lesion.

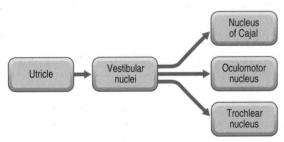

Figure 5.3
Utricular pathways.

Dix–Hallpike manoeuvre

This reproduces the vertigo and nausea of BPPV (Fig. 5.2).

- **Latency**. Vertigo and nystagmus occur 1–2 sec after the head is tilted towards the affected ear. In practice, patients experience vertigo more often on getting out of bed than on lying down.
- **Linear-rotatory nystagmus** is clockwise with left posterior semicircular canal involvement and anti-clockwise with right-sided involvement. Nystagmus is best seen using visual suppression lenses. Freznel spectacles have +30 lenses allowing easy visualization of the patient's eyes but preventing the patient from focusing, thus abolishing visual suppression of nystagmus.
- **Duration** of nystagmus is 10–40 sec, before disappearing.
- **Fatiguability**: vertigo and nystagmus diminish with repeated testing.
- **Reversed direction of nystagmus** (with some vertigo) on sitting up.
- **Atypical features**. If any are present, consider MR brain scanning.

Causes

BPPV may be idiopathic, or may follow head trauma or vestibular neuritis. Untreated, it persists in 30% and returns after variable periods in another 30%.

Management

- **Physical manoeuvres** aim to liberate the debris. These include Epley, Semont (Fig. 5.4) and Brandt–Daroff exercises. With successful treatment, the symptoms settle altogether, 10–20% develop a recurrence and the liberatory manoeuvre needs to be repeated.
- **Vestibular sedatives** are ineffective in treating BPPV and should be avoided.

The Semont manoeuvre (Fig. 5.4) has the advantage of being performed on an ordinary couch without the need for head extension beyond one end. The Semont manoeuvre involves a 180° swing of the head in the plane of the posterior semicircular canal. An aide memoire is to 'go from one ear down to the opposite eye down'.

- Position 1: The patient sits on the couch with the head rotated 45° away from the affected ear. The debris within the semicircular (vertical) canal is not moving: there is no vertigo, as the cupula is not deflected.
- Position 2: This is the equivalent of the diagnostic phase of the Hallpike manoeuvre. The debris sinks to the lowest part of the canal, pulling the cupula downwards: the nystagmus is therefore towards the undermost ear. This causes vertigo after a delay (latency) since the cupula does not move immediately. The vertigo persists until the debris settles and therefore the cupula stops moving. Stay in this position for 3 min.
- Position 3: The patient is swung rapidly, in a single movement, on to the opposite side of the couch and remains there for at least 1 min. The debris moves, again causing nystagmus towards the left ear that is now uppermost. The debris can now enter the utricular cavity and be liberated.

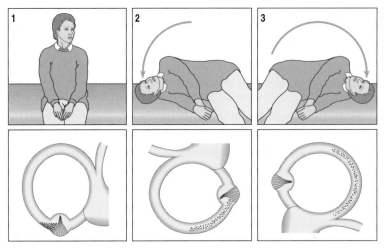

Figure 5.4
The Semont manoeuvre for benign paroxysmal positioning vertigo (BPPV). (Courtesy of AM Bronstein, with permission from ACNR 2005; 5: 13).

If the nystagmus does not beat towards the affected ear, it suggests the debris has moved towards the cupula (ampullopetal) and probably remains within the semicircular canal: the liberatory manoeuvre has failed.

Ménière's syndrome

This well-known condition is frequently diagnosed, though is actually rather uncommon. Most patients given the diagnosis probably have BPPV. It affects people aged 30–50 years and is rare in the elderly. The symptoms are only rarely bilateral. Although there is endolymphatic hydrops ('labyrinthine glaucoma'), there is no known cause and no specific diagnostic test.

Clinical features

Classical triad

1. **Vertigo episodes,** each lasting up to 1 day (24 min–24 h), sometimes with nausea, vomiting, pallor and sweating.
2. **Tinnitus,** which is usually bilateral.
3. **Sensorineural deafness,** progressive and unilateral, initially low-tone and fluctuating, but later global and progressive.

Additional symptoms

- **Before attacks:** ipsilateral ear 'fullness' for minutes or hours.
- **During attacks:** ipsilateral exacerbation of deafness and tinnitus.

Management

ENT specialists are best equipped to manage Ménière's disease.

- **Acute attacks** are treated with orally absorbed prochlorperazine.
- **Prevention** is with dietary salt restriction, betahistine (harmless and sometimes helpful) and avoidance of long-term prochlorperazine.
- **Surgery** is a last resort: saccus decompression or destructive procedures, e.g. intra-tympanic instillation of ototoxic aminoglycosides.

Autoimmune disease presenting like Ménière's disease

This is an autoimmune-mediated audio-vestibular disorder with ocular inflammation e.g. Susacs 'blinding headache falling on deaf ears', Cogan's syndrome.

Clinical features

Manifests as retinal infarction, encephalopathy, deafness and vertigo, probably from autoimmune vasculitis. The vertigo is severe and improves after 1–2 weeks with central and peripheral compensation. Some oscillopsia may remain with quick head movement (corresponding to a persistent positive head thrust). Usually middle-aged female, presenting with bilateral endolymphatic hydrops (often raised ESR).

Management

This includes anti-nausea medication and physical therapy such as Cawthorne–Cooksey exercises. Vestibular physiotherapy can promote compensation, whereas vestibular sedatives may delay this. Steroids are often used to treat autoimmune inner ear disease.

Vestibular paroxysmia

This is similar to trigeminal neuralgia or hemifacial spasm caused by an aberrant vessel irritating cranial nerves. Typically, the condition is characterized by:

- Brief recurrent attacks of vertigo (seconds to minutes).
- Provoked by typical head positions.
- Hyperacusis or tinnitus during and sometimes between attacks.
- Measurable abnormality on auditory or vestibular tests.
- Response to antiepileptic medication, e.g. carbamazepine. Only after failure would surgery be contemplated.

Perilymph fistula
Clinical features

- There is often a history of head trauma or of extreme physical exertion.
- The patient reports episodic vertigo, hearing loss and positional nystagmus of short latency but prolonged duration.
- Tullio phenomenon: vertigo and postural instability provoked by a high intensity auditory stimulus.

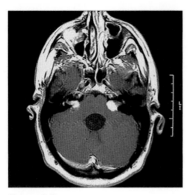

Figure 5.5
MRI showing bilateral acoustic neuromas.

Investigation and management

If the condition persists beyond 2–3 weeks, an exploratory tympanotomy (under local anaesthetic) is indicated. An intra-operative Valsalva manoeuvre can reveal the leaking fistula, which can then be patched.

Migraine

Vertigo may complicate migraine, especially in teenage girls. Migrainous vertigo is often aggravated by changes of head position and may occasionally present as purely positional vertigo. The features distinguishing migrainous vertigo from BPPV are:

- Short duration symptoms with frequent recurrences.
- Onset in childhood.
- Migrainous symptoms during vertigo episodes.

The precise diagnosis depends upon the presence of other brainstem symptoms.

Basilar migraine

The diagnostic criteria include:

- Two or more brainstem aura features, but not motor features.
- Symptoms lasting 5–20 min, but less than 1 h.
- Scotoma, amnesia, dysarthria or drowsiness.

Vestibular migraine

This refers to migraine with episodic vertigo, but without other brainstem symptoms. Most (70%) patients with migraine-related vertigo have headache. Treatment is usually with beta-blockers (atenolol or metoprolol).

Episodic ataxia

Episodic ataxia (types 1 and 2) may present with headache, episodic ataxia and vertigo; a clue may be a family history of ataxia.

Visual vertigo

Exacerbation of dizziness and related symptoms by a stimulating visual environment. This is probably seen in organic and non-organic pathologies as well as normal subjects.

Phobic postural vertigo

This is common and may accompany or follow true postural vertigo. It is characterized by:

- Dizziness on standing or walking.
- Anxiety followed by vertigo.
- Fluctuating dizziness or momentary illusions of body movement.
- Situational attacks, e.g. social gatherings, closed spaces.
- Normal clinical tests.

Oscillopsia

This is an illusion of movement, with objects moving side to side or up and down. It is seen if there is a VOR abnormality and in some forms of nystagmus and related conditions.

Case history outcome

The patient had bilateral vestibulopathy from aminoglycosides. His head thrust test was positive bilaterally and he had difficulty reading while nodding at 1–2 Hz (vestibulo-ocular reflex). This condition is easily overlooked and may be very disabling. There is no safe non-vestibulotoxic dose of aminoglycoside. Management is often difficult, but this patient was helped by vestibular rehabilitation exercises.

- **VOR abnormality** causing oscillopsia follows either bilateral vestibulopathy (Table 5.1) or a central cause such as multiple sclerosis. When patients move their head or body, e.g. walking, they experience visual blurring or the illusion of objects jumping.
- **Nystagmus** can also cause oscillopsia, especially if upbeat, downbeat or pendular.
- **Saccadic interruptions of fixation** may mimic nystagmus and sometimes cause oscillopsia.
  - **Square wave jerks** are repeated, brief, off-target eye movements: they are an exaggeration of normal physiology and usually are asymptomatic.
  - **Opsoclonus** is caused by pause cell dysfunction (Raphe interpositus) and manifests as chaotic eye movement in all directions without inter-saccadic intervals. It suggests brainstem disease, especially from paraneoplasia (breast or visceral malignancy in adults, neuroblastoma in children, giving 'dancing eyes and dancing feet'), encephalitis or demyelination.

- **Ocular flutter**, i.e. opsoclonus confined to horizontal gaze.
- **Superior oblique myokymia** is a benign condition presenting with unilateral torsional oscillopsia causing monocular blurring. The diagnosis may require a slit-lamp examination. The clinical clue is its unilateral nature: cover each eye in turn to confirm this. Carbamazepine may help but some need superior oblique surgery.

KEY POINTS

- Ascertain what is meant by dizziness: the spectrum includes vertigo, pre-syncope, anxiety, off-balance or depersonalization.
- Unilateral sensorineural hearing loss is caused by an acoustic neuroma (Fig. 5.5) until proven otherwise.
- Consider what accompanies the vertigo: abnormal signs apart from hearing loss and provoked nystagmus suggest a central lesion (MRI indicated).
- The Dix–Hallpike manoeuvre is essential, preferably using Frenzel lenses: if nystagmus latency, fatigue and direction are atypical for BPPV, think central.
- Learn how to do canalith repositioning manoeuvre.
- Cerebellar stroke presenting as acute vertigo is easily overlooked: do the head thrust test (normal in cerebellar disease, abnormal with peripheral causes) and examine eye movements and VOR suppression (abnormal in central, normal with peripheral causes).
- Unsteadiness without obvious signs: consider bilateral vestibulopathy and identify drug exposure, particularly aminoglycosides.
- Rare causes of unsteadiness often present as 'dizziness': orthostatic tremor, hydrocephalus and progressive supranuclear palsy.
- Ménière's syndrome is over diagnosed: ENT surgeons should manage true cases.

Further Reading

Bronstein AM. Benign paroxysmal positional vertigo (BPPV): Diagnosis and physical treatment. ACNR 2005; 5(3): 12–14.

Bronstein AM, Brandt T, Woollacott H, Nutt J. Clinical disorders of balance, posture and gait, 2nd edn. London: Hodder Education; 2004.

Dementia and coma

6

Case history

A 75-year-old woman attended a clinic with her husband. Two years before she had become disorientated while on holiday, unable to find the caravan toilet. Her husband described a 3-year history of progressive memory difficulties, e.g. losing things or forgetting where she had parked the car. She no longer read avidly, the same books stayed beside her bed and she no longer followed TV programmes. Her husband now did the shopping, cooking and accounts. She washed herself but needed help to dress, becoming frustrated by putting clothes on back to front. She slept poorly and wandered at night. Her personality and appetite were unchanged and there were no hallucinations. There was no relevant family history.

Her Mini Mental State Examination (MMSE) was 10/30, revealing problems with episodic memory, language, visuospatial function and praxis. Routine tests, including serum B_{12}, thyroid function, VDRL and chest radiograph were normal. MR brain showed generalized cerebral atrophy, particularly affecting the medial temporal lobe. EEG showed loss of alpha activity, with generalized slowing. CSF examination was normal.

INTRODUCTION

Dementia is a sustained memory loss, plus loss of one other cognitive domain, such as language (aphasia), learned motor function (apraxia), perception (agnosia) or executive function (insight, abstraction, planning or problem solving) (DSM-IV 1994). This definition applies principally to Alzheimer's disease where memory is affected early. The exception is frontal lobe dementia where memory may be normal. Dementia is usually, but not always progressive and results in a sufficient change from previous functioning to interfere with social and occupational activities.

CAUSES OF DEMENTIA

The common causes are:

- Alzheimer's disease (AD): 50% of all dementias.
- Vascular dementia: 25%.
- Dementia with Lewy bodies: 15%.

Note that AD often also has a vascular element, so-called 'mixed dementia'.

Dementia is common and set to increase hugely with an ageing population. The prevalence and incidence doubles every 5 years after aged 65 years: prevalence 2% aged 65 years; 35% aged 85 years.

HISTORY TAKING

The history must be taken from the patient and from a witness. Some patients with dementia deny any problems (anosognosia). It is therefore worth telephoning carers for a first hand account. Enquire about day-to-day life, e.g. self-care with washing and dressing, their continence, doing housework, handling accounts and how they spend their days. It is helpful to record specific examples of memory loss and behaviour change to clarify which cognitive domains are affected and to indicate the severity of deficits. Some direct questions (especially to relatives and/or carers) are important to ensure a complete history.

1. **Tempo.** Rapid progression of dementia suggests several diagnostic possibilities (see below).
2. **Other history.** The family history and history of alcoholism are particularly important.
3. **Hallucinations**, especially visual, raise suspicion of dementia with Lewy bodies.
4. **Personality change.** Obsessions, compulsions, or developing a 'sweet tooth' are usually part of a frontotemporal dementia.
5. **Behavioural problems** include wandering, aggression, vocalization and unusual eating habits, including pica. Behavioural problems often lead to institutionalization.
6. **Psychiatric problems.** Depression is commonly associated with dementia and is treatable: relatives will have insight into this.
7. **Who cares?** Clarify who looks after the patient. This is important for both patient safety and carer well being: occupational therapy may help in following this up.

EXAMINATION

General

Look for features of hypothyroidism (slow pulse, facies, slow relaxing reflexes), pernicious anaemia (jaundice, macroglossia), syphilis (pupils, cord signs), HIV (i.v. drug abusers, sexual orientation); check for chronic liver disease (jaundice, spider naevi, palmar erythema, Wernicke/Korsakoff syndrome). Alzheimer's patients may have preserved insight; frontal lobe dementia patients may deny symptoms. Is the patient melancholic (depressive pseudodementia)?

Motor features

Parkinsonism, other movement disorders and ataxia are particularly important and point to several possible causes, many of which are treatable (Box 6.1). AD is rarely associated with significant motor features.

These conditions typically show 'subcortical' cognitive problems characterized by slowness of thought (bradyphrenia), forgetfulness (improved by cueing), perseveration and mental inflexibility. There may be some frontal features but without the other features of frontotemporal dementias (see below).

Box 6.1: *Causes of 'subcortical' dementia with motor features*

Dementias with movement disorder and/or ataxia:
• Vascular dementia.
• Dementia with Lewy bodies.
• Frontotemporal dementias.

Rarer conditions (many potentially treatable):
• HIV dementia.
• Multiple sclerosis.
• Huntington's disease.
• Dentato-rubro-pallido-Luysian atrophy.
• Progressive supranuclear palsy.
• Wilson's disease.
• Cortico-basal degeneration.
• Toxins, e.g. carbon monoxide exposure, heavy metals.
• Neuro-acanthocytosis.
• Hallervorden–Spatz disease.
• Spinocerebellar ataxias.
• Creutzfeldt–Jakob disease.

Specific cognitive deficits

Cognitive function examination is described in Chapter 1. Understanding which cognitive domains are affected is important and can narrow the differential diagnosis. In AD, episodic memory is affected early but working memory is preserved. Confabulation, introducing incorrect or bizarre answers, is a late feature of AD, implying dysexecutive problems.

Semantic dementia

This localizes to the anterior temporal area. The patient has lost information about objects and so cannot name and answers poorly when asked about an object. For example, a gardener may forget flower names, despite good retrieval of other words, and be unable to identify a daffodil or crocus but refer to both only as flowers (category exemplar).

DEMENTIA SYNDROMES

Alzheimer's disease (AD)

AD diagnosis is based upon three clinical criteria:

- **Multiple cognitive deficits:**
  - In memory.
  - Plus one or more of language, praxis, gnosis, executive function.
- **Causing:**
  - Gradual onset and progressive symptoms.
  - Significant impairment and decline in social life or occupation.

- **In the absence of:**
  - Other structural conditions, e.g. hypoxic brain injury.
  - Other psychiatric conditions, e.g. delirium, depression, schizophrenia.

AD is by far the most common dementia (50%); atypical presentations therefore can cause diagnostic difficulty.

Genetics

Familial AD (15% of cases) often presents at a younger age. Autosomal dominant familial AD (FAD) is associated with mutations in three genes:

- **β-amyloid precursor protein** (APP, chromosome 21). There are several mutations with varying phenotypes including hereditary cerebral haemorrhage with amyloid in Dutch families. Increased APP production probably causes dementia in Down's syndrome.
- **Presenilin 1** (PSEN-1, chromosome 14) explains 50% of FAD cases and has a variable clinical spectrum.
- **Presenilin 2** (PSEN-2, chromosome 1) is much rarer (<1% of FAD cases).

The $\varepsilon4$ allele increases the risk of developing late onset AD but there is currently no role for apolipoprotein $\varepsilon4$ allele genotyping (ApoE4, chromosome 19) outside of a research setting.

Dementia with Lewy bodies

The main clinical features are shown in Box 6.2.

Vascular dementia

The main clinical features are shown in Box 6.3.

Frontotemporal dementia

The main clinical features are shown in Box 6.4.

Rapid onset dementia

Box 6.5 gives the major causes of rapid onset dementia.

Box 6.2: Clinical features of dementia with Lewy bodies (DLB)

Dementia, together with one (possible DLB) or two (probable DLB) of the following:

1. Fluctuating cognitive level (the case notes may contain MSU results looking for the cause of recurrent delirium).
2. Visual hallucinations.
3. Motor features of Parkinson's disease.

Note that patients with DLB are exquisitely sensitive to neuroleptics.

Box 6.3: Clinical features of vascular dementia

1. Clinical features
   - **Evidence of stroke**, either on history, physical examination or imaging. Note some strokes are 'silent' or manifest only as reflex asymmetry, pseudobulbar palsy, or 'marche a petit pas'.
   - **Vascular risk factors**, e.g. hypertension. Note these are also risk factors for AD.
   - **Motor features**: gait abnormalities or pseudobulbar signs are common, unlike AD.
   - **Timing**: dementia onset is typically within three months of the stroke.
   - **Radiology**: The topography and severity of stroke changes are variable, ranging from a large discrete middle cerebral artery stroke, to multiple lacunes, to diffuse white matter disease (termed 'leucoaraiosis' if affecting >25% of white matter).

2. Progression
   - **Multi-infarct dementia** typically has a step-wise decline and a history of stroke.
   - **Binswanger disease** shows a progressive deterioration.

3. Rarer vasculopathies
   - **Lupus anticoagulant syndrome.**
   - **Sneddon's syndrome.** Livedo reticularis and stroke associated with anti-phospholipid antibodies (aPL).
   - **CADASIL** (cerebral autosomal dominant arteriopathy with subcortical infarcts and leucoencephalopathy). This is an autosomal dominant condition (notch-3 mutation) characterized by a family history of migraine, stroke, encephalopathy and dementia; it is often mistaken for MS. Imaging shows lesions in the corpus callosum, anterior temporal lobes and external capsule.

4. Management
   Controlling vascular risk factors may help to stabilize or improve cognition.
   - **Blood pressure control** is particularly important. A blood pressure rise (systolic or diastolic) of 10 mmHg increases the vascular dementia risk by 40%.
   - **Aspirin** and other anti-platelet medications are important in secondary prevention.

Beware of dual pathology, particularly vascular dementia and AD.

Creutzfeldt–Jakob disease (CJD)

Clinical features

Sporadic CJD is a rapidly progressive dementia (fatal in <2 years) with two or more of the following:

- Akinetic mutism.
- Myoclonus.
- Pyramidal or extrapyramidal features.
- Visual or cerebellar disturbance.

Other useful pointers are:

- EEG showing background slowing and characteristic periodic complexes.
- CSF assay showing protein 14-3-3.

Normal pressure (communicating) hydrocephalus (NPH)

The main clinical features of normal pressure (communicating) hydrocephalus (Fig. 6.1) are shown in Box 6.6.

Box 6.4: *Clinical features of frontotemporal dementia (FTD)*

FTD accounts for about 10% of dementias.

1. Clinical features
   - **Onset** usually before the age of 65 years.
   - **Behaviour**: impulsive, tactless, inappropriate touching, sexual comments, disregard for personal space, personal hygiene and appearance. Other patients become less spontaneous, lose interest and become apathetic, sometimes with hyperorality and may crave sweets. Behaviour may be perseverative or stereotyped. Some develop preoccupations or compulsions, e.g. hoarding food or avoiding pavement cracks.
   - **Emotions**: Patients typically become emotionally shallow, lacking interest or concern for others. Emotional perception may be disturbed, e.g. for facial expression of anger.
   - **Language**: Patients often show aphasias, stereotypies and surface dyslexias.
   - **Physical signs**: There may be parkinsonism, signs of motor neurone disease (in about 10%), incontinence and primitive reflexes. Oro-facial dyspraxia may be striking, e.g. unable to cough voluntarily (but repeating 'cough') yet reflex coughing is preserved.

Note: Remember motor neurone disease if frontotemporal dementia is suspected.

1. Types
   - **Frontal dementia**: This has the core features above, with personality change, impaired emotion, loss of insight and executive dysfunction.
   - **Primary progressive aphasia**: Speech is non-fluent, with phonemic paraphasias and eventually muteness. There may be oro-facial dyspraxia but other cognitive domains are relatively preserved.
   - **Semantic dementia**. Patients report memory difficulties, but relating to semantic rather than episodic memory. Surface dyslexia is typical and fluency tests are reversed (phonemic better than category fluency).

2. Aetiology
   - There are several possible FTD pathologies, but these correlate poorly with the clinical presentation.
   - Several kindreds with familial FTD and/or parkinsonism (including progressive supranuclear palsy) have mutations on chromosome 17 (tau protein); other are linked to chromosome 3 and 9.

Box 6.5 *Rapid onset dementia (<2 years)*

- Prion disease.
- Cerebral vasculitis.
- Paraneoplastic disease.
- Large decompensated mass, particularly frontal.
- Viral encephalitis (*Note* that dementia is not always progressive).
- Chronic meningitis (e.g. tuberculosis).
- Diffuse malignancy: intravascular lymphoma, carcinomatous encephalitis.

Shunt procedure in NPH

This may be curative, but diagnostic certainty is essential since dilated ventricles from atrophy are common in any dementia. Furthermore, complications occur in up to 40%, especially subdural haematomas. Shunting is most likely to help if:

- The gait problem predominates.
- The dementia is mild and sub-cortical, without cortical difficulties.
- The scan shows dilated ventricles without cortical atrophy or leucoaraiosis.
- Positive Fisher test: CSF withdrawal of 20–30 ml improves timed walking (repeated 2–3 times over 1 week).
- There is an identifiable cause (60% of cases, e.g. previous subarachnoid haemorrhage, Paget's disease).

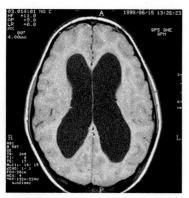

Figure 6.1
MRI scan showing normal pressure (communicating) hydrocephalus.

Box 6.6: Clinical presentation triad of NPH

- Gait apraxia, usually the earliest feature, manifests as a wide-based, slow, short-stepping gait ('sticky feet', 'magnetic gait'). Parkinsonian gait is 'sticky' but narrow-based.
- Dementia is typically sub-cortical, with bradyphrenia, forgetfulness, perseveration, mental inflexibility.
- Urinary incontinence.

PSYCHIATRIC PSEUDO-DEMENTIA

Patients presenting with apparent dementia occasionally have a reversible psychiatric cause. Depression importantly may co-exist with dementia and requires proactive management (see below). There are three forms:

1. **Depression** can be difficult to recognize although usually there are other depressive features. Questions often receive 'I don't know' replies. Patients with depression have 4–5 times the risk of developing dementia in the subsequent 3 years; perhaps the depression unmasks or discloses the dementia, or it may represent a prodrome.
2. **Conversion disorders.** There is typically a disparity between day-to-day function and formal testing. For example the patient may travel alone to the clinic, read books, remain independent and self-caring (shopping, driving), but perform poorly on cognitive tests.
3. **Ganser syndrome.** This is rare, usually in males aged 20–40 years and is characterized by approximate but slightly inaccurate responses to questions (paralogia), e.g. 'How many legs does a cow have?' (Answer 'Five'). 'How many days in a week?' (Answer 'Eight'), etc.

INVESTIGATION

- **Blood tests** including full blood count, ESR, electrolytes, serum B_{12}, thyroid function tests, VDRL, anti-nuclear antibody. Consider HIV and other investigations according to the clinical problem.

- **MR brain scan** is preferable to CT.
- **Electroencephalogram** can help to distinguish FTD from AD: alpha activity is lost early in AD, but preserved in FTD.
- **CSF examination** can help to exclude infective or inflammatory causes (check for oligoclonal bands).
- **Specialized tests**, e.g. genetic testing for Huntington's disease (for chorea and dementia).
- **Biopsy** of brain or leptomeninges may be considered to identify treatable conditions, e.g. cerebral vasculitis/lymphoma.

MANAGEMENT

Care planning

It is important to inform patients and their family and carers about the diagnosis and cause of dementia. Patients and family often feel relief to have an explanation for the symptoms. They need a personalized care plan, including information about specific pharmacotherapies and a discussion about the prognosis.

Behavioural management

Behavioural aspects of dementia are common and include wandering, aggression, abnormal eating habits, disinhibition and non-regular sleeping patterns. Behavioural and psychiatric problems cause the most distress to carers and are the most frequent precipitants of institutionalization. All behaviours can be summarized as '**ABC**':

- The **Antecedent** causes.
- The **Behaviour** itself.
- The **Consequences** of the behaviour.

The causes of behaviour changes can be summarized by '**PAID**':

- **Physical problems**, e.g. pain.
- **Activity**, e.g. carer getting patient dressed.
- **Intrinsic to disease**, e.g. personality change.
- **Delusion**, e.g. theft, hallucinations.

Managing sleep disorder in dementia

General measures

- Encourage diurnal activities.
- Increase social contact.
- Discourage daytime naps.
- Permit sleep only in bed in the dark.
- A large meal for supper rather than lunch.
- A night time sitter to allow the carer to sleep.

Pharmacological measures

- Consider a short course of benzodiazepines.
- For suspected depression, consider a sedating anti-depressant (trazodone) at night.
- If cholinesterase inhibitors are prescribed, a morning rather than evening dose can increase arousal.

Pharmacological

Pharmacological management includes antidepressants, atypical anti-psychotics and cholinesterase inhibitors.

Depression

Depression is common in dementia (perhaps 30–50%), although may be difficult to identify. There are several important features:

- Mood, e.g. appearance, crying, enjoyment.
- Speech, e.g. reduced rate or volume.
- Activity, e.g. pastimes.
- Sleep, usually reduced but may be increased.
- Appetite, e.g. weight loss.

It is worth having a high index of suspicion for depression in demented patients and a low threshold for starting antidepressant medication. SSRIs are usually used, started at a half dose and increased after 1–2 weeks if there are no adverse effects, e.g. paroxetine 10–20 mg after 1 week. Tricyclics are best avoided for several reasons: the anti-cholinergic effects may worsen cognition; they may provoke postural hypotension and they are more dangerous in overdose.

Delusions and hallucinations

Delusions and hallucinations occur with psychosis in up to half of the patients. Visual hallucinations in particular suggest DLB. Psychosis is generally treated with atypical anti-psychotics, e.g. quetiapine, or may respond to cholinergic treatments. Management of psychosis and hallucinations in patients with DLB includes withdrawing dopamine agonists and managing motor features with dopa replacement only.

Cholinesterase inhibitors

Use of cholinesterase inhibitors, e.g. donepezil or rivastigmine, for AD should follow standard guidelines:

1. **Patient selection:** Patients must have a secure diagnosis of AD, with a MMSE of 10–20 and preferably be relatively independent and at home with a carer to supervise.
2. **Discussion of medication side-effects:**

   - Gastrointestinal effects.
   - Cardiovascular (bradycardia, consider an ECG).
   - Insomnia (a morning tablet may be beneficial in somnolent patients).

- Exacerbation of depression (consider an SSRI before treatment).

3. **Monitoring and discontinuation:** Before starting, the patient and family must agree the outcome measures and stopping criteria. Dementia is monitored principally using the MMSE; Clinical Dementia Rating (CDR) complements this, measuring memory, orientation, judgement, problem solving, community affairs, daily activities, hobbies and personal affairs.

Cholinesterase inhibitors offer very modest symptomatic benefits in large clinical trials, delaying symptomatic cognitive decline, although 15–20% of patients show a dramatically favourable response (Fig. 6.2).

Other medication points

- DLB may also benefit from cholinesterase inhibitors, their greater cholinergic deficit suggesting possibly greater benefit than AD.
- Vascular risk factors require treatment in all patients, not only those with vascular dementia.

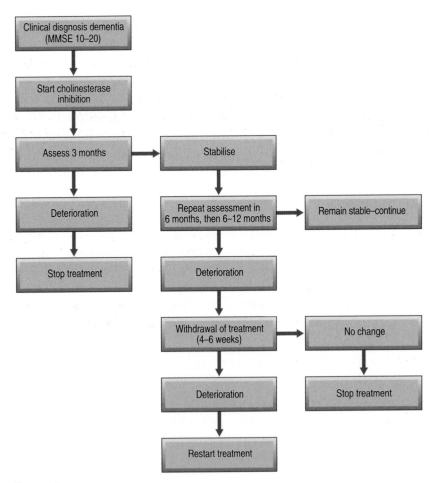

Figure 6.2
Suggested route for prescribing cholinesterase inhibitors.

- Neuroleptics should be avoided in patients with DLB; if necessary small doses of atypical agents should be tried, e.g. quetiapine.
- Cholinesterase inhibitors may also be used for neuropsychiatric problems.

PROGRESSION

Clinical milestones in typical AD are:

- Mild cognitive impairment progressing to dementia.
- Loss of instrumental activities of daily living (ADL).
- Neuropsychiatric symptoms.
- Nursing-home placement.
- Loss of self-care ADLs.
- Death.

PROGNOSIS

The prognosis of dementia is variable. In general, the expected survival for AD is about 8 years. Certain features suggest a worse outlook (Box 6.7). *Minimal cognitive impairment* implies that patients have memory loss over and above that expected for age and educational level; they are normal in other cognitive domains and the problem does not interfere with daily life. These patients can be told they are not demented but they should be offered annual follow-up at a memory clinic. Their risk of developing AD is up to 15% per year.

DELIRIUM

Delirium is common (10–20% of medical inpatients), especially in the elderly. It is easily overlooked, yet has a high mortality and morbidity. Surgery (particularly orthopaedic and cardiothoracic) and ITU are particularly linked to delirium. Distinguishing dementia and delirium can be difficult and they are not mutually exclusive; sometimes the first hint of dementia is a prolonged period of postoperative delirium. The clinical features of delirium (which may help to distinguish it from dementia) are outlined in Box 6.8.

Box 6.7: *Dementia features suggesting a poor prognosis*

- Non-AD dementia.
- Aphasia.
- Vascular disease.
- Extra-pyramidal features.
- Myoclonus.
- Early onset psychosis.
- Unmarried man.
- Older age.
- Psychological morbidity in the carer.

Box 6.8: Clinical features of delirium, distinguishing it from dementia

- **Acute onset.**
- **Fluctuating attention disturbance:**
  - Rambling in conversation, changing subjects, distractible.
  - Cannot maintain concentration, e.g. when attempting serial 7s or counting backwards from 20.
- **Fluctuating behaviour:**
  - Worse at night (ask the nursing staff about this).
  - Disrupted sleep–wake cycle.
- **Fluctuating confusion:**
  - Visual hallucinations are common, classically Lilliputian figures (small men or objects).
  - Confabulation with memory tests.
  - Loss of writing or drawing ability (often profound).
- **Fluctuating arousal:**
  - Hypoactive/hypoalert patients are lethargic, passive, staring, easily sleeping although rousable: these problems are easily overlooked.
  - Hyperactive/hyperalert patients are agitated with prominent autonomic activity; these problems are easily spotted, e.g. in delirium tremens.
- **Delusions:**
  - Capgras syndrome (belief that people, usually relatives, are recognizable but have been replaced).
  - Fregoli syndrome (belief that different people are the same person in disguise).

Causes of delirium

Diffuse changes are the usual cause, relating to neurotransmitter abnormalities, particularly cholinergic deficit or dopaminergic excess.

Focal lesions can cause delirium, especially lesions in the right parietal lobe, prefrontal area, thalamus, basal ganglia (particularly caudate) or fusiform gyrus.

Box 6.9 lists some specific precipitants of delirium.

Management of delirium

- Identify and treat known causes, remembering faecal impaction, urinary and upper respiratory tract infection and pain.
- Consider brain imaging and screening tests covering the precipitants listed in Box 6.9.

Box 6.9: Specific precipitants of delirium

- Infection.
- Metabolic (electrolytes).
- Drugs (particularly anticholinergics and dopaminergic).
- Pain (often under-recognized in postoperative patients).
- Faecal impaction.
- Hypoxia (e.g. lung disease, myocardial infarction, heart failure).
- Sensory deprivation.
- Fragmented sleep.
- Alcohol withdrawal.

- Nurse in a well-lit, quiet room, a safe environment with familiar personal objects, family pictures etc. and, as far as possible, with the same staff looking after patient.
- Haloperidol in small doses (0.5 mg) can be useful (beware Lewy body dementia). However, for delirium tremens use chlordiazepoxide, as haloperidol may provoke dysphoria and lower seizure threshold.

COMA

Physiology

Consciousness incorporates arousal and awareness; these depend upon the ascending reticular activating system and intact cerebral cortex. Space-occupying lesions may interrupt the ascending reticular activating system (extends from caudal medulla to rostral midbrain); however, medullary lesions do not frequently cause coma (Fig. 6.3). Metabolic disturbance and seizure activity are important medical causes; it is also important to identify functional coma.

Causes

- Coma with meningism (Kernig's or Brudzinski's signs):
  - Meningitis.
  - Encephalitis.
  - Subarachnoid haemorrhage.

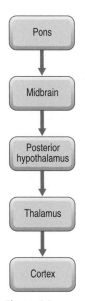

Figure 6.3
Ascending reticular activating system (ARAS).

- Coma without meningism (stiff neck but negative Kernig's and Brudzinski's signs):
  - Foraminal pressure cone (cerebellar herniation).
  - Many metabolic causes (see below).
  - Epilepsy.

Metabolic coma

Metabolic conditions (Box 6.10) are particularly important. Patients with overdose arriving in casualty alive are salvageable no matter what the drug level; this is particularly so with sedative medications. There are specific examination pointers to a metabolic cause.

- **Pupils** are spared in most metabolic coma.
- **Breathing rate** may be high.
- **Oculocephalic reflexes** may be absent.
- **Myoclonus** is common in metabolic coma, especially with CO_2 retention, hepatic and renal coma, as well as some drugs, e.g. antiepileptics, antibiotics (ciprofloxacin) and anti-depressants.

Note: the combination of lost oculocephalic reflex and spared pupil strongly suggests a metabolic rather than a structural cause.

Supratentorial lesions causing coma

Brainstem compression causes coma by pressure on the pontine and midbrain tegmentum, interrupting the reticular activating system.

Supratentorial lesions. Parenchymal lesions e.g. stroke or tumour and extra-axial lesions, e.g. subdural haematoma, can cause brainstem compression through a tentorial pressure cone, either unilaterally (uncal herniation) or bilaterally (central tentorial herniation); both lead to coma.

Box 6.10: Metabolic and diffuse causes of coma

Tissue hypoxia:
- Hypoxaemia.
- Anaemia and carbon monoxide poisoning.
- Ischaemia, e.g. arrhythmias, pulmonary embolus.
- Fat embolus causes hypoxaemia, skin rash, confusion or coma in patients with trauma and bone fractures.
- Histoxic causes, e.g. cyanide poisoning, with inability to utilize oxygen.

Hypoglycaemia:

Diabetic complications, e.g. hyperglycaemic non-ketotic coma and diabetic ketoacidosis.

Wernicke's encephalopathy. If alcoholics are unresponsive to thiamine, consider central pontine myelinolysis.

Liver failure. Consider EEG and serum ammonia.

Renal failure. Note that renal failure patients are susceptible to opiate toxicity, persisting for days.

Poisons and drug overdose:
- Alcohol, methyl alcohol, ethylene glycol: these give a metabolic acidosis.
- Opiate toxicity presents with coma and small pupils.
- Tricyclics poisoning gives anticholinergic effects and arrhythmias.
- Salicylates give a metabolic acidosis, respiratory alkalosis, 'corticospinal tract signs' and asterixis.

Hypertensive encephalopathy often presents with visual symptoms and cortical blindness.

Electrolyte abnormalities including calcium and sodium disorders (Na <125 mmol/L affects consciousness; <120 mmol/L makes seizures more likely).

Central tentorial herniation

This usually develops gradually and signs usually appear in order.

- Pupils:
  - Small and reactive initially.
  - Larger and fixed to light as the compression progresses.
- Ventilation:
  - Sighs and yawns initially.
  - Cheyne–Stokes breathing later.
  - Hyperventilation (pupil usually large) as compression progresses.
- Vestibular ocular reflex with either head movement (oculocephalic) or cold irrigation (caloric):
  - Normal initially.
  - Asymmetric or absent as compression progresses (associated with dilated pupil and hyperventilation).
- Motor features:
  - Asymmetric initially: the patient localizes to pain and shows paratonia or a decorticate (arms flexed, legs extended) posture.
  - Bilateral decorticate posture later (with small pupils and Cheyne–Stokes breathing).
  - Decerebrate (four limb hyper-extension) posture as compression progresses (together with abnormal vestibulo-ocular reflexes, pupils fixed and dilated).

Uncal herniation

This causes a third nerve palsy (the first sign is an ipsilateral dilated pupil) often with hemiparesis. The hemiparesis is usually contralateral, but ipsilateral hemiparesis may result from pressure from the contralateral tentorial edge on the contralateral corticospinal tract (Kernohan's notch).

Infra-tentorial lesions causing coma

Coma is an early feature of infra-tentorial lesions (Fig. 6.4), especially with vascular causes, e.g. pontine or intraventricular haemorrhage.

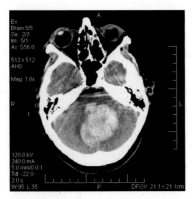

Figure 6.4
CT scan showing posterior fossa haemorrhage.

Clinical features

These depend upon the level in the brainstem affected.

- **Midbrain level lesions** cause bilateral nuclear or infranuclear 3rd nerve palsy with long tract signs.
- **Upper pontine lesions** cause internuclear ophthalmoplegia (assessed with doll's eye or caloric reflexes), small pupils (the parasympathetic 3rd is spared but the sympathetic chain is involved) and facial weakness.
- **Lower pontine lesions** cause several signs:
  - Eye movements are lost horizontally, but exaggerated vertically (the midbrain is spared). This dissociation of vertical and horizontal eye movements points to a structural lesion.
  - Pupils are small but with some retained light reaction (the 3rd nerve parasympathetic is spared).
  - Motor signs are bilateral but often asymmetrical.
  - Ventilation is apneustic or ataxic.

Lower pontine lesions are difficult to distinguish from metabolic coma. The clinician must critically evaluate all the signs and take particular note of the pupils (small but reactive in metabolic coma) and the discrepancy between vertical and horizontal eye movements (suggesting a structural cause). Pontine haemorrhage or infarct is suggested by the rapid onset of coma, pinpoint pupils (the light reaction often returns after 24 h) and fever (pontine: pole axed, pinpoint, pyrexial). If the vascular lesion is confined to the basal pons, the patient may be locked in (see below), often with significant potential recovery.

- **Upward herniation** (cerebellum through the tentorium). With the brainstem pushed upwards, the vestibulo-ocular reflexes may be lost vertically but preserved horizontally. Pupils may be mid-size and fixed.
- **Downward herniation** (cerebellum through the foramen magnum) is often rapidly fatal with compression of the central ventilatory centres.
- **Central pontine myelinolysis** should be considered in alcoholics (although not exclusively) who develop cranial nerve signs, tetraparesis (sometimes locked in) and reduced level of consciousness, but who fail to respond to thiamine.

Locked in syndrome

Although not a disorder of consciousness, this syndrome may easily be mistaken for coma with adverse consequences. Locked in patients are conscious but paralysed (de-efferented) because of a lesion at the ventral pons (or bilateral destruction of corticobulbar and corticospinal tracts in the cerebral peduncles) impairing every voluntary movement except vertical eye movements. The diagnosis can be missed if voluntary vertical eye movement is not assessed in patients who seem unresponsive.

Assessment

The examination in coma can identify the likely cause; the clinician should particularly note the ventilatory patterns and pupil size, corresponding to different levels of brain dysfunction.

Emergency assessment

This involves attention to airway, breathing and circulation, a search for trauma and checking the blood glucose.

History details

These must be obtained from relatives, bystanders, the patient's wallet, or telephoning the family doctor.

General examination

This must include the head and neck, looking for skull fracture, laceration, haematoma (Battle sign), meningism, fundoscopy and auroscopy. Ask the patient to look upwards (may be locked in).

Level of consciousness

Assess this using the Glasgow Coma Scale (GCS) (Box 6.11). Note that coma is defined by the GCS as 2, 4, 2 (no eye opening to command, not localizing pain, not uttering words).

Pupils

The pupils are small in metabolic coma and opiate poisoning. Following most poisonings, the pupils are normal, but with anticholinergics they are large.

Box 6.11: Glasgow Coma Scale

Eye opening…
1. none
2. to pain
3. to command
4. spontaneously

Best motor response…
1. none
2. extension
3. abnormal flexion (shoulder adducted)
4. normal flexion (shoulder abducted)
5. localizing pain
6. spontaneous movements

Best verbal response…
1. unresponsive
2. incomprehensible sounds
3. words, confused
4. words, orientated
5. talking normally

Corneal reflexes

In poisoning, the corneal reflexes are lost early (lost corneals in mild coma suggests overdose and so a good prognosis); for other causes, corneals are retained until late in deep coma (lost corneals in non-overdose coma has a poor prognosis).

Eye position

- Mild eye divergence is normal in coma.
- Gaze away from a hemiparesis suggests a hemisphere cause; gaze towards a hemiparesis suggests a pontine cause.
- Fixed downgaze suggests a metabolic cause or midbrain tectum lesion.

Spontaneous eye movements

- Roving eye movements is non-localizing, but indicates an intact brainstem.
- Spontaneous nystagmus is uncommon in coma because it requires functioning cortex and brainstem.
- Ocular bobbing (eyes drifting downwards) is rare, but may accompany metabolic coma (especially hepatic) and lower pontine lesions.
- Uniocular nystagmoid jerking suggests a mid or low pontine lesion.

Induced eye movements

- Oculocephalic (doll's eye) movements disappear if the pons is depressed or damaged.
- Oculovestibular (caloric) movements show one of four responses:
  1. Nystagmus with fast phase away occurs in awake patients or feigned coma.
  2. Tonic deviation towards the stimulus indicates a supratentorial lesion.
  3. No response or dysconjugate gaze indicates a brainstem lesion.
  4. Tonic upward deviation may follow poisoning.

Breathing

This is often abnormal in coma.

- **Ataxic breathing** (irregular disorganized breathing) is the most common abnormal central breathing pattern and suggests a medullary lesion.
- **Cheyne–Stokes breathing** manifests as hyperpnoea alternating with apnoea. It can occur in normal sleep, with hypoxaemia and with prolonged circulation time (e.g. left ventricular failure). With neurogenic causes (bilateral lesion between the cortex and upper pons) the pattern cannot be broken voluntarily, e.g. by attempting hyperventilation during apnoea. Increased ventilation is due to increased carbon dioxide responsiveness. Ventilation normally continues following hyperventilation, but following forebrain damage or encephalopathy, e.g. hypertensive or uraemic, apnoea develops, causing Cheyne–Stokes breathing.

- **Hyperventilation**. Central neurogenic hyperventilation is caused by an upper brainstem lesion. Patients with metabolic acidosis also hyperventilate. Hyperventilation normally gives low $PaCO_2$ with normal PaO_2; however, some patients have a low PaO_2 implying a pulmonary component, e.g. lung congestion.
- **Apneustic breathing**. Ventilation pauses at the end of inspiration for 2–3 sec. It localizes to the mid or caudal pons, near to the trigeminal motor nucleus.
- **Ondine's curse**. Automatic ventilation fails (medullary lesion, e.g. Wallenburg's syndrome) but voluntary ventilation (cortical projections to the respiratory motor pools via corticospinal tracts) is preserved. Thus the patient may stop breathing when asleep (very rare).

Investigations

Baseline investigations include serum glucose, electrolytes, urine and blood for paracetamol, salicylate and recreational drug levels.

Measurement of arterial blood gas tensions may also help as follows:

- Respiratory alkalosis:
  - Hepatic coma.
  - Salicylate poisoning.
  - Sepsis.
- Metabolic acidosis (rapid breathing):
  - Lactic acidosis.
  - Diabetic ketoacidosis.
  - Salicylate poisoning.
- Alcoholic acidosis:
  - Methyl alcohol (blindness is an early symptom).
  - Ethylene glycol poisoning.
- Others:
  - Consider carbon monoxide levels.
  - Consider fat emboli in young trauma with confusion and fever.

Prognosis

In general, this is difficult to predict. Box 6.12 shows the likelihood of recovery relating to several features.

Case history outcome

The patient had AD. Her early memory problems with involvement of other cognitive domains were sufficient to cause loss of day-to-day function. She was reasonably independent (dressing and washing) and had a carer and so was a candidate for cholinesterase inhibitors. Her behavioural problems (waking and keeping her husband up), justified detailed questions about sleeping patterns, including drinking habits before retiring.

> **Box 6.12: Prognosis of coma**
>
> The following lists the percentage of patients who make a good recovery from coma.
> Aetiology
> - 10% patients (all causes) make a good recovery.
> - 5% subarachnoid haemorrhage.
> - 10% hypoxic–ischaemic episode.
> - 25% metabolic (better prognosis).
>
> Duration
> - Poorer prognosis with longer duration.
> - 2% after 2 weeks.
>
> Brainstem signs
> - Poorer prognosis with loss of brainstem reflexes.
> - 1% with absent brainstem reflexes at 24h.
>
> Depth of coma
> - Poorer prognosis with depth of coma.
> - 20% if opening eyes at 6h; 10% if not opening eyes.
> - 3% if no motor response at 6h; 15% if flexion or better.
> - 8% if no response to sounds at 6h; 30% if responds to sounds.

KEY POINTS

- Obtain a first hand account from a carer.
- Cognitive tests need cooperation: if the patient cannot maintain concentration, e.g. serial 7s, days of week, it is difficult to interpret subsequent findings.
- The tempo of decline is important: rapid progression suggests many important diagnostic possibilities.
- Motor and systemic abnormalities are important, particularly with sub-cortical pattern of dementia: they suggest a range of more treatable causes, including HIV.
- When asking about day-to-day life, remember driving: do passengers feel safe with the patient driving?
- Behavioural and psychiatric aspects of dementia are especially important to carers: there are strategies to cope with these.
- Simple cognitive tests are useful, but remember the MMSE is insensitive to frontal lobe function.
- Normal pressure hydrocephalus is a commonly considered diagnostic possibility. However, the ventricles are capacious in all atrophic brain diseases and shunting has a high morbidity: patient selection is crucial.
- Patients with dementia, especially dementia with Lewy bodies, are particularly sensitive to neuroleptics.
- Give the benefit of the doubt when diagnosing and treating depression in patients with suspected dementia: depression may be difficult to spot in dementia.

- Note the combination of lost oculocephalic reflex and spared pupil strongly suggests a metabolic rather than a structural cause of coma.
- Remember to ask apparently comatose patient to look upwards; they may be 'locked in'.

Further Reading

Bates D. Neurological assessment of coma. J Neurol Neurosurg Psychiatry 2001; 71: 13–17.

Stroke

Case history

A 75-year-old woman presented in coma. She was unresponsive to command, not opening her eyes to noise or pain, and her pupils were unreactive to light. Her right arm and leg were held extended. Both plantars were extensor. She was apyrexial, in sinus rhythm and with normal heart sounds. For 6 months she had become forgetful with several episodes of sudden inability to speak, with right-sided facial numbness lasting for up to 20 min. These had persisted despite aspirin, clopidogrel and warfarin. Her INR was 1.8. CT brain scan showed a large left parieto-occipital lobar haemorrhage.

INTRODUCTION

Stroke is the third leading cause of death worldwide after coronary disease and cancer (incidence 200/100 000 per year) and the most common cause of neurological disability in the developed world. Transient ischaemic attacks (TIAs) are one-quarter as common, and precede 15% of strokes; 25% of strokes occur in people aged <65 years.

STROKE ASSESSMENT

The clinician must address four questions:

1. Was it a stroke/TIA?
2. Where is the damage?
3. What is the damage?
4. What was the cause?

WAS IT A STROKE/TIA?

Stroke is a sudden onset ('at a stroke') focal neurological deficit of presumed vascular aetiology, characterized by:

- Loss of function, i.e. numbness and/or weakness rather than tingling and/or shaking.
- Maximum at onset, i.e. not progressive.
- Focal (see below).

With these criteria met, the diagnosis is 80% accurate. Box 7.1 gives the differential diagnosis.

TIA diagnosis is more challenging, relying more upon the history than signs and with a broader differential diagnosis. In the Oxfordshire Community Stroke Project (OCSP), 62% of TIAs from primary care had a different diagnosis including the following:

- **Migraine with aura** is the most common cause of 'TIA' in younger people. It is 2500 times more common than TIA in 40 year olds, and still 15 times more common in 70 year olds.
- **Giant cell arteritis** is the major differential diagnosis of amaurosis fugax (see Ch. 14 for others).
- **Critical carotid artery stenosis** may give runs of TIAs, often amaurosis fugax. These may be associated with limb jerking mimicking a focal seizure.
- **Capsular warning syndrome** causes brief, recurrent, stereotyped attacks, e.g. recurrent hemiplegias without cortical features. It is related to lacunar ischaemia (small vessel disease), from stenosis and hypoperfusion in small penetrator vessels. It is easily overlooked as either non-vascular or psychological.
- **Non-focal symptoms**, e.g. isolated dizziness or confusion are commonly misdiagnosed as TIA.

TIAs are important because the early stroke risk is high (8–12% at 7 days; 11–15% at 28 days). TIA patients therefore need rapid assessment, definitely within 7 days. Box 7.2 gives factors that increase the stroke risk following TIA.

Box 7.1: Differential diagnosis of stroke

- Metabolic/toxic encephalopathy, e.g. hypoglycaemia.
- Functional (non-organic).
- Seizures, e.g. with Todd's paresis.
- Migraine.
- Structural cause, e.g. meningioma, subdural haematoma.
- Encephalitis or abscess.
- Head injury.
- Hypertensive encephalopathy.
- Multiple sclerosis.

Box 7.2: TIA: factors increasing stroke risk

- Brain rather than retinal TIA (reflecting emboli size).
- Older age.
- Widespread, e.g. peripheral, vascular disease.
- Carotid stenosis >80%.
- Increasing TIA frequency in the previous 3 months.

WHERE IS THE DAMAGE?

Clinical localization

The OCSP derived a useful guide:

- **Exclusive carotid territory**, e.g. monocular blindness or language abnormality (dominant hemisphere).
- **Definite vertebrobasilar territory**, e.g. tetraparesis, diplopia, ataxia, cortical blindness, or vertigo.
- **Either anterior or posterior territory**, e.g. unilateral sensory or motor problems, dysphagia, dysarthria, homonymous hemianopia.

Stroke patterns

The OCSP derived several stroke syndromes, allowing classification of 99% of strokes.

Total anterior circulation syndrome (TACS)

TACS comprises 20% strokes with new onset of:

- Hemiparesis (with or without sensory loss) involving at least two body areas (face, arm or leg).
- Homonymous hemianopia.
- Higher cortical dysfunction, e.g. language, neglect.

Drowsiness is usual but beware the 'walking TACS', with only slight motor loss: such patients may have a posterior circulation infarction with secondary internal capsule or thalamus disruption.

Partial anterior stroke syndrome (PACS)

PACS comprises 30% strokes with new onset of:

- Any two of the three TACS criteria.
- Isolated cognitive deficit.
- Predominant proprioceptive abnormality in one limb.
- Isolated symptoms in one limb.

General rule: only one limb with upper motor neurone problems, think cortical.

Lacunar stroke (LACS)

LACS comprises 25% strokes, with four main patterns:

1. **Pure motor hemiparesis**: 50% of lacunar strokes (internal capsule or pons).
2. **Hemisensorimotor**: 35% of lacunar strokes (pons, internal capsule, or corona radiata).

3. **Ataxic hemiparesis** (dysarthria and a clumsy hand): 10% of lacunar strokes (pons *and/or* internal capsule).
4. **Pure hemisensory**: 5% of lacunar strokes (thalamus).

Posterior circulation stroke (POCS)

These comprise 25% of strokes and overlap with lacunar strokes.

- **Brainstem strokes,** many named eponymously, are useful for learning anatomical relationships.
- **Cerebellar strokes** may be subtle, e.g. patients feeling 'off balance', but the underlying infarct may be surprising large. Consider possible embolic sources. Also beware the potential for these strokes to cause obstructive hydrocephalus.
- **Thalamic infarcts** present in several ways:
  - 'Diencephalic amnesia', with confusion, dysphasia (left thalamus), and neglect (right thalamus). This starts suddenly and does not progress (unlike Alzheimer's disease).
  - Hypersomnolence.
  - Eye movement disorders, e.g. supranuclear gaze problems.
  - Pupil abnormalities.
  - Depressed consciousness.
  - Motor and sensory signs.
  - Ataxia, e.g. dentato-rubro-thalamic pathway.
  - Movement disorders, implying associated basal ganglia involvement, e.g. chorea, hemiballism, dystonia.

General rule: Strokes presenting in an unusual way (confusion or 'stroke somewhere, stroke nowhere'): think thalamus or cerebellum.

WHAT IS THE DAMAGE?

The main question is whether the cause is infarct (80%) or haemorrhage (20%, including 5% from subarachnoid haemorrhage). Haemorrhage is proportionately more common in Asians and blacks (30–40%). All stroke patients require early plain CT brain scanning to assist the diagnosis.

CT brain scan (Fig. 7.1)

The appearances depend upon the timing of imaging.

- **Within the first week,** plain CT distinguishes haemorrhage (Fig. 7.2) from ischaemia.
- **In the second week,** the infarct initially is hypodense, and later fades, becoming isodense ('fogging').
- **After 2 weeks,** the infarct becomes more hypodense and easier to see.
- **After several weeks,** CT cannot distinguish haemorrhage from ischaemia.

Contrast is not recommended, unless there is a possible alternative diagnosis, e.g. abscess.

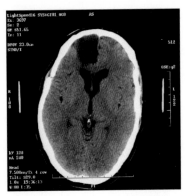

Figure 7.1
CT scan showing frontal ischaemic infarct.

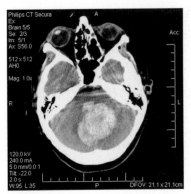

Figure 7.2
CT scan showing posterior fossa haemorrhagic stroke.

WHAT WAS THE CAUSE?

The exact cause remains uncertain in 40% of strokes despite extensive investigations.

Atherothrombosis (thrombo-embolic) disease

This causes 45–50% of strokes.

Large vessel atherosclerosis

This form of arteriosclerosis is characterized by fatty and necrotic material accumulation in the arterial wall (Greek *athere* – porridge). Atherosclerotic plaques can become inflamed (mediated by oxidized LDL cholesterol in the fatty core) causing plaque rupture and consequent platelet-mediated thrombosis and coagulation. Thus, atherosclerosis is often acute-on-chronic, with rupture or inflammation causing series of TIAs and a high immediate incidence of stroke. Note that cardiac events occur in 3–5% or TIA patients per year, but do not cluster.

Small vessel disease

Disease of vessels <500 µm diameter shows on cerebral imaging as periventricular white matter rarefaction (leucoaraiosis) (Fig. 7.3). There are several causes:

- **Lipohyalinosis** is subintimal thickening with foamy macrophages, causing occlusion. It may cause 60% of lacunar infarctions, sometimes with haemorrhages.
- **Atherosclerosis** (microatheroma) is the same process as in large arteries, and causes 30% of lacunar infarctions.
- **Arteriolosclerosis** gives a uniform concentric arteriolar wall thickening, especially in diabetes mellitus and hypertension.

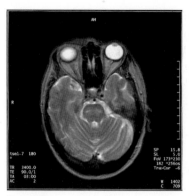

Figure 7.3
MRI showing deep white matter disease.

- **Unusual causes** are relevant if the patient is young and neither diabetic nor hypertensive. They include inflammatory vasculopathies, CADASIL (see Multiple sclerosis), Spatz–Lindenburg disease and many others. Often, elderly patients have coexistent amyloid angiopathy.

Cardiac causes

Cardiac emboli cause 20% of strokes.

Atrial fibrillation (AF)

About 20% of elderly stroke patients have AF. Box 7.3 outlines the main risk factors for stroke in these patients.

Endocarditis

Infective endocarditis must be considered in all strokes. Non-infective endocarditis is commonly overlooked.

Box 7.3: AF and stroke risk

Overall risk is 5% per year, i.e. six times more than patients in sinus rhythm.
- **High risk**: 6–12% per year:
  - Age >65 years, with hypertension or diabetes mellitus.
  - Previous TIA or stroke.
  - Heart failure.
  - Thyrotoxicosis.
  - Echocardiogram shows left atrial thrombus.
- **Moderate risk**: 3–5% per year:
  - Age <65 years, with hypertension or diabetes mellitus.
  - Age >65 years, with no other risk factors.
- **Low risk**: 1% per year:
  - Age <65 years, with no other risk factors.

- **Marantic endocarditis** (marasmus: wasting) accompanies underlying malignancy (emboli may precede tumour diagnosis). The vegetations are usually on the atrial side of the mitral valve, whereas infective endocarditis usually affects the ventricular side.
- **Libmann–Sacks endocarditis** accompanies SLE (see Antiphospholipid syndrome) and although embolism is rare, the brain is the most likely target.

Other valvular abnormalities

Rheumatic and prosthetic valve abnormalities carry major thromboembolism risk (see Ch. 15).

Vasculopathies

Vasculopathies (either inflammatory or non-inflammatory) cause 5% of strokes.

Inflammatory vasculopathies

These have three patterns of presentation:

1. Stroke with encephalopathic features.
2. Multiple sclerosis-like conditions.
3. Space-occupying lesion.

Some inflammatory vasculopathies have features outside the CNS:

- **Systemic features** reflect systemic vasculitis. Remember to analyse the urine and consider a formal glomerular filtration rate if the creatinine is borderline or high.
- **Giant cell arteritis (GCA)** can cause stroke, often involving the posterior circulation. Box 7.4 gives the GCA diagnostic criteria.
- **Specific patterns** occur with rare vasculopathies, e.g. Susac's syndrome of deafness, blindness and headache.
- **Infections.** Stroke may result from infective meningitis causing vasculitis as blood vessels traverse the meninges, e.g. TB, syphilis or cryptococcus.

Box 7.4: Giant cell arteritis

The diagnosis needs three or more of the following:
- Age >50 years (usually 70+ years).
- New onset of headache.
- Tender or pulseless temporal arteries.
- Elevated ESR (note some have normal ESR, so check CRP).
- Abnormal temporal artery biopsy.

Non-inflammatory vasculopathies

These are rare congenital or inherited conditions:

- Moya moya disease (Japanese: 'puff of smoke', refers to the angiogram appearance) is a relatively common cause of stroke in children.
- Fabry's disease: males with rash, pain (small fibre neuropathy), and stroke: easily mistaken for CADASIL on imaging grounds.
- Ehlers–Danlos syndrome.
- Fibromuscular dysplasia.
- Pseudoxanthoma elasticum.
- Marfan's syndrome.

Trauma (dissection)

This is an important cause of young-onset stroke. Even trivial trauma such as cervical manipulation or yoga can precipitate arterial dissection. Dissections are usually sub-intimal with ischaemic symptoms arising as the thrombosed blood embolizes; occasionally they may be subadventitial and present with bleeding (subarachnoid haemorrhage). Dissection may be seen (but sometimes missed) with Doppler/duplex ultrasound; vertebrobasilar ultrasound is technically more difficult. MRI (T1 axial) may show a narrowed arterial lumen with a rim of high signal thrombus, but intra-arterial angiogram is the gold standard.

Haematological

Antiphospholipid syndrome

- **Lupus anticoagulants** are immunoglobulins that interfere with phospholipid binding and the formation of prothrombin activator (a complex of calcium ion, factors Xa and V, and the phospholipid, platelet factor III). *In vitro* there is slowed thrombin formation and prolonged clotting.
- **Anticardiolipin antibodies** are different and detected by immunoassay.

Lupus anticoagulants and anticardiolipin antibodies may co-exist in 60% of antiphospholipid syndrome cases, but 40% have only one.
Clinical features include:

- **Pro-coagulant state** (70% have venous thrombosis, 30% arterial), the most common arterial site being the cerebral circulation.
- **Migraine-like headaches.**
- **Livedo reticularis.** Sneddon's syndrome is stroke plus this rash.
- **Recurrent miscarriages.**

Thrombophilia

Primary pro-coagulant states cause 5% of strokes, e.g.

- Factor V Leiden deficiency (prevalence 5%).
- Prothrombin G20210A (prevalence 1%).

These usually cause venous events and therefore are incidental to arterial ischaemic strokes: most stroke patients do not need thrombophilia testing. However, note that women heterozygous for factor V Leiden on the oral contraceptive pill have up to 40-fold risk of thrombosis, i.e. the risk is multiplicative.

Venous infarcts

Venous infarcts present according to the thrombus location.

- **Stroke presentations** are the most common, particularly in young women (F:M ratio is 3:1). They may be accompanied by seizures. Imaging typically shows a lesion not conforming to an arterial territory, more swollen than an arterial infarct, and containing 'finger-like' haemorrhages.
- **Idiopathic intracranial hypertension** (IIH) presentation from intracranial venous thrombosis is the reason for imaging (CT or MR venogram) all IIH patients.
- **Focal presentations**, e.g. cavernous sinus thrombosis.
- **Reduced conscious level** following several days of headache. This is easily misdiagnosed as encephalitis, and note that lumbar puncture may be contra-indicated owing to cerebral oedema.
- **Thunderclap headache.** (Mimicking SAH).

It is important to search for underlying causes before anticoagulating with warfarin (see below).

Pregnancy

Stroke complicates about 1 in 3000 deliveries. There are many potential mechanisms, particularly cardiac, venous thrombosis, dissection, or rarely embolic (air, fat, or metastatic choriocarcinoma).

Intravascular lymphoma

This rare but progressive condition presents with progressive CNS deficit (paraparesis or dementia) often with rash and elevated serum lactate dehydrogenase.

Mitochondrial cytopathy

MELAS (mitochondrial encephalopathy with lactic acidosis and stroke-like episodes) presents as stroke episodes with other mitochondrial features, e.g. deafness, short stature, seizures. The strokes themselves are often occipital, and not conforming to a vascular territory. Diffusion weighted MRI can distinguish mitochondrial strokes (vasogenic oedema) from ischaemic strokes (cytotoxic oedema).

Cholesterol embolization

This resembles a vasculitis with skin and kidney infarcts plus stroke-like events and confusion. Eosinophilia and low serum complement may suggest a vasculitis, but skin biopsy demonstrates cholesterol emboli. It occurs either spontaneously or following surgical procedures.

Haemorrhagic strokes

There are several causes.

- **Hypertension.** Most haemorrhagic strokes occur in hypertensive people with small vessel disease (lipohyalinosis). They mostly involve areas supplied by small arteries, e.g. putamen, thalamus and pons.
- **Clotting problems,** e.g. low platelets, warfarin, etc.
- **Amyloid angiopathy** is the most common cause of lobar haemorrhage in the elderly. It presents often with cognitive problems and recurrent transient events, including positive sensory problems, mimicking ischaemic TIAs. Beware this diagnosis, particularly as aspirin is not the best treatment.
- **Vascular abnormalities** should be considered in younger stroke patients – even if drugs such as cocaine seemed to precipitate the event – since a surprising number have underlying arteriovenous malformations, usually in a lobar location.
- **Malignancy,** and particularly kidney, lung, choriocarcinoma and melanoma metastases, may give lobar haemorrhages.
- **Venous thrombosis** (see above).
- **Trauma.** This may be occult, especially in the elderly.
- **Vasculitis** (see above).
- **Haemorrhagic transformation** of an infarct is particularly likely in embolic strokes where, as the embolus disperses, the soft infarct is re-perfused at arterial pressure. CT scanning of the initial infarct is the only reliable way to distinguish haemorrhagic transformation from a primary intracerebral haemorrhage: another reason to perform imaging early.

CLINICAL DIAGNOSIS

Diagnosing haemorrhagic stroke

Check the blood pressure and think of clotting, including bleeding time.

- **Young person:** consider drugs and arteriovenous malformation. Illicit drugs (cocaine and amphetamines) are a factor in many young strokes. Test for cocaine metabolites (present in urine for 36–48 h) and opiates. Hydrochloride cocaine is particularly associated with haemorrhagic stroke, whereas alkaloidal cocaine gives an equal risk of ischaemic and haemorrhagic stroke. Note that cocaine causes stroke through acute hypertension (spontaneous haemorrhage or rupture of underlying vascular malformation), but also through vasculitis or cardiogenic sources (infective endocarditis or cardiomyopathy).

- **Middle-aged person:** the most likely cause is small vessel hypertensive disease.
- **Older person:** consider amyloidosis.
- **Neglect:** note that scurvy can present with haemorrhagic stroke.

Diagnosing ischaemic stroke

The main causes are atherosclerotic, embolic or small vessel disease, but there are several reasons for diagnostic confusion.

- **Young person:** consider dissection, cardiac source, illicit drugs (cocaine).
- **'Funny' strokes,** e.g. preceded by fever, headache or other systemic or neurological problems: consider vasculopathy (inflammatory or non-inflammatory), infective endocarditis or mitochondrial cytopathy.
- **Vasculitic stroke** may be mimicked by cholesterol embolization, intravascular lymphoma, endocarditis (infective and non-infective), lupus anticoagulant and haemolytic–uraemic syndrome (often with thrombotic thrombocytopenic purpura, so check the platelet count and renal function).
- **Subarachnoid haemorrhage** causing vasospasm occasionally presents only with delayed ischaemic stroke. Clearly, the history is crucial: the headache may be remembered later, e.g. onset during exertion.

Investigations

CT brain scan is essential in all new onset stroke and TIA (see above).

Simple investigations

These should be considered for all stroke/TIA patients.

- Full blood count.
- Glucose.
- Renal profile.
- Chest radiograph.
- Electrocardiogram.

Carotid ultrasound scan

This can identify and quantify carotid artery stenosis, which is significant if ipsilateral to the TIA. It is indicated if the patient:

- Has had a non-disabling carotid artery event.
- Is willing to have surgery.
- Is well enough for surgery.

Carotid ultrasound scanning can estimate the degree of stenosis and may detect a dissection. However, ultrasound may miss dissections that start distal to the internal carotid origin. For dissection, axial MRI of the neck vessels is the imaging modality of choice or CTA/MRA should be performed.

Echocardiogram

It is important to consider a possible embolic source for stroke. Consider an echocardiogram if there is:

- A young patient.
- A non-lacunar infarct.
- Abnormality on clinical cardiac examination.
- Abnormality on ECG or chest radiograph.

MRI

It could be argued that MRI has little or no role in the management of acute stroke at the time of writing. However, if thrombolysis becomes widely established as an acute treatment, this will change as diffusion weighted imaging can distinguish TIA from established infarction and act as a guide to therapy.

Deterioration in stroke

Early deterioration (first week)

This usually has a neurological cause.

- Cerebral oedema, especially following large strokes, and worst at the third day.
- Haemorrhagic transformation, especially following embolic infarction. Usually, however, this occurs without new symptoms.
- Incorrect diagnosis (see Box 7.4).
- Seizures.
- Early further stroke is fairly common (see above).

Late deterioration (after first week)

This includes either new weakness or an old infarct 're-presenting', and usually has non-neurological causes.

- Medications, e.g. benzodiazepines.
- Anaemia.
- Infections, e.g. pneumonia from aspiration.
- Depression.
- Electrolyte disorders, e.g. dehydration.
- Deep venous thrombosis with pulmonary embolus.
- Pressure sores.

PROGNOSIS

- **Recurrence:** 30% of stroke patients have a further stroke before 5 years: 90% are of the same pathological type.

> **Box 7.5:** *Presenting features suggesting a poorer prognosis*
>
> - Decreased level of consciousness.
> - Bilaterally extensor plantar responses.
> - Incontinence.
> - Dense hemiplegia.
> - Gaze paresis.
> - Pupil abnormalities.
> - Cardiac failure.
> - Atrial fibrillation.

- **Dependence:** 30% of stroke patients are dependent at 1 year.
- **Mortality:** 30% of stroke patients are dead at 1 year and 60% at 5 years.

Box 7.5 gives the presenting features associated with a poorer prognosis.

MANAGEMENT

Early management emphasizes the prevention of further strokes.

Stroke units

Stroke units are the most effective proven intervention for acute stroke. Ideally, there should be a stroke unit in all district general hospitals. Patients managed on acute stroke units have:

- Lower mortality (3% absolute risk reduction).
- Fewer requirements for institutional care (2% absolute risk reduction).
- Less long-term dependency (5% absolute risk reduction).

Stroke units:

- Facilitate accurate diagnosis and early investigations.
- Offer potential for acute medical treatment (see below).
- Focus early attention on physiological changes, e.g. adequate hydration, blood glucose and oxygenation and prevention and management of infections.
- Encourage early mobilization and splinting, hence preventing contractures or shoulder subluxation on the hemiparetic side.
- Facilitate multidisciplinary liaison through case management in a 'geographically defined' area. This includes planning discharges. The team includes doctors, nurses, physiotherapists, occupational therapists, speech and language therapists, psychologists and others.

Exceptions to stroke management in hospital include patient preference or patients with significant co-morbidities.

Thrombolysis

Early thrombolysis may benefit patients, based upon 2889 patients in eight randomized controlled trials of rt-PA (tissue plasminogen activase), but it is still unclear how generalizable the trials results will be. rtPA is now licensed in the UK for administration within 3 h of acute stroke (ongoing trial IST-3 uses rtPA within 6 h). The evidence shows benefits but also risks.

Benefits

Death or dependency at follow-up was significantly better in the thrombolysis group (51%) compared with controls (57%): i.e. 57 more per 1000 were alive and independent (126 per 1000 among those randomized within 3 h).

Risks

Symptomatic intracranial haemorrhage (fatal and non-fatal) was significantly higher in treated patients than controls (10% vs 3%), i.e. 73 additional haemorrhages per 1000. **Deaths from all causes** during follow-up did not differ significantly (15% treatment vs 13% controls; 18 additional dead for every 1000 treated).

Secondary prevention

- **General measures.** The success of secondary prevention depends upon the patient's understanding of the relevance and necessity of controlling vascular risk factors.
- **Evidence-based interventions.** Long-term measures for secondary prevention of stroke should be evidence-based if possible. Stroke, unlike cardiovascular disease, is very heterogeneous (small and large vessel disease, and some with an embolic source), often limiting the applicability of trial results.

Anti-platelet drugs

- **Aspirin.** The IST and CAST trials showed the benefit of aspirin in early stroke: with 10 deaths or recurrent strokes prevented for every 1000 patients treated. There were no significant adverse events in those subsequently shown to have had a haemorrhagic stroke. Aspirin is prescribed at 300 mg/day for 2 weeks and 75 mg/day thereafter.
- **Clopidogrel** gives similar benefit. It causes less gastrointestinal haemorrhage and dyspepsia than aspirin, but more diarrhoea and rashes.

Combining several randomized controlled trials (20 000 patients) of antiplatelet therapy following TIA and stroke showed a 22% reduction in subsequent serious vascular events (36 events per 1000 people on treatment for 2.5 years; 51 per 1000 in controls). Antiplatelet therapies cause a tiny excess of intracranial haemorrhage (1 per 1000 over 3 years), but overall the benefit to 15 people per 1000 outweighed this risk.

Heparin alone does not decrease the risk of death or stroke (IST) following carotid artery TIAs.

Aspirin failures

Some patients develop TIA or stroke while on aspirin. It is worth considering a cardiac embolic source, e.g. performing a 24-h ECG for paroxysmal AF. There are two main treatment options:

1. **Add long-acting dipyridamole.** The European Stroke Prevention Study 2 (ESPS-2) showed aspirin 200 mg and dipyridamole 25 mg gave greater benefit than either aspirin alone (50 mg) or dipyridamole alone (450 mg). Systematic reviews, however, showed little benefit, suggesting the results reflected either dipyridamole's anti-hypertensive effects, or insufficient aspirin in monotherapy. The ESPRIT trial has shown benefit in combining aspirin and dipyridamole after stroke.
2. **Switch to clopidogrel.** The CAPRIE study showed reduced relative risk of stroke, MI or vascular death. The MATCH study showed that adding aspirin to clopidogrel gave no additional stroke risk benefit and more haemorrhage risk than clopidogrel alone.

Anticoagulation in atrial fibrillation

The IST trial of AF treated with heparin showed a recurrent stroke risk of 2.8% in the first 2 weeks and 4.9% on placebo. This significant reduction was negated by increased haemorrhage in the anticoagulated group, with no overall decrease in stroke or death among AF patients given heparin acutely. A pragmatic approach is to withhold warfarin for 10–14 days following AF-related stroke, but this varies with the infarct size and blood pressure control; e.g. with a small stroke and well-controlled blood pressure, start warfarin in 2–5 days.

Antihypertensive medication

Blood pressure (BP) is the single most important modifiable risk factor for stroke. The relative risk reduction of primary stroke is 35–40%, seen following either a systolic reduction of 10–12 mmHg or a diastolic reduction of 5–6 mmHg. The PROGRESS trial (6100 patients from 172 centres) showed that blood pressure reduction with an angiotensin-converting enzyme (ACE) inhibitor (perindopril) alone or combined with a diuretic (indapamide) benefited all recent stroke patients irrespective of blood pressure: recurrent ischaemic and haemorrhagic stroke reduced from 14% in placebo to 10% on treatment. The HOPE trial (Heart Outcomes Prevention Evaluation) evaluated 9297 patients with vascular disease (mainly coronary disease) and showed the stroke risk was 32% lower in treated (ramipril) patients compared to placebo. Patients who cannot tolerate ACE inhibitors benefit from other BP lowering agents, according to the British Hypertension Society's AB/CD rule.

- Younger patients, with their relatively higher renin levels, benefit from A (ACE inhibitors) and B (β-blockers).
- Older patients, with generally low renin levels, benefit from C (calcium antagonists) and D (diuretics).

The target BP is <140/85 mmHg (<130/80 mmHg for diabetics).

Caution

Cerebral autoregulation is disturbed after a stroke so lowering BP too early may cause hypoperfusion. In general, delay BP treatment for 1 week after a stroke except in 'malignant' hypertension, i.e. those with BP of >200–220 mmHg systolic and 120–130 mmHg diastolic. In those with occlusive carotid disease, do not lower the BP below 115/75 mmHg.

Statin therapy

The Heart Protection Study (HPS) showed that in patients with coronary heart disease, stroke/TIA or diabetes, simvastatin 40 mg/day reduced the risk of stroke and myocardial infarction and revascularization by 25%. Statins should be given for fasting cholesterol levels of >3.5 mmol/l, but note that an individual's overall risk is more important than the absolute cholesterol level.

Carotid endarterectomy

The characteristics suggesting a favourable outcome for carotid endarterectomy in patients with ipsilateral carotid artery stenosis of >50% are best expressed as the number needed to treat (NNT) to prevent one stroke at 5 years.

- **Timing of surgery from last symptoms**: <2 weeks: NNT=5; >3 months: NNT=125.
- **Age**: aged >75 years: NNT=5; aged <65 years: NNT=18.
- **Sex**. Men: NNT=9; Women: NNT=36.

This implies that the operation should be performed within 2 weeks; guidelines aiming for operations within 6 months need revising.

Cerebral venous thrombosis

Anticoagulant therapy (intravenous heparin or subcutaneous nadroparin followed by warfarin (INR 2–3)) gives a 16% reduced relative risk of death or dependency compared with placebo. It appears safe to anticoagulate patients with only modest haemorrhage on their scans, although the data are not extensive. Locally injected thrombolytic therapy may help those with a poor prognosis (particularly depressed level of consciousness), but without any supportive trial data.

HISTORY AND EXAMINATION TIPS

History

- **Three questions**: Is this a stroke? Where is it? What caused it?
- **Stroke symptoms** are sudden-onset and negative.
- **Risk factors** for all strokes include smoking, hypertension and diabetes. For young strokes, ask about illicit drugs.
- **Migraine** is more common than stroke at all ages. TIAs have a large differential diagnosis.

Examination

- **General examination** is important: blood pressure (both arms in posterior circulation strokes), peripheral pulses and bruits.

Investigation

- **Early plain CT** on all strokes.
- **Image TIAs**, particularly those involving the anterior circulation. Occasional scans before endarterectomy show glioma.
- **Beware pro-coagulopathies.** A thrombophilia screen is essential for venous thrombosis stroke but many apparent positives following arterial stroke are red herrings.

Management

- **Short term. Do the basics well:** this is why stroke units are so effective. Attend to fluid balance, temperature, glucose (physiological variables), speech and language therapy, physiotherapy and watch for depression (occurrence is not influenced by the lesion site).
- **Long term. Think secondary prevention:** this is easy to overlook.
- **TIAs: think surgical.** Anti-platelet medications may be needed in combination; if not a surgical candidate but the TIA symptoms persist, consider warfarin. But with persisting TIA, before each treatment change, reconsider the diagnosis.
- **'Funny strokes'**, e.g. confusion only or 'stroke somewhere: stroke nowhere', think thalamus or cerebellum, and note these can be fatal and often have an embolic source.

Case history outcome

The several TIA-like episodes were unusual, coming on slowly over minutes. The diagnosis was cerebral amyloid angiopathy, a common cause of lobar haemorrhage in the elderly, particularly parieto-occipital. Her INR was slightly elevated but this alone was not the explanation since the haemorrhage risk in a pooled analysis of patients with mildly elevated INRs (2.0–4.2) was low, with only four haemorrhages in 1889 patient years. Amyloid angiopathy may explain many warfarin-related intracerebral haemorrhages. The transient attacks may have been ictal or due to migraine-related spreading depression of neuronal activity. Distinguishing transient attacks related to amyloid angiopathy from arteriosclerotic TIAs is important since anti-platelets drugs and anticoagulation are potentially harmful. A gradient-echo MRI can identify old cortical haemorrhages supporting a clinical impression of amyloid angiopathy.

KEY POINTS

- After acute stroke do the basics well; hydration, nutrition, metabolic status.
- Prescribe 300 mg aspirin and dipyridamole to all acute ischaemic strokes.
- All patients should have a CT brain scan within 48 h of acute stroke or TIA.
- Carefully select patients who might benefit from carotid endarterectomy and refer to surgical units with broad experience.

- Arterial dissection is a relatively common cause of strokes in young patients; other common causes in the young are drug-related and cardiac.
- Think of venous sinus thrombosis in 'atypical' strokes.

Further Reading

Langhorne P, Dennis MS. Stroke units. Lancet 2004; 363: 834–835.

Myelopathy and ataxia

Case history

A 54-year-old woman presented with an 8-week history of pain in the soles, extending to her legs and buttocks. She reported occipital headaches with nausea and vomiting. Three weeks earlier she had developed visual problems affecting the left eye. Examination showed a pyramidal pattern of limb weakness, with absent lower abdominal reflexes and extensor plantar responses. Joint position and vibration sense were reduced, but pinprick perception was relatively preserved. Her CSF contained 20 lymphocytes/mm^3, with positive oligoclonal bands. Her chest radiograph demonstrated bilateral mediastinal lymphadenopathy.

MYELOPATHY

Spinal cord disease (myelopathy) must be promptly recognized, as there are many treatable and reversible causes. The following features suggest myelopathy.

- Bilateral leg weakness, with or without arm involvement.
- Impaired sphincter function.
- Back pain, or pain in the girdles, chest, or abdomen.
- Sensory involvement in the lower limbs, particularly if the reflexes are present.
- Bilateral extensor plantar responses with no signs above the neck (e.g. normal neck flexion).
- Brown–Séquard distribution: impaired position sense on the hemiparetic side, impaired spinothalamic sensation on the contralateral side.

Having established that the problem is a myelopathy, the clinician must establish the height (spinal level) and the depth (extent of cord cross-section involvement) of the lesion and whether it is intrinsic or extrinsic.

Spinal level

For most cord lesions, the clinical motor and sensory levels localize the lesion. The sensory level is the lowest spinal dermatome with normal sensation. Remember that the clinical (motor or sensory) level may be several segments below the actual lesion, especially in the early stages.

Lesions high in the cord may cause particular diagnostic difficulty.

- Craniovertebral junction myelopathy (foramen magnum level) typically causes:
  - Involvement of the arms and/or legs.
  - Neck pain.

- Downbeat nystagmus (Daroff's sign).
- Facial numbness: remember angle of jaw C3, behind ear C2.
- High cervical myelopathy typically causes:
  - Arms more affected than legs.
  - Wasted hands.
  - Loss of position sense especially in the hands (sensory ataxia and pseudoathetosis).

Intrinsic lesions

Intrinsic lesions include syrinx, demyelinating plaque, or intrinsic tumour. Several clinical pointers suggest that a lesion is intrinsic.

- **Reflex arc interruption.** The old rule that one cannot diagnose a syrinx without reflex loss has proven often incorrect with MRI, but it is still a useful starting point.
- **Spinothalamic features** lead to painless cuts or burns.
- **Wasting and fasciculation** due to anterior horn cell dropout.
- **Horner's syndrome** due to involvement of the descending sympathetic pathway.
- **Pyramidal signs.** Corticospinal tract involvement is less severe than in extrinsic cord compression.
- **Early bladder involvement.**
- **Normal position sense.** Syrinx, tumours and cord infiltration tend to spare the dorsal columns, whereas in MS there is dorsal column involvement.
- **Late symptoms.** MR scanning may show the lesion is large before symptoms appear.

Extrinsic lesions

The most common extrinsic compressive lesion is cervical spondylosis. Several pointers suggest that a lesion is extrinsic.

- **Root pain** (worse on lying flat) due to venous distension.
- **Corticospinal** motor problems predominate.
- **Late bladder and sensory symptoms:** their appearance indicates imminent irreversible myelopathy.

A common clinical problem is to distinguish spondylotic from MS myelopathy. Box 8.1 provides some clinical pointers to this.

Box 8.1: Distinguishing cervical spondylotic myelopathy from MS myelopathy

- Aged >50 years: spondylosis is much more likely.
- Sensory features: Early and rapid onset suggests MS; later and more restricted onset suggests spondylosis. Both cause dorsal column symptoms including tight feelings around the joints or hands (like wearing boxing gloves).
- Early bladder involvement suggests MS.
- Lhermitte's symptom occurs in both, but more commonly in MS (also in B_{12} deficiency, arachnoiditis and post radiation myelopathy).
- Reflexes: A brisk jaw jerk suggests MS (lesion above mid-pons); an inverted supinator jerk favours cervical spondylosis.
- Cranial nerve signs: optic disc pallor, dysconjugate eye movements, or altered colour vision all favour MS.

> **Box 8.2: Scan-negative myelopathies**
>
> There is a wide differential diagnosis, which can be narrowed by taking account of the clinical context.
> - **Demyelination**, especially primary progressive MS (see text and Ch. 10).
> - **Motor neurone disease**, especially primary lateral sclerosis (see Ch. 11).
> - **Vascular causes** (see text).
> - **Radiotherapy** (see text).
> - **Nutritional**. B_{12} is the most common deficiency, but others include lathyrism (pyramidal tract dysfunction caused by eating chickpeas during times of starvation), konzo (spasticity cassava-related) and Strachan's syndrome (neuropathy, optic neuritis).
> - **Genetic causes:**
>   - Hereditary spastic paraparesis (family history and preserved superficial abdominal reflexes).
>   - Leucodystrophies, e.g. adrenoleucodystrophy: check for very long chain fatty acids, especially in males.
>   - Dopa-responsive dystonia (see Ch. 9).
> - **Infective causes**, including syphilis, HIV, HTLV-1.
> - **Intracerebral**. The main diagnostic puzzles occur with a parasagittal meningioma or with bilateral anterior cerebral artery ischaemia following anterior communicating artery aneurysm rupture.
> - **Paraneoplastic** (see text).

Box 8.2 outlines the common causes of 'scan-negative' myelopathy.

Demyelination

Multiple sclerosis

MS myelopathy gives predominantly sensory symptoms. Primary progressive or secondary progressive MS affects mainly the spinal cord: in older people, this may be difficult to distinguish from cervical spondylotic myelopathy.

Transverse myelitis

- **Aetiology:** This is caused by a T-cell mediated immune response and often follows a viral infection (30%). Clinical clues include bullous myringitis (mycoplasma), palatal petechiae (Ebstein–Barr virus) or skin rashes (enterovirus). It also occurs with heroin abuse and in SLE.
- **Clinical features:** The onset may be sudden (usually a few days) causing profound weakness and sensory loss: it is sometimes a devastating illness. By contrast, MS has a less severe and rapid onset with less severe acute disability. The thoracic cord is affected in 80%.
- **Investigations:** MR imaging in transverse myelitis often shows a long (several vertebrae) signal lesion; in MS the signal change is often confined to one vertebral level. CSF abnormalities include pleocytosis but not generally oligoclonal bands.
- **Prognosis:** Poor prognostic signs include rapidity and severity of disability, pain at onset and delayed SSEPs. CSF abnormalities do not correlate with severity.

Devic's disease

Devic's disease is distinct from MS and presents with simultaneous optic neuritis and myelopathy; a serum autoantibody marker is now available. Brain MRI is normal. Cord MRI usually shows 'long' lesions affecting several cord segments. Other causes of this combination are MS, SLE and neurosarcoidosis.

Vascular myelopathy

Some vascular conditions present as scan-negative myelopathies. They are often diagnoses of exclusion.

Spinal cord infarction

Cord infarctions are rare compared with cerebral infarctions.

- **Anatomy:** The (single) anterior spinal artery arises from the vertebral arteries opposite the odontoid peg and runs in the ventral midline from foramen magnum to the filum terminale. It receives 5–10 unpaired feeder (radiculomedullary) arteries with a characteristic 'hairpin' appearance. The paired posterior spinal arteries are fed at nearly every spinal level and form a rich (radiculospinal) anastomosis (Fig. 8.1). Thus spinal infarctions usually spare the posterior columns.
- **Clinical features:** Back pain is common (80%) and is usually thoracic: small and large infarcts are equally painful. The characteristic presentation is with a painful paraparesis, initially flaccid, with dissociated sensory loss and sensory level at about T10.

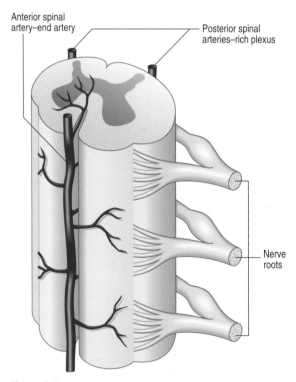

Anterior spinal artery–end artery

Posterior spinal arteries–rich plexus

Nerve roots

Figure 8.1
Segmental blood supply of the spinal cord. Infarction usually spares the dorsal cord causing dissociated sensory loss.

- **Mechanisms:** Thrombotic causes are the most common, especially in patients with vascular risk factors. Emboli are either arteriosclerotic (especially in elderly vasculopaths) or fibrocartilaginous (in young women and usually cervical). Dissection of the vertebral artery can cause spinal infarction, owing to the origin of the anterior spinal artery. Vasculitic infarctions used to occur frequently with syphilis.
- **Prognosis:** This relates mainly to the severity at presentation, the presence of proprioceptive problems and bladder involvement.
- **Imaging** may show a cord infarction, typically with an 'owl's eye appearance'. There may be an infarct in the adjacent vertebral body.
- **Watershed infarctions** typically follow a severe hypotensive episode, usually with additional cerebral features of hypoperfusion. The lesion is often at T4 level owing to the anatomy of the artery of Adamkiewicz (watershed area).

Foix–Alajouanine syndrome

An arteriovenous fistula (Fig. 8.2) in the lower thoracic cord or dura may cause Foix–Alajouanine syndrome (described in 1926). The arterial side transmits high pressure first to the venous system (causing back pain) and then to the venous plexus draining the cord (preventing cord perfusion and causing infarction and flaccid paraparesis). Thrombosis is not a feature until late. The presentation may be apoplectic in 10–20%. It classically affects men (M:F ratio 4:1) aged 30–70 years. The MRI is often 'negative' though careful inspection may reveal dilated vessels around the cord; CSF protein is often raised and occasionally there are increased cell numbers.

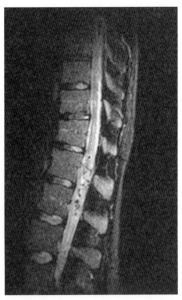

Figure 8.2
MRI showing spinal arteriovenous fistula.

Spinal extradural haematoma

Typically, this is of sudden onset and is painful. It may follow anticoagulation though most cases are idiopathic.

Cancer associated myelopathy

Primary spinal tumours

These include sarcomas, myeloma or plasmacytoma and haemangioma (incidental in 10% of the population).

Metastatic

Five percent of patients dying from cancer have symptomatic metastatic spinal cord compression; 70% have asymptomatic spinal metastases at autopsy.

- **Primary tumours:** The most common primaries are breast, bronchus, prostate, kidney and thyroid. Breast and lung cancers often metastasize to the thoracic spine following its venous drainage. Prostate often affects the lumbosacral spine where the seeded tumour cells release osteoclastic factors.
- **Spinal metastases:** 60% are thoracolumbar, 30% are lumbosacral. Tumour cells extend into the posterior elements causing pain, pathological fracture and compression. Less commonly, tumour cells directly extend epidurally without concomitant pathological fracture.
- **Clinical features:** Pain is the most common symptom, worse on lying flat due to epidural venous plexus distension and often present for several weeks to months. Two-thirds of patients are non-ambulant when diagnosed.
- **Investigations:** Plain radiograph changes develop when 50% of bone is lost. Plain films and bone scans do not show cord compression: MR is the optimal imaging modality, but need to image the entire neuraxis because 30% have multi-level disease.
- **Management:** In principle, even patients with disseminated malignancy should be treated urgently as even if they are paraplegic, it is worth attempting to salvage sphincter function.
  - Dexamethasone at an initial bolus of 16 mg relieves pain (daily regimens vary to 16+ mg/day, but most prefer lower doses).
  - Radiotherapy results in one-third of non-ambulant patients regaining walking ability; melanoma and renal secondaries are often radio-resistant.
  - Surgery followed by radiotherapy is worth contemplating for a solitary metastasis. Spinal stability is important: two of the three columns (anterior vertebral body, posterior vertebral body and spinal arch) are needed to preserve stability.
  - Chemotherapy is logical and considered when tumour is not radiosensitive.

Paraneoplastic

Paraneoplastic myelopathy is rare and usually occurs with other paraneoplastic disorders.

Radiation myelopathy

The likelihood of myelopathy relates to the radiation dose exposure. However, 5% of radiation myelopathy occurs following doses <5000 cGy.

- **Onset:**
  - Acute. Within hours.
  - Early. 4–6 months, with prominent sensory features and often good recovery.
  - Late. This is typically bimodal (12 months and again around 24 months, but up to 10 years), although can be progressive from the start. There are early sensory features, but later motor problems.
- **Clinical features:**
  - Sensory features are more prominent than motor.
  - Spinothalamic features dominate at first, e.g. cold feelings and numbness.
  - Lhermitte's symptom occasionally occurs.
  - A purely lower motor neurone syndrome may occur: wasting and weakness without upper motor neurone signs.
- **Distinction from cord compression:**
  - Cord compression gives localized back pain and prominent motor symptoms.
  - Radiation myelopathy gives little pain and prominent sensory symptoms.
- **Investigations:**
  - MRI shows signal change in the marrow with cord T2 signal change or atrophy.
  - CSF is usually normal, but can show raised protein or a mild pleocytosis.

Chemotherapy myelopathy

Myelopathy may follow either intravenous (e.g. cisplatin) or intrathecal (e.g. methotrexate or cytarabine) chemotherapy.

Infection and spinal abscess

Consider this particularly in diabetics, dialysis patients and drug abusers.

- **Clinical features:** These are variable, but there is usually back pain (worse at night) with myelopathy or radiculopathy. There may be few systemic signs: apyrexial in 50%, normal ESR in 20%. Search for an infection source, e.g. catheter, infective endocarditis.
- **Pathogenesis:** The infection typically begins in the vertebral end plates, later extending to the epidural space. Less frequently, there are vertebral fractures with retropulsion of infected debris. Investigations: MRI shows inflammation in the disc space and adjacent vertebral body.
- **Management** includes surgery (debridement and tissue culture) and medications (intravenous antibiotics for 4–6 weeks).
- **Spinal tuberculosis** presents variably and may mimic a spinal tumour. 1% of patients with TB have bone involvement, usually spinal. The infection may extend beneath the anterior ligament to adjacent segments and track to form a psoas cold abscess.

Bladder function

Normal bladder function relies on three reflexes.

- Vesicosympathetic.
- Vesicoparasympathetic.
- Vesicopudendal (S3) Onuf's nucleus, supplying the external urethral sphincter.

Stretch receptors fire in proportion to bladder distension. Voluntary inhibition of stretch reflex is mediated by the hypothalamic and pontine centres; frontal inhibitory fibres descend next to corticospinal pathway.

A lesion anywhere from frontal lobe to sacrum can disrupt bladder function.

The treatment of an upper motor neurone bladder depends upon the bladder abnormality.

- **Residual volume <100 mL.** Anticholinergic drugs, e.g. oxybutynin 2.5 mg twice daily or imipramine 75 mg twice daily. Note side-effects of dry mouth, visual disturbance and constipation.
- **Residual volume >100 mL.** Intermittent self-catheterization (ISC), often combined with anticholinergic treatment, is indicated. ISC is clean but non-sterile, with reusable catheters. The main limitation is patient non-acceptance or impaired manual dexterity.

ATAXIA

The nature of ataxia is discussed elsewhere (see Ch. 2).

History

The clinician should note three specific aspects:

1. **The speed of onset** gives the biggest clue to the aetiology (Box 8.3).
2. **The age of onset.** Among those with chronic ataxia, young onset often suggests autosomal recessive conditions, e.g. Friedreich's ataxia; older onset suggests either an autosomal dominant spinocerebellar ataxia or multiple systems atrophy.
3. **The family history.** If there is no family history, the chance of a positive spinocerebellar ataxia mutation is low.

Examination

- **Eye movements** are often abnormal, especially with broken pursuit movements, failure to inhibit the vestibular ocular reflex, or saccadic dysmetria (either hypermetric or hypometric saccades). There may also be interruption of fixation with square wave jerks (also seen in other conditions, e.g. parkinsonian syndromes), ocular flutter or opsoclonus (think paraneoplastic).
- **Gait.** Ask the patient to walk heel to toe. Truncal instability may be the only features of a vermis lesion, e.g. from alcohol. Truncal instability with eye movement abnormalities

Box 8.3: Aetiology of ataxia relating to speed of onset

- **Hyper-acute:**
  - Stroke: ischaemic or haemorrhagic.
- **Acute:**
  - Miller Fisher syndrome of areflexia and ophthalmoplegia.
  - Demyelination, often with other signs or suitable history.
  - Hydrocephalus.
  - Central pontine myelinolysis, caused by rapid serum sodium changes (low sodium causes cerebral oedema). The condition's first appearance coincided with the 'plastic revolution'; Wernicke's disease often accompanies myelinolysis (30% at post-mortem).
  - Space occupying lesions in the posterior fossa, e.g. tumour or abscess.
  - Toxins: Antiepileptic medications, worming tablets, or solvents (the latter may give a neuropathy and rash around the nose and mouth).
- **Intermediate:**
  - Alcohol and Wernicke's disease (most do not have the classical triad of ophthalmoplegia, ataxia and confusion).
  - Paraneoplastic. These patients often have other signs.
  - Prion diseases.
- **Chronic:**
  - Genetic conditions. This large group of disorders is detailed in Box 8.4. Genetic ataxias are either of early onset (aged <20 years, e.g. Friedreich's ataxia) or of late onset (aged >20 years, e.g. other spinocerebellar ataxias).
  - Multiple systems atrophy (see Ch. 9). This is the most common explanation for older onset non-genetic ataxia.
  - Vascular conditions, e.g. siderosis, presents with cognitive problems, deafness and anosmia.
  - Deficiencies, especially of vitamin E or zinc. Vitamin E deficiency can resemble Friedreich's ataxia, though often with titubation.
  - Prion disease. Ataxia may be an isolated feature of sporadic CJD (Brownell–Oppenheimer variant) and is characteristic of variant and iatrogenic (e.g. growth hormone induced) CJD, as well as some genetic prion diseases.
  - Wilson's disease (see Ch. 9). The ataxia may leave the gait relatively unaffected but often with titubation.
  - Progressive myoclonic ataxia. Search particularly for mitochondrial cytopathy, Unverricht–Lundborg disease and coeliac disease.
  - Other mitochondrial cytopathies, including NARP-neuropathy, ataxia and retinitis pigmentosa (where there may be maculopathy).
  - Hypothyroidism is a rare cause of ataxia, but worth checking.

suggests Wernicke's disease. In late onset cerebellar ataxia, look for extrapyramidal signs suggesting multi-system atrophy, e.g. a narrow walking base despite ataxia. However, very ataxic patients have little arm swing anyway.

- **Intention tremor.** The tremor becomes worse when the target is approached and may over- or under-shoot (dysmetria, c.f. saccadic dysmetria).
- **Dysdiadochokinesis** is a break down of rhythmic, rapid alternating movements. The clinician may even 'listen' to cerebellum by observing disrupted rhythm during rapid alternating movement. Watch the movements: they may become rotatory in cerebellar disease. For example, ask the patient to rotate their wrists with their palms facing their body and their elbows flexed. In cerebellar lesions, there may be a jerky quality with flexion/extension of the wrist. The wrist may also be dorsiflexed with fingers flexed. *Comparison* may be possible by asking the patient to make a series of dots with a pencil within a 1 cm diameter circle, the number falling outside the area being compared.

Box 8.4: *Genetic ataxias*

1. Early onset (aged <20 years): mostly autosomal recessive
   - Friedreich's ataxia (incidence 1 in 100 000) is caused by a GAA repeat on frataxin gene chromosome 9. The age of onset is usually 8–15 years, but may be much later. The clinical features include ataxia, pyramidal tract signs, sensory neuropathy (often absent SAPs electrophysiologically), cardiomyopathy (ECG shows wide-spread T wave inversion; echocardiogram is indicated), scoliosis, pes cavus, optic atrophy and deafness. Some 10% develop diabetes mellitus and 20% more have impaired glucose tolerance.
   - Cerebrotendinous xanthomatosis. This is a mitochondrial sterol-27 hydroxylase deficiency involving bile salt metabolism. The clinical features include xanthomata, neuropathy, cataracts and occasional palatal myoclonus. The serum cholesterol is low or normal and cholestanol is raised. T2 MRI brain shows symmetrical high signal lesions in the cerebellar deep white matter.
   - Hartnup disease.
   - Leucodystrophies, e.g. metachromatic or Krabbe.
   - Abetalipoproteinaemia and hypolipoproteinaemia.
   - Refsum's disease.

2. Late onset (aged >20 years): mostly autosomal dominant
   - Autosomal dominant cerebellar ataxias type 1 (ADCA 1) manifest as ataxia, variably associated with extrapyramidal features, dementia, ophthalmoplegia and neuropathy. The underlying gene abnormalities include spinocerebellar ataxia (SCA) genes 1, 2, 3, 12, 17 (mostly CAG repeats).
   - ADCA 2 (SCA7) manifests as ataxia with pigmentary maculopathy. Note that NARP has a similar phenotype.
   - ADCA 3 (SCA6) manifests as ataxia alone.

- **Dysarthria.** Say, 'baby hippopotamus' or 'British Constitution'. In cerebellar dysarthria, the syllables are broken up. Dysarthria is useful in distinguishing motor from sensory ataxia (as is Rombergism and eye movements).
- **Pendular reflexes** are rare.

Case history outcome

This patient had neurosarcoidosis. Neurological involvement develops in 5% of sarcoidosis patients: half are older women. Neurosarcoidosis involves particularly the meninges and cranial nerves 7, 8 and 2; it may also present as a space-occupying lesion or as MS-plus. Some 10% have raised serum calcium; CSF shows raised protein in 50–70%, pleocytosis in 50%, positive oligoclonal bands in 30% and raised CSF ACE in 70%.

KEY POINTS

- In myelopathy, the sensory level may not correspond to the lesion level.
- Wasted hands with arms involved more than legs (especially with altered position sense) suggests a high cervical cord lesion.
- Intrinsic lesions have early sensory and bladder features; extrinsic have early motor features.
- An extrinsic lesion with sensory (and bladder) features spells impending doom.
- Intrinsic tumours spare the dorsal columns; inflammatory lesions do not.
- Vascular myelopathy is often a diagnosis of exclusion; it is rare now that syphilis is rare.

- Cancer myelopathy must be distinguished from radiation myelopathy: radiation myelopathy is less often painful, more symmetrical and involves several segments on MRI.
- Scan-negative myelopathy, remember MND or parasagittal lesion.
- Rehabilitation and continuing care are essential for myelopathy patients.

Further Reading

Muzaimi MB, Thomas J, Palmer-Smith S et al. Population based study of late onset cerebellar ataxia in south east Wales. J Neurol Neurosurg Psychiatry 2004; 75: 1129–1134.

Movement disorders

9

Case history

A 17-year-old girl with cerebral palsy described worsening gait and became wheelchair bound. She reported leg stiffness, which did not vary in severity. Her cognitive function was normal. Her mother, who also had longstanding mild leg stiffness, stated that her daughter's problem had begun around aged 5 years. She had walked when age 1 year and had normal speech and language. Examination showed equinovarus foot deformities and persistent big toe extension. There was no tremor. Her tone was increased in all limbs (extrapyramidal and possibly dystonic) and her reflexes were brisk.

INTRODUCTION

The spectrum of movement disorders is very broad and includes tremor, tics, restless legs, parkinsonism, chorea, dystonia, ballism and myoclonus.

TREMOR

Tremor is a regular, rhythmical oscillation of a body part. The key clinical questions are: 'What are the characteristics of the tremor?' and 'Are there associated neurological signs?'

Characteristics

- **Rest tremor**, with the patient resting, supine and completely supported by the couch (implies idiopathic Parkinson's disease, IPD).
- **Kinetic (movement) tremor** has several forms:
  - **Postural tremor** on extending the arms forwards (implies physiological tremor or essential tremor).
  - **Intention tremor** and other cerebellar signs: tremor appears or worsens as the visual target is approached.
  - **Task-specific tremor**, e.g. primary writing tremor (usually at a later age than writer's cramp). Some have a family history or remote history of trauma.
  - **Simple kinetic tremor** appears during movement but is not target-directed.
  - **Isometric tremor**, e.g. orthostatic tremor giving unsteadiness when standing still but normal when walking. The tremor is fast (14–16 Hz) and audible with a stethoscope over the standing patient's patellae (helicopter noise).

- **Midbrain or rubral tremor** occurs at rest, on posture and worsens with movement. Other signs are common, e.g. hemiplegia or 3rd nerve palsy. Rubral tremor may respond to levodopa.
- **Palatal tremor** is a rhythmic movement of soft palate and pharynx sometimes with oscillation of external ocular muscles and diaphragm. Primary forms have young onset (about 30 years), often 'clicking' sound in ears and normal MR brain scan. Secondary causes give older onset, have no auditory clicking and MRI is abnormal: lesion within 'Guillain–Mollaret triangle' (inferior olive, red nucleus and dentate nucleus) and olive hypertrophy.

Associated signs

- Dystonia: dystonic tremor.
- Tachycardia: thyroid disease.
- Areflexia: neuropathies, particularly demyelinating (chronic inflammatory demyelinating polyradiculo neuropathy, CIDP, 3% have tremor; especially IgM paraproteinaemic CIDP; tremor also in Charcot–Marie–Tooth disease, CMT). The mechanism may be a delayed afferent feedback loop, causing mis-timed corrective movements.

Essential tremor (ET)

- ET is commonly misdiagnosed as IPD: this is particularly likely because postural tremor is common in IPD. However, ET is 10 times more common (population prevalence c.2%) so most tremors will be ET not IPD. Box 9.1 outlines some of the major differences helpful in distinguishing the two.

Management

The best medications are β-blockers (propranolol up to 320 mg/day: check for asthma history first) or primidone (50 mg at night initially; maximum 750 mg). Gabapentin or topiramate may help. Wrist weights can dampen oscillations.

Box 9.1: *Features distinguishing ET from IPD*

- The tremor duration at first consultation is far longer in ET (5–7 years) than in IPD (2 years); 20% of ET has onset aged <30 years.
- ET involves the upper limbs (e.g. holding a cup), head (yes–yes or no–no tremor) or voice. IPD rarely involves the head or face but jaw tremor common. (Isolated head tremor is often a form of dystonic tremor.)
- ET may respond to alcohol (50–75%), but so do others including IPD postural tremor and essential myoclonus.
- ET is symmetrical; IPD is often asymmetrical.
- ET does not have a rotational element, whereas IPD tremor does.
- ET may show apparent cogwheel rigidity, but rest tremor and bradykinesia unusual.
- IPD patients may have mirror movements. Observe both hands, ask patient to sequentially press fingers to thumb, watch other (passive) hand and look for involuntary movements replicating active movements (common in normal children).
- IPD postural tremor is sometimes 're-emergent'. These patients have a resting tremor, which disappears when they hold their arms outstretched but reappears after a latent period at the same frequency as the resting tremor.
- Olfaction is normal in ET, but impaired in IPD.

Psychogenic tremor

Psychogenic tremor often starts suddenly, is intermittent, changes (in amplitude or frequency) with a load, is distractible and entrains to the frequency of other limb if the patient is asked to perform tapping movements etc.

TICS

Clinical features

- Tics are suppressible (unlike myoclonus).
- Patients may describe a sensation just before a tic ('like a sneeze').
- Some have obsessive–compulsive disorders (OCDs) or attention deficit hyperactivity disorder (ADHD).
- Transient motor tics are common in childhood (15% of boys have tics lasting <1 year).
- Gilles de la Tourette syndrome is not uncommon (onset is before aged 18 years). Multiple motor tics and later (aged 11–13 years) vocal tics develop but classical coprolalia is rare.

Underlying causes

Tourettism may follow cerebrovascular disease, e.g. caudate infarcts; tics may be part of degenerative conditions, e.g. HD. It is important to look for other features, especially in late onset forms.

Management

This may include clonidine (particularly in OCDs), sulpiride or pimozide – but note these are all associated with long-term problems.

RESTLESS LEGS SYNDROME

This common (under-recognized) disorder occurs in 5–15% of adults.

Causes

The main associations are with pregnancy (symptoms resolving after delivery), iron deficiency and renal failure; there is a strong genetic influence.

Clinical features

Diagnostic features are:

- An urge to move the limbs.
- Dysaesthesia.
- Symptoms worse in the evening.
- Symptoms worse at rest.
- Partial relief with activity.

Supportive features are:

- Dopamine responsiveness.
- Periodic limb movements in sleep.
- Sleep disturbance.
- Family history.
- Normal examination (although 5–9% of patients have small-fibre sensory neuropathy).

Differential diagnosis

- **Akathisia.** History of neuroleptic or dopaminergic use; no diurnal variation.
- **Painful legs and moving toes.** Evidence of neuropathy, spinal root disease and varicose veins; no relief with movement.
- **Vesper's curse.** Transient lumbar canal stenosis from lumbar vein distention due to cardiac failure.
- **Peripheral neuropathy.**

Management

Consider underlying causes, e.g. anaemia investigations (oral iron); stop aggravating medication, e.g. anti-depressants, calcium antagonists, caffeine. Then decide with the patient whether a medication trial is warranted.

- **Dopamine agonists**, e.g. cabergoline 0.5–4 mg nocte.
- **Opiates**, e.g. oxycodone.
- **Anti-epileptics**, e.g. gabapentin.
- **Benzodiazepines**, e.g. clonazepam.
- **Others**, e.g. clonidine, baclofen.

IDIOPATHIC PARKINSON'S DISEASE

IPD is common and frequently misdiagnosed (50% in primary care, up to 10% in movement disorder clinics). The diagnosis rests upon **core features**, but the clinician must identify **non-motor features** and watch for 'red flags'.

Core features

Parkinsonism comprises rest tremor, rigidity and bradykinesia.

Tremor

- **Rest tremor** (4–6 Hz) is the first symptom in 75% of patients, but remains absent in 20%. It is abolished by posture or voluntary movement, predominantly involves the upper limbs and occasionally the chin and lower lip, is typically unilateral and intermittent at the onset, worsens with anxiety and disappears in sleep.
- **Postural tremor** (6–8 Hz) is often less prominent, present on maintaining a posture, worsened by anxiety and may improve with alcohol.

Rigidity

This is present in 97% of IPD patients at diagnosis. It is unchanged by speed or direction of passive movement.

- **'Lead pipe' rigidity** increases throughout movement.
- **'Cog-wheel'** rigidity has tremor superimposed and is best found at the wrist.
- **Froment's sign:** arm rigidity enhanced by the patient moving the contralateral arm.
- **Wilson's sign:** poor arm swing on passive shoulder rotation.

Hypokinesia and bradykinesia

- **Hypokinesia** is poverty of movement, e.g. unilateral loss of arm swing when walking.
- **Bradykinesia** is slowed movement. Note pyramidal problems also cause slowed movement, although without progressive loss of amplitude. Patients with IPD attempting repetitive movements with the more severely affected hand commonly show mirror movements in the less affected hand.
- **'Freezing'.** Patients may describe difficulty moving when encountering an external stimulus, e.g. passing through a door.

Postural instability

This is a late feature of PD (usually after 8–10 years). Postural instability and falling occurring early (within 2 to 3 years) is a 'red flag' and suggests progressive supranuclear palsy.

- The **'pull test'** is best to demonstrate this.

Non-motor features

Psychiatric manifestations

- **Depression** is common in IPD, but treatment can cause problems. SSRIs may exacerbate tremor and must be used with caution if prescribed with selegiline, owing to the risk of serotonin syndrome. Drugs with anticholinergic properties in theory may exacerbate dementia.
- **Enhanced mood.** Levodopa promotes elevated mood, even mania. Patients may show punding (stereotyped repetitive manual handling of objects), increased sexual appetite, gambling, or wandering (homeostatic dysregulation syndrome).
- **Dementia** in IPD is common (prevalence 20%). The clinical features include a subcortical dementia (slowed thought, forgetfulness, perseveration, mental inflexibility), fluctuating cognition, visual hallucinations and increased neuroleptic sensitivity (see Ch. 6).

Other features

- **Hypersalivation:** sugar-free chewing gum may help.
- **Autonomic involvement:** There may be mild detrusor hyper-reflexia or postural hypotension; both may be exacerbated by dopamine agonists and levodopa.
- **Aches and pains,** e.g. frozen shoulder, result mainly from rigidity.
- **Sleep disturbance:** This results from restless legs (levodopa-induced) and discomfort from being 'off'. However, REM sleep behaviour disorder (REM parasomnia) occur in IPD and Parkinson-plus syndromes: a change from normal suppression of motor activity in REM sleep may lead patients literally to act out their dreams; it responds to clonazepam.
- **Reduced sense of smell** is well recognized in IPD and may be useful in distinguishing this from essential tremor.

'Red flags'

Several clinical features should prompt clinicians to question the diagnosis of IPD.

- Rapid progression.
- Early postural instability (within 2–3 years of onset) or falls (especially backwards) suggest progressive supranuclear palsy (PSP); falls in IPD usually occur only after 8–9 years.
- Early autonomic symptoms (incontinence, postural dizziness) suggest multiple system atrophy (MSA).
- Poor levodopa responsiveness.
- Symmetry of signs is unusual in IPD.
- Absence of rest tremor.
- Supranuclear ophthalmoplegia: this strongly suggests PSP.
- Pyramidal signs including pseudobulbar findings suggest PSP, cerebrovascular disease or NPH.
- Cerebellar features suggest MSA.
- Hand contractures or cool peripheries suggest MSA.
- Wheelchair-bound.

Investigations

IPD is diagnosed clinically, so investigations are to exclude other causes.

- **CT brain scan** may exclude small vessel disease, benign tumour involving the basal ganglia (e.g. frontal meningioma) or hydrocephalus.
- **Functional imaging** is not generally used. Positron emission tomography (PET) uses several tracers taken up by nigrostriatal dopaminergic neurones, e.g. ^{18}F-6-fluorodopa. Single photon emission tomography (SPECT) is similar but cheaper and more available, but lacks spatial resolution.
- **Olfactory testing.** 'Scratch and sniff' smell tests may help in distinguishing IPD (where olfaction is frequently impaired) from essential tremor.
- **Other tests.** Consider Wilson's disease (copper studies) or Huntington's disease (gene testing) in young-onset parkinsonism.

- **Apomorphine testing** has little role in diagnosis.
- **Levodopa trial** over several weeks is worthwhile, more to explore a potential treatment of related conditions than as a diagnostic test. PD-plus conditions may respond to levodopa although usually only partially and temporarily.

Pathology

In IPD, the midbrain substantia nigra shows >80% neuronal loss. Lewy bodies, the pathological hallmark of IPD, are rounded, eosinophilic, ubiquitin-positive, hyaline inclusions found in nigral neurons of all patients and in cortical neurons of most.

Parkinsonism: other causes

The clinician should distinguish IPD from other causes of Parkinsonism on clinical grounds. Box 9.2 lists the features supporting a diagnosis of IPD.

- **Essential tremor.** This causes particular diagnostic difficulty if asymmetrical and disabling, especially as postural tremor also occurs in IPD. Box 9.1 outlines the main clinical features distinguishing ET from IPD.
- **'Parkinson-plus' syndromes.** This comprises multiple systems atrophy (MSA), progressive supranuclear palsy (PSP) and corticobasal degeneration (CBD) (detailed below).
- **Cerebrovascular disease.** Typically this gives lower body parkinsonism.
- **Neuroleptics** commonly cause parkinsonism (see below); culprits can include prochlorperazine given for dizziness.
- **Significant head trauma**, e.g. in boxers.
- **Heredo-degenerative conditions**, e.g. young-onset Huntington's disease (Westphal variant), Wilson's disease.
- **Hypoxic or toxic encephalopathies**, e.g. from heavy metals or methanol.
- **Liver disease and hypoparathyroidism** may cause parkinsonism.
- **Rapid-onset** parkinsonism suggests prion disease or other infections (e.g. Japanese B encephalitis), extrapontine myelinolysis, or toxin/drug exposure.

Management

Current management of IPD is symptomatic rather than neuroprotective or restorative. The clinician and patient must consider the crucial question: 'Is any treatment needed?' If the patient's symptoms justify it, there are several options.

Box 9.2: Clinical features supporting the diagnosis of IPD

- Progressive symptoms.
- Excellent levodopa response, maintained for >5 years.
- Levodopa-induced dyskinesias (40–80% after 5 years).
- No alternative explanation following investigation.
- Unilateral onset, with persistent asymmetry.

Levodopa

Levodopa has a dramatic symptomatic benefit in IPD and has been widely used since the 1970s.

- **Prescribing:** Start with a low dose of levodopa with a breakdown enzyme inhibitor (e.g. Sinemet LS), taken with food. Combine domperidone with levodopa for several days to reduce nausea and peripheral effects, e.g. hypotension; continue domperidone if necessary. Slow release formulations are useful for overnight treatment but are best avoided in the daytime as dyskinesias may worsen.
- **Motor complications** of levodopa develop in 10% per year. They include dyskinesias (chorea, dystonia) and response fluctuations (on/off) sometimes swinging unpredictably from immobile to mobile. Long-term motor complications lead many clinicians to delay introducing levodopa, particularly in young patients (<75 years). Long-term toxicity concerns have been allayed by the ELLDOPA trial, showing no convincing evidence of *in vivo* toxicity.

Dopamine agonists (DAs)

- **Efficacy:** DAs give fewer motor complications (dyskinesias) than levodopa, but are less effective and have more short-term adverse events (somnolence, constipation, nausea, hallucinations). DAs are commonly prescribed to patients likely to require anti-parkinsonian medication for many years (e.g. those aged <75 years), to delay motor complications. However, it is acceptable to use levodopa provided the patient understands the balance of symptom benefit versus the risk of long-term side-effects.
- **Adverse events:** Ergot DAs in particular are associated with potentially serious fibrotic and serosal complications, including cardiovascular valvopathy, lung fibrosis and retroperitoneal fibrosis.

Apomorphine

Apomorphine is a DA used in advanced IPD. It has poor bioavailability and often causes severe nausea and postural hypotension. It is usually prescribed only from specialist clinics, with ongoing nurse specialist supervision.

- **Indication:** Apomorphine may help control refractory motor fluctuations in late IPD. It is usually given intermittently for refractory 'off' periods.
- **Administration:** Given subcutaneously, rotating injection sites. Patients requiring >6 injections per day may benefit from continuous subcutaneous infusion, started in hospital at 2 mg/h, but most eventually require 50–200 mg/day.
- **Side-effects and monitoring:** Apomorphine can stain clothes, cause sleepiness and induce panniculitis at injection sites. Three-monthly blood counts are indicated because haemolytic anaemia may occur.
- **Amantadine** may help apomorphine-induced dyskinesias. An amantadine trial is usually 100–300 mg/day for 6 weeks, while reducing other medication.

Other medications

Several other medications are available for management of IPD. IPD management will be clearer following completion of the PD-MED trial: early IPD randomized to monotherapy levodopa, selegiline or DA; late IPD randomized to adjuvant therapy with a COMT inhibitor, MAO-B inhibitor, or DA (Fig. 9.1).

Surgery

Surgery is not a cure: patients need continued medication even following successful surgery. Patient selection is important. Consider referring patients before there is very advanced disability, provided they show dopamine responsiveness and no significant cognitive or psychiatric problems. Patients with postural instability or bulbar dysfunction respond poorly to surgery.

- **Lesional surgery.** Long-term adverse events have largely curtailed this approach.
- **Deep brain stimulation** induces a functional lesion either through a depolarizing block, or perhaps through the preferential activation of inhibitory neurones. Bilateral sub-thalamic stimulation can give sustained benefit.
- **Newer techniques.** Glial cell line-derived neurotrophic factor (GDNF) directly infused into the brain and stem cell transplantation have exciting preliminary results and are the focus of further research.

PARKINSON PLUS SYNDROMES

Multiple systems atrophy (MSA)

MSA comprises 10–15% of patients diagnosed as IPD. The onset is usually in the early 50s and almost all begin >30 years. The median survival is about 8 years.

Clinical features

Core features include combinations of:

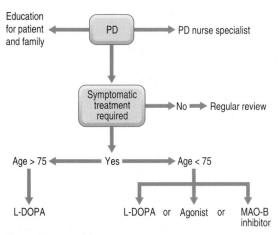

Figure 9.1
Management of early Parkinson's disease.

- Parkinsonism (almost all).
- Autonomic abnormalities (almost all).
- Cerebellar ataxia (50%).
- 25% of MSA patients with parkinsonism have no additional pyramidal or cerebellar problems.

Typical autonomic features include impotence and urinary incontinence (sometimes preceding motor features by several years), sighing, cool hands and skin blanching on pressure.

Additional features include:

- Dystonia, e.g. axial dystonia (antecollis or 'Pisa syndrome') and laryngeal dystonia (high voice, stridor and sleep apnoea).
- Pyramidal features, especially hyper-reflexia and extensor plantars, rarely weakness and spasticity.
- Dyskinesias, especially facial, with levodopa treatment.
- Cognitive dysfunction.
- Hand contractures.
- REM sleep parasomnias.

Dementia is not a feature of MSA.

Investigations

The MR brain scan (Fig. 9.2) may show the 'hot-cross bun' sign (high signal in the pons on T2 weighting). Anal sphincter electromyography may be abnormal (in IPD it is usually normal). However, note false positives following childbirth and perianal surgery (e.g. for piles).

Management

This is mainly symptomatic and depends upon the clinical features.

1. **Autonomic symptoms:** Consider specific management of postural hypotension and impotence.
2. **Parkinsonism:** Amantadine 100mg three times daily for a one-month trial and continued if beneficial. Levodopa may be effective but not to the same extent as in IPD.

Progressive supranuclear palsy (PSP)

This elderly-onset (>50 years) condition, also known as Steele–Richardson–Olszewski syndrome, presents as supranuclear gaze palsy (particularly for downgaze), early-onset falls (particularly backwards and with injury) and progressive dementia. The response to levodopa is partial and short-lived. The usual survival is about 6 years. A 'full house' of PSP is very striking (Fig. 9.3).

Clinical features

- **Supranuclear vertical gaze palsy.** This characteristic feature may be absent on first presentation and sometimes delayed by several years. The initial finding is saccade slowing. If the

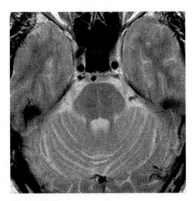

Figure 9.2
MRI showing pontine high signal change in multiple systems atrophy (MSA).

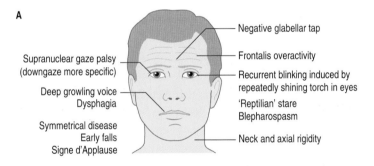

A

Supranuclear gaze palsy
(downgaze more specific)

Deep growling voice
Dysphagia

Symmetrical disease
Early falls
Signe d'Applause

Negative glabellar tap

Frontalis overactivity

Recurrent blinking induced by
repeatedly shining torch in eyes

'Reptilian' stare
Blepharospasm

Neck and axial rigidity

B

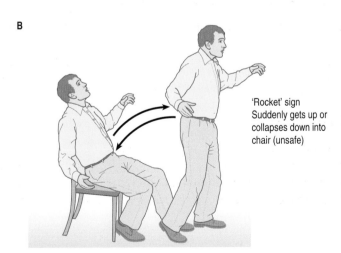

'Rocket' sign
Suddenly gets up or
collapses down into
chair (unsafe)

Figure 9.3
Clinical features of progressive supranuclear palsy (PSP). (a) Symmetrical disease, early falls and *signe
d'applause*. (b) 'Rocket' sign. Suddenly gets up or collapses down into chair (unsafe!).

patient's neck is rigid, the examiner can use Bell's phenomenon to elicit upgaze, e.g. ask the patient to close eyes and then the examiner opens the eyelids; should see the whites of the eyes in normals but not PSP. The 'messy tie' sign results from inability to look down at a plate.

- **Postural instability** occurs early (within 2–3 years) causing frequent falls, especially backwards. There is particular difficulty with walking downstairs owing to difficulty looking downwards.
- **Facial bradykinesia.** The 'Mona Lisa stare' is characterized by raised eyebrows; blepharospasm and reduced blink rate (<4/min).
- **Rigidity.** This is symmetrical and axial more than appendicular. Retrocollis is characteristic.
- **Bulbar features.** The voice may be deep and growling, with pseudobulbar palsy signs. Significant dysphagia is more often the terminal event than in MSA.
- **Perseveration.** Although the glabellar tap is often negative, the patient keeps blinking to a torch shone in the eyes. The '*signe d'applause*' is continued clapping when asked to clap three times (perseveration).
- **Rare features** include prominent dyspraxia (particularly frontal lobe apraxia) or palatal myoclonus.

Pathology

The substantia nigra shows neuronal depletion and basophilic globose neurofibrillary tangles in the surviving nigral cells.

Investigations

The MR brain scan typically shows midbrain 'Mickey Mouse ears' (Fig. 9.4). The anal sphincter EMG may be abnormal.

Management

- **Rehabilitation:** Home adaptations; falls cause morbidity – so a wheelchair should be considered at an early stage.

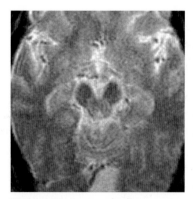

Figure 9.4
MRI in progressive supranuclear palsy (PSP) showing midbrain 'Mickey Mouse ears'.

- **Medications:** The response to levodopa is partial and short-lived. It is worth trying amantadine for the parkinsonism.

Corticobasal degeneration (CBD)

Clinical features

The main clinical features are:

- Asymmetrical akinetic-rigid syndrome, sometimes with myoclonus.
- Apraxia including involuntary unilateral limb movements: 'alien limb' with 'a will of its own'.
- Cognitive problems (early or late), often with focal features, e.g. parietal or frontal.
- Higher cortical sensory abnormalities.
- Difficulty initiating saccades.

Pathology

There is asymmetrical substantia nigra degeneration with tau-positive astrocytic plaques and ballooned achromatic neurons. Such CBD pathology also occurs in frontotemporal dementia. Conversely, the CBD syndrome may occur without typical CBD pathology.

CHOREA

Clinical features

Chorea is an irregular, involuntary, purposeless, non-rhythmic movement disorder. The patient appears fidgety, something often noticed first by family members. The movements may be partially suppressed or incorporated into a semi-purposeful movement, e.g. touching the hair or face, thereby 'camouflaging' the condition.

- **Distribution:** Huntington's disease (HD) chorea affects the upper limb and all the face; tardive dyskinesias affect mainly the lower face. Hemichorea suggests an underlying brain lesion.
- **Motor impersistence** often accompanies chorea, e.g. inability to maintain tongue protrusion ('trombone tongue') or steady grip ('milkmaid's grip').

Several features associated with chorea may suggest the aetiology:

- **Seizures.** Consider dentato-rubro-pallido-Luysian atrophy (DRPLA)
- **Cognitive decline** suggests HD and is often subcortical, with psychiatric and behavioural aspects. Beware of anosognosia (e.g. HD patients may deny all problems). Variant CJD may also present with chorea.
- **Positive family history.** Consider HD and DRPLA.
- **Blindness and/or deafness.** Short stature. Consider mitochondrial cytopathy.
- **General findings.** Skin rash (consider lupus), tachycardia (thyrotoxicosis), splenomegaly (Niemann-Pick type C (NPC), Gaucher's disease).

- **Gait** is disproportionately affected in HD, more than by chorea alone.
- **Ataxia.** Consider NPC, DRPLA, Friedreich's ataxia.
- **Eye movements.** Particularly supranuclear gaze problems (vertical in NPC; horizontal in Gaucher's disease). HD patients have difficulty initiating saccades and suppressing unwanted saccades, making fundoscopy difficult.

Huntington's disease (HD)

This is a progressive (autosomal dominant) disease with chorea, dementia and psychiatric features.

- The prevalence is 1 in 10 000.
- The movement disorder includes chorea, tics, dystonia and parkinsonism.
- Dysarthria is common at presentation.
- Swallowing difficulties develop in middle and late disease: remember to weigh HD patients.
- The diagnosis is by genetic testing: CAG repeat on chromosome 4p16.3.
- General measures include education and consideration of family and carer needs. The swallowing and psychiatric manifestations (particularly depression) are treatable.
- Chorea is treated **only** if disabling or contributing to weight loss: sulpiride (200–400 mg/day) or tetrabenazine (12.5 mg/night, increased to 12.5 mg weekly; maximum 50 mg/day); alternatively use clonazepam.

Dentato-rubro-pallido-Luysian atrophy (DRPLA)

This rare condition, another autosomal dominant CAG repeat, presents with:

- Progressive myoclonic epilepsy.
- Ataxia.
- Chorea and dementia (like HD but with epilepsy).

Systemic lupus erythematosus (SLE)

This is a common cause of chorea in young women.

- SLE typically presents during or shortly after pregnancy.
- The pathogenesis is either a vasculopathy or antibody-mediated.
- Anti-cardiolipin antibodies and/or lupus anticoagulant are often found.
- SLE-related chorea may remit, so do not rush to treat.

Sydenham's chorea

This is a common explanation for generalized chorea in children.

- Group A streptococcal infection is the underlying cause.
- Late recurrences comprise 20%, e.g. from the contraceptive pill or pregnancy.

- The pathogenesis reflects antibody cross-reactivity between streptococcus and the basal ganglia: basal ganglia antibodies may be positive.
- Psychiatric problems, including obsessive–compulsive disorder, are grouped together as PANDAS (paediatric autoimmune neuropsychiatric disorders associated with streptococcal infection).

Neuroacanthocytosis

This heterogenous group of disorders is characterized by:

- Acanthocytes on a fresh blood film (>3% is abnormal; repeat three times if negative).
- Normal serum lipoprotein electrophoresis (unlike abetalipoproteinaemia, which also has peripheral acanthocytes).
- X-linked inheritance, recessive or dominant, e.g. the XK gene (McLeod phenotype), VPS13A and junctophilin-3.
- Several movement disorders occur, including chorea and orofacial dyskinesias.
- Axonal peripheral neuropathy and/or myopathy may occur (raised serum creatine kinase).
- Imaging shows cerebral and caudate atrophy, sometimes with white matter disease.

Miscellaneous

Other causes of chorea include vascular lesions and tumours (of the caudate and other basal ganglia), thyrotoxicosis, polycythaemia, metabolic problems (sodium, calcium) and drugs (levodopa, oral contraceptives, phenytoin).

DYSTONIA

Dystonia is a sustained muscle contraction, often with twisting postures or repetitive movements (including tremor). It is often misdiagnosed as functional.

Distribution

- **Focal** dystonia involves one body part. Dystonia in adults usually presents focally in the head, neck or upper limb, e.g. blepharospasm, torticollis, spasmodic dysphonia, or writer's cramp and rarely (10–20%) spreads elsewhere. Dystonia in children starts usually in the lower limbs, e.g. a foot. The nearer the ground the onset, the more likely it is to generalize (90% with leg onset).
- **Segmental** dystonia involves two or more contiguous parts, e.g. arm and neck.
- **Multifocal** dystonia involves two non-contiguous areas.
- **Hemidystonia** suggests an underlying brain lesion.
- **Generalized** dystonia is usually of childhood-onset.

Provoking factors

Dystonia is often provoked by certain actions.

- **Walking.** It is essential to see the patient walk. In idiopathic torsion dystonia, couch examination may be normal yet with very abnormal gait.
- **Task-specific.** Examination depends on the distribution of symptoms, e.g. with dystonia only when writing, observe writing arm movements, but note the other arm is often affected ('overflow dystonia').

Relieving factors

- Torticollis may show *geste antagoniste*: temporary relief by slight facial touch.
- Generalized dystonia worsening with walking may improve with running or walking backwards.

Aetiology

Primary dystonia has no additional neurological abnormality except occasional dystonic tremor.

- **Idiopathic generalized dystonia** (AD, DYT-1 chr 9 – GAG deletion) is the most common in childhood. It presents with foot dystonia that often later generalizes.
- **Focal dystonia**, e.g. spasmodic torticollis, is the most common in adults and is genetically determined.

Dystonia-plus has additional neurological abnormalities, e.g. myoclonus or parkinsonism.

- **Dopa-responsive dystonia** (DRD) is extremely important. It is either autosomal dominant (guanosine-5-triphosphate cyclohydrolase deficiency) or autosomal recessive (tyrosine hydroxylase deficiency). Occasionally DRD may present to adult clinics with 'cerebral palsy,' isolated foot dystonia (an odd distribution for adult onset dystonia), or a tremor predominant Parkinsonian syndrome. It responds dramatically to levodopa and may not be associated with long-term complications of levodopa therapy.

Secondary (non-genetic) dystonia implies dystonia is the sole manifestation of an underlying disorder.

- **Drugs**, e.g. neuroleptics, prochlorperazine, metoclopramide (see below).
- **Stroke**, including hypoxic-ischaemic cerebral palsy.
- **Demyelination** may cause fixed or paroxysmal focal dystonia.

Heredodegenerative dystonia implies dystonia as part of a widespread underlying process and includes some eminently treatable aetiologies.

- HD or DRPLA.
- Neuro-acanthocytosis.
- Neurodegeneration with brain iron accumulation (NBIA), acaeruloplasminaemia, neuro-ferritinopathy (Fig. 9.5a,b), pantothenate kinase associated neurodegeneration (PANK).

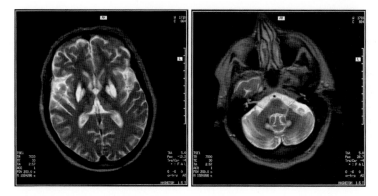

Figure 9.5
Neuroferritinopathy. (a,b) MRI (T2 weighted) showing high signal surrounded by low signal change (iron deposition) in basal ganglia and dentate regions.

- Mitochondrial cytopathy.
- Kuf's (adult Batten) disease: unlike childhood onset, vision may be normal.
- Wilson's disease (see below).
- Niemman–Pick type C (NPC) and Gaucher's disease (GD) have cognitive problems, ataxia and supranuclear gaze palsies (see chorea).
- Leucodystrophies, especially metachromatic form (arylsulphatase A deficiency).

Management

Explanations bring understanding and often relief, especially if the symptoms had previously been perceived as psychological.

Specific strategies are sometimes available, e.g. writing dystonia responds better to using thick pens than to medication or injections.

Genetic counselling is important in any autosomal dominant disorder, but information is often imprecise owing to the relatively low gene penetrance.

Medications

- **A levodopa trial** (Sinemet 275 mg twice daily for 8 weeks) is essential, especially in childhood-onset or generalized dystonia, to exclude dopa-responsive dystonia.
- **Anticholinergics**, e.g. benzhexol, improve dystonia in about 40%, but doses are limited by side-effects, especially dry mouth and sphincter dysfunction.
- **Botulinum toxin** is the treatment of choice for focal dystonia. The benefit is sustained for 2–3 months and side-effects are surprisingly infrequent.

Surgery

- **Stereotactic thalamotomy** is a last resort for disabling dystonia.

BALLISM

Sub-thalamic lesions (stroke or other pathology) may cause hemiballism, a violent unilateral movement disorder. It affects the trunk and so appears to be bilateral. Neuroleptics or sodium valproate may help.

MYOCLONUS

These are sudden shock-like muscle contractions (positive myoclonus) or sudden loss of muscle tone (negative myoclonus).

Clinical points

Types

- **Cortical myoclonus** is often distal and stimulus-sensitive (action myoclonus).
- **Brainstem reticular reflex myoclonus** is triggered by distal touch.
- **Spinal myoclonus** may be either segmental (myotomal) or propriospinal. Propriospinal myoclonus (repetitive flexion jerks of the body) often appears only when supine, or is provoked by eliciting lower limb reflexes. It must be distinguished from *axial dystonia* and *stiff person syndrome*, which are neither position dependent nor stimulation-provoked.
- **Hyperekplexia** manifests as an excessive startle response to stimuli such as touch over the mantle area (but not spontaneously). Tonic spasms may follow hyperekplexia jerks.
- **Asterixis** (Greek asterigma: without support) is a negative myoclonus (loss of tone) particularly associated with metabolic encephalopathy. The outstretched hands show a sudden flap (asymmetric and not rhythmic) with brisk flexion and slower extension.

Distribution

- **Distal** involvement suggests cortical myoclonus, owing to the large representation of the hand in the motor cortex.
- **Proximal and distal** large body jerks suggest brainstem reticular reflex myoclonus or hyperekplexia.

Triggers

- Provocation by **arm or hand movement** (action myoclonus) suggests a cortical origin.
- Provocation by **auditory stimuli** (usually large jerks) suggests brainstem reticular reflex myoclonus.

Specific syndromes

- **Essential myoclonus** is an autosomal dominant condition with onset before aged 20 years. It affects mainly the head and resembles a fast head tremor. There are no other neurological problems.
- **Repetitive focal twitching** of the fingers or hands is probably a form of cortical myoclonus (*epilepsia partialis continua*). It is usually secondary to a vascular or neoplastic cortical abnormality. The EEG may be normal.

Investigations

- **Electroencephalogram.** Cortical spikes correlate with the myoclonus, e.g. preceding a hand jerk by 20 msec and lasting <70 msec (suggests cortical myoclonus).
- **Electromyography** also informs about the spread and latency of jerks in other myoclonic conditions.
- **Somatosensory evoked potentials** may be 'giant' in cortical myoclonus.
- **Bloods:** urea and electrolytes and liver function tests.
- **Chronic myoclonus:** investigate for neurodegenerative conditions (see below).
- **Rapid deterioration** with myoclonus: investigate for prion disease, encephalitis or paraneoplastic syndromes.

Causes

Cortical

- **Degenerative conditions**, e.g. Alzheimer's disease, Huntington's disease.
- **Progressive myoclonic epilepsies**, e.g. mitochondrial cytopathy, Unverricht–Lundborg disease, Lafora body disease.
- **Progressive** myoclonic ataxias, e.g. coeliac disease, mitochondrial cytopathy.

Brainstem reticular reflex myoclonus

- Uraemia.
- Hypoxic encephalopathy.
- Encephalitis.

Hyperekplexia

- Hereditary, e.g. abnormality of the alpha-1 subunit of the glycine receptor.
- Symptomatic, e.g. infective, paraneoplastic or hypoxic encephalopathy.
- Sporadic.

Management

- Clonazepam is effective for most myoclonic conditions.
- Valproate is effective with cortical and brainstem reticular reflex myoclonus.
- Piracetam is effective only in cortical myoclonus.

SPECIFIC MOVEMENT DISORDERS

Stiff person syndrome (SPS)

1. **Stiffness** of axial muscles (giving lumbar spine hyperlordosis) and of the proximal legs.
2. **Spasms**, often precipitated by noise or touch and typically with blood pressure changes and diaphoresis. These may be severe enough to result in fractures.
3. **Causes:**
   - **Autoimmune.** SPS is associated with other autoimmune conditions: 30% have diabetes mellitus, 60% have anti-GAD (glutamic acid decarboxylase) antibodies. GAD is involved in the synthesis of GABA, an inhibitory transmitter.
   - **Paraneoplastic.** This is rare: <5% of SPS patients have anti-amphiphysin antibodies. Paraneoplastic SPS may also manifest as progressive encephalopathy with rigidity and myoclonus (PERM).
   - **Idiopathic.** No identified autoimmune conditions or antibodies.
4. **Management**
   - **Immune modulation** with intravenous immunoglobulin, plasma exchange, steroids.
   - **Restoration of GABA** with benzodiazepines, valproate, baclofen.

Paroxysmal dyskinesia

Dyskinesias which fluctuate include:

- **Paroxysmal non-kinesigenic dyskinesia** manifests as long attacks (4 h) of dyskinesia precipitated by coffee, alcohol, stress or fatigue. Some respond to clonazepam.
- **Paroxysmal kinesigenic dyskinesia** begins aged 5–15 years and manifests as very brief dyskinesias (seconds to a few minutes) induced by movement. It often responds to carbamazepine.
- **Paroxysmal exercise-induced dyskinesia** manifests as dyskinesias, particularly of the lower limbs, induced by exercise (even chewing gum) or water (cold shower).

Wilson's disease (WD)

Clinical features

- **Age of onset** is typically 6–40 years (may be later).
- **Liver disease.** A liver presentation is most common before puberty and neurological presentations after puberty. Some 25% of WD patients have a liver history, e.g. unexplained haemolytic anaemia or hepatic jaundice.
- **Movement disorder.** A wide range occurs, including tremor, parkinsonism, dystonia, chorea, ataxia, or titubation with little gait abnormality.
- **Neuropsychiatric** features are common.
- **Ophthalmic.** Look for Kayser–Fleischer rings (Fig. 9.6): refer suspected WD patients to an experienced ophthalmologist.

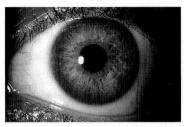

Figure 9.6
Kayser–Fleischer rings in Wilson's disease.

Investigations

- Serum caeruloplasmin is usually low (but is an acute phase protein so false negatives occur), serum copper is high, normal or low; liver biopsy (dry weight) and urinary copper are high.
- Aminoaciduria may occur.
- Management is with chelating agents, e.g. penicillamine and best undertaken by centres with particular expertise. Starting treatment may cause temporary clinical worsening.

Drug-induced movement disorders

Most drug-induced movement disorders are reversible, although tardive dyskinesia often persists following drug withdrawal.

Dystonia

- **Acute**. Neuroleptic exposure can precipitate acute dystonic reactions within 1–2 days, e.g. oculogyric crisis (forced upward deviation of the eyes) or cervical dystonia e.g. torticollis. Young males are the most vulnerable. Anticholinergics (benztropine or trihexyphenidyl) are usually effective and should be continued for 3–4 days.
- **Chronic**. Tardive dystonias occur in 2% on neuroleptics and may be focal, e.g. writer's cramp, torticollis.

Parkinsonism

This may be indistinguishable from IPD. It results from dopamine antagonists (e.g. tetrabenazine) or dopamine depleting agents (e.g. reserpine). Some 10–15% of psychiatric patients, especially women, develop parkinsonism, usually within a few months (90% by 3 months). The management plan should be:

- Withdraw the neuroleptics (if possible).
- Anticholinergics or amantadine for symptom relief (if needed).
- Levodopa is effective, but may worsen the psychiatric condition.
- Patients may need chronic therapy, but attempt withdrawal of amantadine/anticholinergics etc. after 3 months.

Akathisia

- Restlessness (differential diagnosis of restless legs).
- Acute or tardive reaction neuroleptics.
- Management: reduce or stop neuroleptics and consider β-blockers (propranolol), amantadine, anticholinergics or clonazepam.

Neuroleptic malignant syndrome (NMS)

Clinical features

1. Fever (low- or high-grade).
2. Autonomic instability (arrhythmias).
3. Rigidity and other movement disorders (0.2% of patients exposed to neuroleptics).
4. Confusion.

Investigations: The serum creatine kinase is often raised.

Management: Stop the neuroleptics, re-hydrate and carefully monitor renal function. DAs (bromocriptine) or levodopa are helpful; also consider benzodiazepine or dantrolene.

Prognosis: NMS is an emergency with 20% mortality.

Tardive dyskinesia

- This occurs in 20% of patients exposed to neuroleptics for >3 months.
- It is more common in older women and those with a history of head injury or alcohol exposure.
- Orolingual dyskinesias: repetitive protrusion of the tongue or chewing occur, but are more stereotyped than chorea.
- Spontaneous dyskinesia occurs in 5–10% of elderly patients.
- Management is difficult. Stop the neuroleptic if possible. A higher potency dopamine antagonist may suppress the dyskinesias, reflecting dopamine receptor denervation hypersensitivity. Clonazepam, baclofen, valproic acid may help, or occasionally tetrabenazine or reserpine.
- About 50% improve, some only after 1 year.

HISTORY TAKING

In addition to a full neurological history, particular aspects are important:

- **A drug history** is important for any movement disorder. Many drugs cause tremor, e.g. valproate, lithium, asthma inhalers, antidepressants, metronidazole, thyroxine, statins, steroids, cyclosporine. Neuroleptics can cause Parkinsonian tremors and tardive tremors, often of the chin. Neuroleptic exposure is relevant in most movement disorders, e.g. tic disorders (tardive tics) and tremor (Parkinsonian or tardive tremor).
- **Tremor:** symmetry, duration (ET vs IPD), family history, alcohol, anxiety, caffeine, diurnal variation, contraindication to beta blocker, anxiety. Does the tremor come and go, change with a load, is it distractible, does it entrain? (suggests psychogenic tremor).

- **Parkinsonism:** asymmetry of onset (IPD vs parkinsonism), more slowing than tremor, neuroleptics history, walking, turning, turning in bed, rising from a chair, writing, speech. Ask the partner whether the patient thrashes around violently when dreaming.
- **Dystonia:** provoking factors (especially medications), diurnal variation, family history, previous trial of levodopa.
- **Chorea:** pregnancy, pill, thyroid status, behaviour, dementia, family history, rheumatic fever, epilepsy.
- **Myoclonus:** provoking factors, family history.

EXAMINATION

For all movement disorder patients

- **Observe the movement.** Consider (with permission) a video, then identify any accompanying signs.
- **Weigh** patients with chronic neurological illness, especially IPD and HD.
- Exclude **Kayser–Fleisher rings** in any young-onset movement disorder.
- Watch the patient **walk**.
- **Cognitive assessment.** Remember also that the basal ganglia are not just involved in movement: there are behavioural and cognitive aspects to most movement disorders. Some cognitive assessment is essential in patients with parkinsonism.

Specific conditions

- **Tremor:** rest, postural, intention, look for symmetry.
- **Parkinsonism:** tremor, rigidity, bradykinesia, symmetry, dementia, eye movements, autonomic tests, cognitive function, cerebellar features. Watch the patient walk down the outpatient corridor – there is often insufficient space in the consultation room – and watch the patient come through the door. Ask patient to write in medical notes: is their writing smaller compared with old samples of writing, e.g. diaries. Consider olfactory testing (scratch and sniff) if suspecting IPD. Measure autonomic function.
- **Dystonia:** jerky tremor, *geste antagonistique*.
- **Chorea:** eye movements in HD; cognitive function.
- **Myoclonus:** stimulus or noise-sensitive.

Case history outcome

This patient had dopa-responsive-dystonia (DRD). Levodopa gave a dramatic improvement within 1 week. She had Parkinsonian features and dystonic legs, including a 'striatal toe'. DRD mainly affects females (3:1). There may be diurnal variation with sleep benefit (this is seen with other dystonias and is not invariably present in DRD). It is vital to consider because it is dramatically treatable: both mother and child improved remarkably.

KEY POINTS

- Isolated tremor is much more likely to be benign than IPD.
- Parkinson's tremor comprises both rest and postural tremors.
- Red flags suggesting diagnoses other than IPD include symmetry of signs, early falls and early dementia.
- A trial of levodopa is essential in patients with dystonia.
- Think of Wilson's disease in all young onset movement disorders (<50 years).
- Depression is a common treatable cause of cognitive dysfunction in HD.
- Young onset HD may present with parkinsonism and seizures.
- DRPLA is the second most common familial chorea.
- A neuroleptic history is essential in all movement disorders.
- A drug and toxicology history is essential in movement disorders.
- Dystonia is commonly misdiagnosed as functional.

Further Reading

Morris H. Genetics of Parkinson's disease. Ann Med 2005; 37(2): 86–96.

Multiple sclerosis

Case history

A 40-year-old woman presented with a 5-day history of altered sensation in both legs. Over the following days she developed right eye visual blurring, occasional incontinence and hand tingling. She became profoundly weak, essentially bed-bound. There was no significant previous history. On examination, higher cortical function was normal. Visual acuities (Snellen chart) were 6/60 (right) and 6/5 (left) with a right central scotoma. There was spasticity in her arms and legs. Her legs were very weak, with an inability to lift them off the bed. Her plantar responses were extensor. All sensory modalities were impaired to T4 (right) and T10 (left). General examination was normal. She later recalled a previous episode at age 27 years of visual problems in which her right eye was sore to move for 2 weeks.

INTRODUCTION

Multiple sclerosis (MS) is common (about 1:800 in the UK, though less in equatorial countries) and makes up a considerable proportion of a neurologist's workload. It normally presents at age range of 20–50 years. MS is characterized by central white matter demyelination. Some sites are more commonly affected, particularly the optic nerves, cervical spinal cord and the brainstem. This means that 'white matter' features such as optic neuritis, internuclear ophthalmoplegia (see below), sensory cord symptoms, weakness and ataxia are more common than 'grey matter' features such as chorea, dystonia, aphasia, apraxia, agnosia and epilepsy. MS usually follows a relapsing–remitting course with recovery dependent upon remyelination, resolution of inflammation, modification of sodium channel numbers and distribution and neural plasticity.

HISTORY AND EXAMINATION

Careful documentation of previous symptoms provides first-hand evidence of dissemination in time and space.

Visual

Visual loss. 20% of MS patients present with optic neuritis and 60% have acute optic neuritis at some stage of the illness. Sub-clinical optic neuritis is very frequent. Optic neuritis presents with mild pain, worse with movement and visual blurring. Most patients have a central scotoma and two-thirds show visual field defects in the unaffected eye. The optic disc is swollen in one-third (the remainder have inflammation further back in the optic nerve). There may be a Marcus–Gunn pupil (and swinging flashlight sign) and defective colour vision. The vision typically worsens for 1–2 weeks, the nadir being 1–7 days. Most patients recover, with only 5% having acuity of <6/60.

Diplopia is common in MS; it is important to identify whether it is (or was, since it may have recovered) horizontal or vertical and the direction of gaze it was in. An INO often causes horizontal diplopia, worse on looking laterally; sometimes there is oscillopsia through ataxic nystagmus (a subtle residual INO often leaves only nystagmus in the abducting eye). Occasionally, nuclear or infranuclear 3rd, 4th or 6th nerve palsies, gaze palsies and (less commonly) the one-and-a-half syndrome may occur (see Fig. 2.12b).

Sensory

Altered sensation, for example facial numbness, is not necessarily accompanied by definite signs. A definite and constant sensory level is unusual in MS; it should raise the possibility of alternative or additional pathology.

- **Regional sensory loss.** Lower limb tingling or numbness might start in a foot, ascend over a few days, then cross to affect the other limb. There may be no associated bladder or motor disturbance and the patient may dismiss it as 'one of those things', especially as most resolve spontaneously. Upper limb symptoms may affect one or both arms similarly, sometimes sparing the trunk and legs; a high cervical plaque is likely.
- **Useless hand (Oppenheim).** A high cervical cord lesion involving the dorsal columns, gives loss of vibration and joint position sense (often with pseudo-athetoid movements). Usually one hand is affected but sometimes both. Improvement usually occurs 6–9 months after the onset. Hand function should be tested, e.g. buttoning a shirt, since there may be a disparity between minimal abnormalities on examination and function.
- **Paroxysmal sensory symptoms.** It is worth specifically asking directly about three paroxysmal features that are seldom volunteered.
  - **Trigeminal neuralgia** is described in Box 10.1.
  - **Lhermitte's symptom,** where neck flexion provokes brief paroxysms of tingling sensations radiating down the back or arms.
  - **Uthoff's phenomenon,** where a transient worsening of symptoms coincides with body temperature increases through exercise (as originally described) or hot bath (hence hot bath test).

Box 10.1: Trigeminal neuralgia (TN)

- 5% of MS patients.
- TN with onset aged <50 years is usually symptomatic, e.g. MS; TN with onset aged >50 years is usually idiopathic (presumed microvascular compression).
- TN distribution is usually the 2nd/3rd division (maxillary/mandibular), it is odd to affect the 1st (ophthalmic) division.
- Examination is normal in idiopathic TN, e.g. normal corneal reflexes.
- Bilateral in 30% MS cases; 5% of idiopathic cases.
- Autonomic features are absent in TN. If present, consider trigeminal autonomic cephalgias, e.g. SUNCT (short-lasting unilateral neuralgiform pain with conjunctival injection and tearing), which often affects the 1st division.

Motor

Spasms are exacerbated by irritation so look out for nociceptive stimuli, e.g. a urethral sore with catheter, pressure sores, toenail problems, infections, toothache, etc.

Paroxysmal motor symptoms. Tonic spasms are unilateral spasms, often painful and lasting for less than 1 min. They are not startle-induced but can be precipitated by hyperventilation or movement. Paroxysmal dysarthria or paroxysmal weakness are other examples.

An **upper motor neurone syndrome** (Box 10.2) affecting one or all limbs and comprising several positive and negative features, results from involvement of the corticospinal and parapyramidal tracts (i.e. rubrospinal, tectospinal, vestibulospinal, reticulospinal). Paraparesis or tetraparesis are more common than hemiparesis in MS.

Superficial abdominal reflexes are traditionally lost early in MS in contrast to other conditions such as motor neurone disease (MND) or hereditary spastic paraparesis, where they tend to be preserved.

Depressed reflexes are found in 10%, because the dorsal root entry zone may be affected.

Pressure palsies may develop in vulnerable and immobile patients.

'Non-organic' motor signs, e.g. Hoover's sign, may be seen in MS; clinicians must therefore be wary about diagnosing illness as 'non-organic'.

Brainstem features

- **Ataxia** is common, but is rarely the sole manifestation of MS.
- **Swallowing and respiratory symptoms** are common (45% of patients) and result from disruption of the lower brainstem nuclei or supranuclear connections. The clinician should watch the patient drink water and enquire about recent chest infections.
- **Eye movement abnormalities** (see above).

Box 10.2: *Upper motor neurone (UMN) syndrome*

Negative features
- Weakness.
- Lost dexterity.
- Fatigue.

Positive features
- **Passive response to proprioceptive stimulation**:
  - Clonus.
  - Exaggerated tendon jerks.
  - Increased tone (velocity dependent).
- **Passive response to nociceptive stimulation**:
  - Extensor plantars.
  - Flexor spasms.
- **Active (during movements)**:
  - Co-contraction of agonist and antagonist muscles during movement.
  - Associated reactions (spasm/dystonia) during movement.

- **Other cranial nerve abnormalities** are less common, but include fascicular 3rd nerve palsy, 6th nerve palsy or a lower motor neurone 7th nerve palsy (approximately 4%).
- **Facial myokymia** (wriggling movements beneath the skin) suggests intrinsic brainstem disease.

Sphincter dysfunction

Bladder control is affected at some point in 80% of patients; 10% have problems at diagnosis but only in 1% is it a presenting complaint.

Bowel function is often affected, particularly constipation. Bowel incontinence is surprisingly common, occurring more than once weekly in 25% of patients.

Cognition

Mood may be affected and depression reasonably common; contrary to previous beliefs, euphoria is unusual. Measurable cognitive changes develop in half of MS patients, and in 5% this is a major impairment. It is usually sub-cortical, characterized by bradyphrenia, perseveration, mental inflexibility and with other frontal lobe problems. The MMSE is therefore relatively insensitive to MS-related cognitive problems.

Fatigue

This is defined as a lack of physical or mental energy that interferes with usual or desired activities. Most (75–90%) patients describe tiredness during their illness, although rarely present with it. They may refer to a feeling of lassitude or to muscle fatigue with repetitive movements (part of the upper motor neurone syndrome: see Box 10.2). Remember that depression, anaemia, dysthyroid disease and sleep disruption (through pain or spasticity) are reversible causes of fatigue.

MAKING THE DIAGNOSIS

MS remains a clinical diagnosis but paraclinical tests (MRI brain, CSF analysis and evoked potentials) remain important. The McDonald diagnostic criteria are summarized in Box 10.3. It is worth emphasizing a few aspects:

1. The diagnosis requires dissemination in space and time (clinically or radiologically).
2. The diagnosis requires objective clinical signs and not just historical symptoms.
3. There must be no better explanation than MS to explain the clinical picture.
4. Relapses must last longer than 24 h. Body temperature should be normal during relapses.
5. Relapses must be separated by one month or more from the start of the first to the onset of the second.

Most patients with MS have brain imaging abnormalities (95%); it is therefore still possible to have MS with a normal scan, particularly with the progressive form; additional

---

Box 10.3: *McDonald criteria for MS diagnosis*

Essentially these criteria use clinical and MR evidence to identify at least two lesions disseminated in space and two lesions disseminated in time.

MS may be diagnosed with:
1. Two or more attacks, with clinical signs of two or more lesions.
2. Two or more attacks, with signs of one lesion, plus MRI evidence of dissemination in space (below).
3. One attack, with two or more abnormal signs, plus MRI evidence of dissemination in time (below).
4. One attack with one abnormal sign, plus MRI evidence of dissemination in space and time.

MRI evidence of dissemination in space requires any three of:
• Gadolinium enhancing lesion or 9 hyperintense lesions on T2 imaging.
• One infratentorial lesion.
• One juxta-cortical lesion (involving U-fibres).
• Three periventricular lesions.

MRI evidence of dissemination in time requires one of:
• New gadolinium enhancing lesion within 3 months of symptoms onset.
• New T2 lesions on subsequent scans.

Insidious onset (primary progressive) requires:
• Positive oligoclonal bands.
and
• Dissemination in space judged by any one of:
  • 9+ T2 weighted brain lesions.
  • 2+ cord lesions.
  • 4–8 brain lesions with one cord lesion.
  • <4 brain lesions with one cord lesion plus abnormal visual evoked potentials.
and
• Dissemination in time judged by either of:
  • The criteria above.
  • Progression for 1 year.

---

investigation with cord imaging, CSF examination and evoked potentials are worth considering (Figs 10.1, 10.2, 10.3).

Vascular or demyelinating MRI lesions

Demyelination is favoured by lesions which are:

• Distributed in the cord, corpus callosum, or U-fibres (i.e. juxtacortical).
• Ovoid with their long axis pointing towards cortex (Dawson's fingers).

GIVING THE DIAGNOSIS

It is standard practice to inform patients of the diagnosis when it is known and to share a strong suspicion of the diagnosis with them. This needs to be done by someone aware of the clinical problems and investigations results and, if appropriate, with a family member or someone to offer immediate support. Ideally, an MS specialist nurse should be included. Discussion of clinically isolated syndromes, e.g. optic neuritis, should note the possibility of MS: 50% will develop MS. Knowledge of the natural history is helpful in discussion (Box 10.4 and Table 10.1 give prognostic indicators).

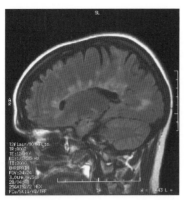

Figure 10.1
MRI brain showing demyelinating plaques in MS.

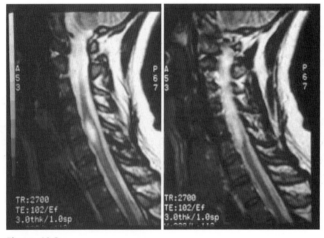

Figure 10.2
(a,b) MRI cord showing high signal lesion.

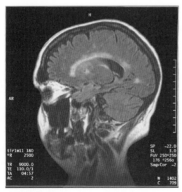

Figure 10.3
MRI brain showing vascular lesions.

Box 10.4: MS natural history

- 70% begin as relapsing–remitting; 15% begin as progressive.
- Secondary progressive MS (following relapsing–remitting) occurs 10–15 years after the onset, a similar age as the onset of primary progressive MS.
- Benign MS occasionally occurs. Pathological changes of MS are found in 1:500 of non-neurological autopsies. Benign MS cannot be diagnosed early since late deterioration (>25 years after presentation) is possible regardless of the prognostic features.
- Morbidity. After 15 years, patients have a 50% chance of walking without aids.
- The Kurtzke scale (EDSS) is the most commonly used disability measure. It measures mainly mobility and is insensitive to dementia or blindness. (EDSS 3: mild disability; EDSS 6: walks 100 m with aids; EDSS 8: bed-bound; EDSS 10: dead).
- Survival is good: life expectancy is reduced by 5–7 years, equivalent to smoking 20 cigarettes daily. The suicide risk is increased, particularly in those isolated socially.
- Pregnancy is protective but there is an increased relapse risk post-partum.
- Vaccination does not significantly affect the natural history and should be given as needed.

Table 10.1: MS prognosis

Poor prognosis	Good prognosis
Male	Female
Old age	Young age
Early disability to EDSS 3	Long interval to reach EDSS 3
Short inter-attack intervals	Long inter-attack intervals
High frequency of early relapses	Low frequency early relapses
Polysymptomatic	Monosymptomatic
Early motor or cerebellar features	Early sensory or vision symptoms

DIFFERENTIAL DIAGNOSIS

MS diagnostic criteria are appropriate only if there is no better explanation for the clinical picture.

Structural disorders

Brainstem

- **Foramen magnum lesions**, particularly meningiomas and Chiari malformation, cause fluctuating symptoms and signs and can cause diagnostic confusion.
- **Intrinsic brainstem lesions** such as glioma and central pontine myelinolysis often do not cause sensory problems, whereas brainstem MS often does.

Spinal cord

There are many causes of chronic progressive myelopathy besides relapsing–remitting MS.

- Progressive MS (see McDonald criteria).
- Spinal cord compression (tumour, disc, etc.).
- Spinal arteriovenous malformation (including dural AV fistula).

- Chiari malformation.
- Syringomyelia.
- HTLV-1 (note: oligoclonal bands may occur).
- Motor neurone disease (especially primary lateral sclerosis).
- Other neuro-inflammatory disorders.
- Other neurovascular diseases.
- Vitamin B_{12} deficiency.
- Genetic disorders, including hereditary spastic paraparesis.

Other neuro-inflammatory disorders

Acute disseminated encephalomyelitis (ADEM)

Box 10.5 outlines the main features distinguishing MS from ADEM.

Sarcoidosis

Some 5% of sarcoidosis cases have neurological complications (both peripheral and central), the most common being facial palsy; 30% of neurosarcoidosis cases have meningeal gadolinium enhancement on MRI. Carefully search for rashes, particularly erythema nodosum and seek an ophthalmology opinion (iritis). CSF is abnormal in 80%; raised protein, increased CSF ACE (questionable utility) and positive oligoclonal bands (50%). Consider a gallium scan and ideally obtain a biopsy, e.g. of rash, lung, conjunctiva, or lymph node.

Behçet's disease

This presents with focal neurological signs, meningism, or raised pressure headache (secondary to venous thrombosis). The diagnosis requires >3 episodes of oral ulceration plus two of the following: genital ulceration, skin lesions, positive pathergy test (read at 24–48h, often negative in Caucasians), iritis or retinal abnormalities. Oligoclonal bands are rare in Behçet's disease.

Sjögren's syndrome

This presents with the triad of dry mouth and eyes (sicca) occurring with another connective tissue disorder. Optic nerve involvement may be prominent and develop early. Anti-Ro and La antibodies are helpful but not always positive.

Box 10.5: Acute disseminated encephalomyelitis (ADEM) vs MS

- **Age:** ADEM often in childhood.
- **Encephalopathy** (fever, headache, seizures, meningism and bilateral optic neuritis) is more likely with ADEM.
- **Preceding illness or immunization** is more likely with ADEM.
- **MR brain scan** in ADEM shows oedema and lesions involving both grey and white matter and of the same age (with gadolinium). MS has more periventricular lesions and of different ages (some lesions are new and enhance with gadolinium, others are old and do not); T1 MRIs have black holes in MS.
- **Oligoclonal bands** are less common in ADEM and disappear with time.

Infections

Indolent infections including HTLV-1, HIV, Whipple's disease, syphilis or Lyme disease may resemble MS and oligoclonal bands are often positive.

Diffuse neurovascular disease

Vasculitis. This has three classical presentations.

1. MS type illness, but with headache, obtundation and systemic features including weight loss (these are unusual in primary CNS angiitis).
2. Encephalopathy.
3. Space occupying lesion.

A tissue diagnosis is ideal, from brain (if other organs are not involved) or other involved organ in systemic vasculitis. Brain biopsy gives serious morbidity in up to 2% of cases. Biopsy is positive in 70–80%. Unexpected pathology is sometimes found with or without vasculitis, e.g. low-grade infections (toxoplasmosis), lymphoma, or MS. Thus, many clinicians are reluctant to treat cerebral vasculitis without a tissue diagnosis.

Systemic lupus erythematosus. Although a neurological presentation is rare (3%), 50% lupus patients during their illness develop headache, seizures, psychiatric problems and occasionally a severe myelopathy. An ANA is therefore indicated in undiagnosed encephalopathy or myelopathy (significant titre is >1:160).

CADASIL (Cerebral Autosomal Dominant Arteriopathy with Subcortical Infarcts and Leucoencephalopathy) is an autosomal dominant condition, caused by a mutation in the Notch-3 gene on chromosome 19q12. Patients present with migraine headaches, small vessel strokes and sub-cortical cognitive problems or encephalopathy. Imaging (Fig. 10.4) often reveals white matter disease, particularly in the anterior temporal area and less specifically the external capsule.

Cardiac embolic disease is uncommon but treatable: remember to do an echocardiogram looking for marantic or infective endocarditis, or atrial myxoma.

Genetic causes

- Friedreich's ataxia and other spinocerebellar ataxias should not cause diagnostic confusion. Many can be diagnosed using a blood test.
- Leber's hereditary optic neuropathy occurs mainly in males (4:1); women may present with an MS-like illness associated with severe optic neuritis (Harding's syndrome).
- Leucodystrophies may mimic progressive MS. Adrenoleucodystrophy (X-linked recessive, so predominantly in males) is the most common; typically, the 'very long chain fatty acid' levels are elevated.

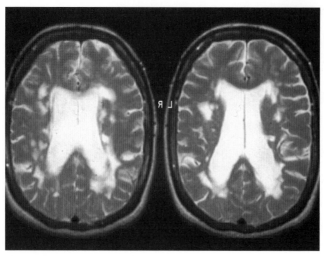

Figure 10.4
MRI brain showing typical (florid) lesions in cerebral autosomal dominant arteriopathy with subcortical ischaemic leucoencephalopathy, CADASIL.

MANAGEMENT

Acute relapse

Corticosteroids accelerate recovery but do not influence the long-term outcome (Box 10.6). Oral or intravenous corticosteroids may be given for relapses. Intravenous methylprednisolone is the appropriate choice for significant motor relapses, brainstem problems or severe optic neuritis.

Symptomatic treatment

A multidisciplinary approach is central to symptom management. This should include focused history and examination, education, specialist therapy input and (finally) pharmacological treatment.

Box 10.6: Summary of findings from Beck's (1992) study into natural history of optic neuritis

Multicentre (15) trial; 457 patients with acute, isolated, unilateral optic neuritis (onset in previous 8 days); no existing diagnosis of MS. Randomized into three groups:

- i.v. methylprednisolone 1 g for 3 days, then oral prednisolone 1 mg/kg per day for 11 days.
- Oral prednisolone 1 mg/kg per day for 14 days.
- Oral placebo for 14 days.

At 6 months, the i.v. methylprednisolone group showed faster recovery, but at 1 year, there was no benefit. At 2 years, the i.v. methylprednisolone group had less MS development; at 5 years this was no different. At 10 years, 38% of patients had developed MS; the risk was 56% in those with 1+ brain lesions but only 22% in those with normal initial MRI.

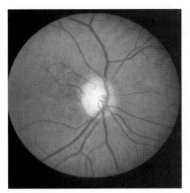

Figure 10.5
Optic neuritis from treatment trial.

Spasticity

When assessing patients with spasms or tone problems, try to identify a nociceptive trigger such as urinary infection or a pressure sore. Therapy and education are important, e.g. a standing programme. Pharmacological measures (Box 10.7) may also be needed as part of the multidisciplinary approach.

Fatigue

If there are no exacerbating or contributory causes (see above), advise energy-conserving measures, e.g. pace yourself through the day, resting when necessary. Drug therapy can sometimes help and includes selective serotonin reuptake inhibitor (SSRI) (e.g. fluoxetine 20 mg daily), amantadine (100–200 mg daily) or modafinil (100–200 mg daily).

Bladder, bowel and sexual dysfunction

Urinary: A useful algorithm has been devised for urinary incontinence – check residual volume with ultrasound. If significant, the patient needs ISC plus bladder stabilizers (anticholinergics). If non-significant, give anticholinergics only.

Bowel: Constipation is often managed by polyethylene glycol, an iso-osmotic laxative, started twice daily with a maintenance dose of once daily.

Box 10.7: *Anti-spasticity medications*

- **Baclofen** ($GABA_b$ agonist): start 5 mg t.d.s., maximum 60–120 mg daily. Drowsiness and weakness are side-effects.
- **Tizanidine** (B_2 adrenergic agonist): start 2 mg t.d.s., maximum 24–32 mg daily. Check liver function tests weekly for 1 month and then monthly for 6 months.
- **Dantrolene sodium** works peripherally and can complement baclofen or tizanidine. Watch for hepatotoxicity.
- **Benzodiazepines:** clonazepam is particularly useful for nocturnal spasms.
- **Botulinum toxin** may help a localized problem, e.g. adductor spasm.
- **Surgery** includes baclofen pumps for intrathecal delivery.

Sexual: It is important to recognize both direct neurological impairments and indirect impairments through social, psychological or other physical problems. Referral to a sexual dysfunction clinic is often helpful. Sildenafil is very helpful in MS (both men and women may benefit). Prostaglandin E1 (alprostadil) given urethrally is an alternative.

Ataxia

This is difficult to manage and a frustrating complication. Steroids can hasten recovery from ataxic relapses. Propranolol, isoniazid (with pyridoxine) and ondansetron have been tried with variable benefit.

Paroxysmal symptoms and pain

Pain has many causes and many are not from the MS, e.g. bursitis or toothache. Carbamazepine remains the drug of choice for trigeminal neuralgia, tonic spasms and other transient symptoms. Pain may be part of an upper motor neurone syndrome. Neuropathic pain is generally treated with tricyclic anti-depressants, anti-epileptics, opiates or topical agents, e.g. capsaicin.

Disease modifying treatments

Beta interferons (Betaseron, Avonex and Rebif) and glatiramer acetate have been shown to reduce the relapse frequency by 30% in selected MS patients. This selected sub-group comprises 10% of patients who meet all the following criteria:

- ≥18 years of age.
- No specific contraindications, e.g. pregnancy or lactation.
- Walks independently, preferably 100 m without assistance (EDSS <5.5).
- Two or more clinically significant relapses in the previous 2 years. Preferably these should be confirmed by neurological examination or from another source, e.g. general practitioner's records.

Patients prescribed either interferon or glatiramer require regular follow-up. Interferon users need blood counts and liver function tests at months 1, 3, 6, 9 and 12 and thereafter 6-monthly. Before starting interferons, a protein electrophoresis must exclude a paraprotein, which could interact with interferon. Side-effects of both interferon and glatiramer include headache, flu-like symptoms (requiring paracetamol or NSAIDs) and injection site reactions. Take care when treating patients who are depressed.

The stopping criteria should be discussed at the beginning. These might include:

- Two disabling relapses in the previous year.
- Secondary progression over 6 months.
- Inability to walk for 6 months or more.

Progressive MS. Disease modifying medications are not used for primary progressive MS. They may be used in secondary progressive MS if relapses still occur, according to the following guidelines:

- >18 years of age.
- No specific contraindications.
- Able to walk 10 m with or without assistance.
- Two or more disabling relapses in the previous 2 years.
- Increased disability due to disease progression in the ≥2 previous years.

Isolated syndromes are not usually prescribed disease-modifying medications in the UK.

Other disease modifying medications include:

- **Azathioprine.** A meta-analysis has shown modest but significant effects on relapse rates (Yudkin 1991).
- **Mitoxantrone**, an anthracenedione cytotoxic agent has been used in relapsing–remitting and secondary progressive disease. The major side-effect is cardiotoxicity.
- **Anti-α_4 integrin antibody** (Antegren), a humanized monoclonal antibody, administered monthly, reduces clinical and radiological disease activity in relapsing–remitting MS.
- **Campath** is an antibody currently on trial in MS.

Case history outcome

This patient had multiple sclerosis (MS). She presented dramatically and there were concerns about a diagnosis of ADEM. However, she remembered a previous episode of optic neuritis and had several clinical and paraclinical features making MS more likely. She was therefore given intravenous corticosteroids. Early consideration was given to disease modifying treatment.

KEY POINTS

- MS is a clinical diagnosis although para-clinical tests are helpful.
- Sensory symptoms without signs and motor signs without symptoms are characteristic of MS.
- Progressive MS is the most common cause of scan negative myelopathy in the UK.
- Red flags for dual cord pathology include: nerve root pain, a fixed sensory level, or segmental muscle wasting.
- Progressive MS: before diagnosing, consider HTLV-1 (there may be positive oligoclonal bands) and primary lateral sclerosis.
- Visual loss: if progressing for >2 weeks, consider optic nerve compression.
- Before diagnosing MS, consider B_{12} deficiency, hereditary spinocerebellar ataxias (including Friedreich's ataxia), Chiari malformation and systemic lupus erythematosus.
- In encephalopathic presentations (seizures, fever, headache, meningism), consider vasculitis, ADEM or infections, e.g. infective endocarditis.
- Age-related MRI vascular white matter changes can resemble demyelination. If in doubt, check CSF and VEPs.
- Vasculitis and/or sarcoidosis usually require a tissue diagnosis, even a brain biopsy.
- When discussing the diagnosis, know the details including all relevant results; understand the natural history but remember limitations of prognostic prediction.
- Structured rehabilitation is important, emphasizing the role of other therapists and of education as well as therapeutics.

Further Reading

Coles A, Compston A. Multiple sclerosis. Lancet 2002; 359(9313): 1221–1231.

Beck RW, Cleary PA, Anderson MM Jr et al. A randomized, controlled trial of corticosteroids in the treatment of acute optic neuritis. The Optic Neuritis Study Group. N Engl J Med 1992; 326(9): 581–588.

Neuromuscular disorders

Case history

A 23-year-old woman was referred urgently with a suspected a 3rd nerve palsy. She reported intermittent painless diplopia for several months and slurred speech on the telephone in the evening. Examination showed right-sided partial ptosis with incomplete and fatiguable eye movements bilaterally. Her shoulder abductors and finger extensors became weaker with repeated movements (see below).

MYOPATHY

Inflammatory

Inflammatory myopathies are generally rare, characteristically cause more weakness than pain and affect the pelvic girdle more than the shoulder. Inclusion body myositis is the exception with more distal muscle involvement (see below).

Clinical spectrum

- **Dermatomyositis (DM).** This is a humorally-mediated, complement-dependent attack on muscle capillaries by B-cells and CD4+ T cells. 20% of adults have underlying malignancy, so consider screening. A lavender coloured rash appears on sun-exposed areas (heliotrope), e.g. cheeks and hands (knuckles, Gottron's sign and mechanic hands).
- **Polymyositis (PM)** has cell-mediated muscle damage (CD8+ T cells) usually without underlying cancer but often with other connective tissue diseases.
- **Inclusion body myositis (IBM)** is the most common myopathy in those >50 years. The quadriceps and long finger flexors are most often affected, with considerable focal atrophy. Facial weakness and dysphagia may be early features. Pathologically there are intramuscular protein aggregates and a cytotoxic CD8 lymphocytic response. The inflammation may be an epiphenomenon. IBM responds poorly to immunosuppression.
- **Infective**, e.g. HIV, HTLV-1.
- **Connective tissue diseases**, e.g. systemic lupus erythematosus.
- **Drugs**, statins, AZT.

Diagnosis

- **Serum creatine kinase** (CK) is usually significantly elevated, e.g. up to 50 times normal. However, in IBM the level is only 3–5 times normal.

- **Electromyography** is useful for confirming myopathy, often showing spontaneous activity. IBM often shows additional neurogenic changes.
- **Muscle biopsy** should be performed if immunosuppression is contemplated. There is no 'gold standard', some inflammatory myopathies may have almost normal biopsies, so a thorough work-up is important.

Outcome

This is influenced by lung involvement (10% with DM or PM; often with anti Jo-1 antibodies), cardiac muscle involvement and underlying malignancy.

Management of DM/PM

The aim is control rather than cure.

- **Corticosteroids** (prednisolone 60 mg/day) are useful if the diagnosis is definite; if the CK falls to normal, then reduce by 5 mg every 2 weeks on alternate days (aiming for 10–20 mg alternate days); sometimes initially loaded with 1 g methylprednisolone for 3 days. Clinical state and CK level help decisions upon dosage reduction.
- **Azathioprine** is often started simultaneously (see Myasthenia gravis).
- **Consider** other treatments including cyclophosphamide and intravenous immunoglobulin.
- **Remember** that 'treatment resistant' DM/PM is usually caused by IBM.

Metabolic

- **Mitochondrial disorders** are more common than generally realized (1/100 000). Look for the other features (eye muscle involvement, short stature, deafness etc.).
- **Glycogen storage diseases**, e.g. McArdle disease (myophosphorylase deficiency) causes early cramps in exercise and may present late with fixed weakness. The CK is usually high. Rhabdomyolysis may occur (renal failure in 50% of these). 'Second wind' is the improvement in cramps after exercise (normal muscle uses fatty acid at rest, glycogen in early exercise and fatty acid in prolonged exercise; after switching to fatty acids and with exercise-related improvement in blood supply, the symptoms improve).
- **Lipid abnormalities.** Carnitine palmitoyltransferase deficiency causes pain and rhabdomyolysis after prolonged exhaustive exercise, particularly if fasted (e.g. a long run on an empty stomach) or sometimes with infection.

Dystrophy

Dystrophinopathies

Duchenne and Becker (Xp21 dystrophies). Dystrophin is a sub-sarcolemmal structural protein, part of the anchor connecting actin to the extracellular matrix (particularly laminin). Becker may present in adult practice with limb-girdle weakness, pseudohypertrophy of the calves and cardiomyopathy (sometimes isolated cardiomyopathy). There is not always a family history (30% are new mutations). Earlier intervention in Duchenne dystrophy with spinal surgery (to prevent scoliosis), corticosteroids (to slow disease progression) and assisted nocturnal ventilation have led to a marked increase in survival, with many Duchenne patients now living to aged 30 years and beyond.

Myotonic dystrophy

There are two forms: DM type 1, the common form, and DM type 2 (or PROMM: proximal myotonic myopathy). Both are autosomal dominant and both are systemic disorders with cataracts, diabetes mellitus, problems with gastrointestinal motility, daytime somnolence, cognitive slowing and frontal balding. The facial weakness is often marked although the ptosis usually receives more attention. In DM type 1 there is distal wasting of the arms and legs. In PROMM myotonia is more prominent and there is no distal wasting, few cognitive problems and no severe congenital form of the condition. Myotonia rarely requires treatment, but mexiletine sometimes helps (can prolong the QT interval). Genetic studies show an expanded CTG repeat on chromosome 19 in DM 1 and a CCTG expansion on chromosome 3 in DM type 2.

Facioscapulohumeral muscular dystrophy (FSHMD)

FSHMD is autosomal dominant (incidence 1:20 000) and fully penetrant by aged 30 years, although patients sometimes first notice their problem later in life. There is prominent facial muscle involvement (ask about whistling ability). The upper arms are affected but deltoid is spared, with characteristic scapular winging on arm abduction, Beevor's sign (upward deviation of umbilicus on asking patient to sit up when supine) and horizontal scapulae with extra axillary skin crease. Sometimes the distal lower limb muscles are involved (foot drop). Occasionally it is asymmetrical, or with deafness or retinal problems (Coat's syndrome); sometimes pain is prominent. A genetic test is now available.

Limb–girdle dystrophy

This is a heterogeneous group of rare, inherited conditions (usually autosomal recessive). There is usually no facial involvement, but there may be a cardiomyopathy or ventilatory failure. The spectrum of disorders includes fukutin, calpain, dysferlin and sarcoglycanopathies; genetic testing may help in some forms. Diagnostic confirmation usually still requires a muscle biopsy with detailed histopathology.

Dystrophy with early contractures

Dystrophy patients with early contractures (Fig. 11.1), e.g. limiting neck flexion or elbow extension: consider Emery–Dreifuss (EDMD; important because of cardiac involvement) or Bethlem myopathy (no cardiac involvement).

Endocrine and toxic

Endocrine

Several endocrine conditions have associated myopathy, particularly Cushing's disease, thyroid disease (hyper- and hypo-), acromegaly and osteomalacia.

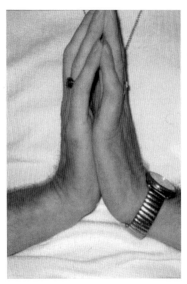

Figure 11.1
Patient with Emery–Dreifuss and finger contractures.

Alcohol

There are two types.

1. Acute painful myopathy after a binge in chronic drinkers.
2. Chronic painless myopathy, often exacerbated by hypokalaemia.

Drugs

Statins. Myalgia is common with statins; patients should be warned to report muscle pain. Statin myopathy is more likely with diabetes mellitus, dysthyroid disease, amiodarone, cyclosporin and grapefruit juice. If the symptoms are tolerable and the CK normal with no weakness, continue the statin. If the CK is >10 times normal, the statin is usually stopped even if asymptomatic.

Corticosteroids. EMG should distinguish inflammatory myopathy from steroid myopathy (no spontaneous activity).

Others. Ipecac (also causes cardiomyopathy), colchicine (particularly renal patients), vincristine, the anti-retroviral AZT and many others.

History

The history in suspected muscle disorder must include several specific aspects.

- **Early life features**. Enquire about strength as a child, running, jumping, myotonic symptoms and myoglobinuria (tea-coloured urine).
- **Proximal muscle weakness**. In the arms this may present, e.g. with difficulty applying shampoo; in the legs there may be difficulty descending as well as ascending stairs.
- **Cramps** occurring with exercise; a history of contractures is important.

- **Myoglobinuria.** Myoglobin, an oxygen-binding muscle protein, leaks with muscle necrosis. Rhabdomyolysis follows toxin exposure (e.g. alcohol), trauma, compression, infection, heat stroke and malignant hyperthermia and occurs with metabolic muscle conditions (see below). Fasting (e.g. religious reasons) may provoke symptoms.
- **Family history** is important; but note that inherited dystrophies may arise through new mutations (e.g. 30% of Duchenne and FSHMD).
- **Respiratory and cardiac.** Dyspnoea from muscle weakness occurs on exertion or on lying flat. Sleep-related breathing disorders may occur. The heart is often involved in muscle disease; right heart failure may present with ankle oedema.
- **Anaesthetic problems.** Duchenne, carnitine palmitoyltransferase deficiency and central core disease can cause malignant hyperthermia with anaesthetics, e.g. halothane or neuromuscular blocking agents.
- **Rash** typically accompanies dermatomyositis.

Examination

- **Systemic features.** Consider the cataracts, frontal balding and cognitive problems of myotonic dystrophy.
- **Muscle inspection** and palpation for atrophy and hypertrophy.
- **Limb weakness.** In most myopathies, the pelvic muscles are affected more than the shoulder girdle. Upper limb weakness characteristically involves the neck, shoulder and upper arm; lower limb weakness affects mainly the pelvic muscles. Ask the patient to rise from a chair with the arms crossed. Gowers' sign (timed) is useful in children. In IBM, weakness characteristically involves the long forearm flexors and the quadriceps.
- **Facial weakness** characterizes myotonic dystrophy, FSHMD, myasthenia gravis and Kennedy's disease.
- **Contractures.** 'Early contractures' occur in EDMD. 'Late contractures' occur in many myopathies, but often only after becoming wheelchair-bound, e.g. in Duchenne dystrophy.
- **Abdominal paradox** implies diaphragmatic weakness.
- **Myotonia** is often worse in the cold and distally and is enhanced by hand immersion in ice. 'Warm-up' phenomenon is myotonia improvement on repetitive use.
- **Paradoxical myotonia** (paramyotonia congenita) worsens with repetitive movement, e.g. opening and closing eyes forcefully increases eyelid myotonia, eventually inducing inability to open the eyes.
- **Action myotonia.** Ask the patient to grip tightly for 20–30 sec and then let go.
- **Percussion myotonia.** Tap the muscle with a hammer and observe muscle 'heaping'.
- **Neuromyotonia** has only action myotonia and no percussion myotonia.
- **Respiratory involvement.** Ventilatory muscle involvement is characteristic of myotonic dystrophy, limb–girdle muscular dystrophy (LGMD), Duchenne/Becker muscular dystrophies (DMD/BMD), acid maltase deficiency, nemaline myopathy, inflammatory myopathies, mitochondrial cytopathy and amyloidosis (may have pseudohypertrophy).
- **Cardiac involvement** is characteristic of myotonic dystrophy (note prolonged PR interval), EDMD, desminopathy, some LGMD and DMD/BMD.

Investigations

- **Serum creatine kinase** (*Note*: not creatinine kinase) is raised in many myopathies, particularly dystrophies and inflammatory myopathies.
- **Neurophysiology.**
- **Muscle biopsy.** Consider carefully if this would help. Select a weak muscle that is not completely atrophic or end-stage. Needle biopsies are easier to organize but may give poorer samples than neurosurgical open biopsy.
- **Genetic analysis,** for periodic paralysis, myotonic dystrophy, FSHMD, BMD/DMD.
- **Ischaemic forearm exercise test.** If glycogen cannot be metabolized (e.g. McArdle's disease) ammonia rises (normal) but lactate does not. Take care with this test owing to the risk of compartment syndrome.

Box 11.1: *Respiratory assessment of neurological patients*

Acute
Forced vital capacity (FVC); normal is 70–75 ml/kg. If FVC drops rapidly or reaches 15 ml/kg (cannot count to 10 in one breath), consult ITU urgently. Aim to avoid last minute problems and intubation at night in sub-optimal conditions.

- Patients may not look distressed despite dangerous hypoventilation because of facial weakness.
- Patients may be bent forward (minimizing gravity on the diaphragm) with rapid shallow respirations.
- The FVC result may be underestimated (poor mouthpiece seal): attach a well fitting facemask to the spirometer.

Others. A general examination and chest radiograph should be included.

Chronic
Symptoms. Diaphragmatic weakness leads to nocturnal ventilatory problems, disturbed sleep, vivid dreams, morning headache, daytime somnolence, poor concentration, orthopnoea and dyspnoea after immersion in water (pressure on the diaphragm).

Signs
- **When supine**, the diaphragm normally descends and abdomen moves out on inspiration at rest. A weak diaphragm moves paradoxically upwards, so the abdomen moves inwards.
- **In REM sleep**, the intercostals and accessory muscles are suppressed; breathing is solely with the diaphragm. With diaphragm weakness, there is nocturnal hypoventilation or apnoea.
- **The jugular venous pressure** may be elevated.

Investigations
- **FVC supine and upright**. With diaphragmatic weakness, FVC falls by >25% from sitting/standing to lying.
- **Overnight oxygen saturation** falls <88% for 5 consecutive min.
- **Arterial PaCO$_2$** rises >45 mmHg (6.0 kPa).
- **Bicarbonate** may rise (compensating for CO$_2$ retention).

Management. If there are symptoms suggesting chronic ventilatory muscle weakness, supported by test results, consider discussing non-invasive ventilation. Significant bulbar problems make non-invasive ventilation difficult, but do not necessarily preclude it.

Box 11.2: *Swallowing assessment*

- Patients must be alert (GCS >13/15), sitting up, not breathless and able to cough.
- Swallow 3–4 ml of water from a spoon, observe for coughing and/or altered (wet, gurgly) speech.
- If satisfactory, swallow 50–150 ml of water as quickly (but safely) as possible. Time it and count the swallows (normal male 20 ml/sec, 20 ml/swallow; female 10 ml/sec, 10 ml/swallow); again listen to speech afterwards.
- If abnormal, then put nil by mouth, arrange speech and language therapist assessment and discuss alternative feeding methods.

NEUROMUSCULAR JUNCTION DISORDERS

Myasthenia gravis (MG) and Lambert–Eaton myasthenic syndrome (LEMS) cause weakness through disrupted neuromuscular transmission. Less common are botulism (resembles Guillain–Barré syndrome (GBS)) and hypermagnesaemia (resembles LEMS and seen in renal patients given magnesium laxatives or eclampsia patients given magnesium).

Acetylcholine binds, allowing sodium ion inflow to muscle fibres (Fig. 11.2a). If sufficient acetylcholine is released and there are enough acetylcholine receptors, then the inflowing sodium ions take the muscle membrane potential above threshold, depolarizing the muscle with contraction. Acetylcholine release is calcium dependent; calcium influx is temporary and diffuses away in 100–200 msec.

If the motor nerve is repeatedly excited (repetitive stimulation), acetylcholine (quanta) release reaches its nadir at the fifth stimulus (Fig. 11.2b). Then secondary vesicle stores are mobilized, halting the decline. The muscle membrane and endplate potential (EPP) change with the amounts of acetylcholine released but still exceed the threshold potential; thus, muscle action potentials are still initiated. This is the safety margin (the ratio between EPP and the threshold for action potential initiation).

Whatever causes the neuromuscular pathology (pre- or post-synaptic) the safety margin is reduced since either insufficient acetylcholine is released (pre-synaptic) or there are too few receptors (post-synaptic) (Fig. 11.2c). Thus, the threshold for action potential initiation is not always exceeded and sometimes muscle contraction fails. Since the EPP naturally declines on the fifth in a series of repetitive stimuli, more myofibres within a muscle will fail at approximately the fifth stimulus (see normal physiology). As myofibres drop out, the compound muscle action (sum of all myofibres) potential declines; this manifests as the decremental response of LEMS, MG or botulism.

The LEMS antibody is directed against the calcium channel; insufficient calcium accumulates to ensure acetylcholine vesicles are released (Fig. 11.2d). The calcium diffuses away after 100–200 msec, but following maximum voluntary contraction or rapid stimulation (stimuli arriving at <100–200 msec intervals, i.e. 5–10 Hz) there is insufficient time for calcium to diffuse. Calcium therefore accumulates, increasing the vesicle numbers released, so increasing strength and CMAP size.

Myasthenia gravis (MG)

MG is not rare (prevalence 1:10 000, equivalent to MND in the over 60s). Both sexes have a bimodal age of onset; females more commonly have onset aged 15–40 years and males between 50 and 70 years. The biggest obstacle to the diagnosis is omitting to think of it. MG is particularly under-diagnosed in the elderly. A recent study of 2000 people aged >60 years found 0.7% prevalence of anti-acetylcholine receptor (AChR) antibodies; half of those with positive antibodies had been labelled as stroke or TIA.

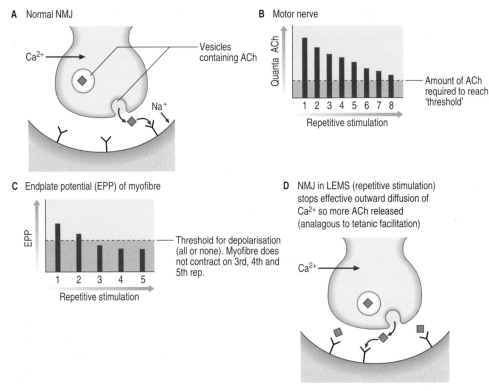

Figure 11.2

Disorders of neuromuscular junction. (a) Normal nerve–muscle junction (NMJ). Nerve–muscle junction with acetylcholine vesicles ('quanta'). (b) Normal physiology of motor nerve. (c) Endplate potential (EPP) of myofibre. (d) Potentiation. NMJ in Lambert–Eaton myasthenic syndrome (LEMS) (repetitive stimulation). Stops effective diffusion of Ca^{2+} so more ACh released (analogous to the effect of facilitation).

History

Myasthenia: The weakness distribution is 'top down'. Note symptoms of diurnal variability, diplopia, ptosis, dysarthria, dysphagia and dyspnoea. Enquire about ability to whistle, blow balloons, suck a straw or roll the tongue. Consider other autoimmune conditions, e.g. thyroid disease. The drug history should include penicillamine, anti-arrhythmics and antibiotics.

Note that in MG:

- Hoarseness and non-dysarthric whispering do not occur.
- Dysarthria almost invariably accompanies dysphagia.

LEMS: The diagnosis is frequently overlooked in the early stages. Patients describe non-specific variable proximal leg weakness. Ask whether hot weather/hot baths exacerbate weakness and whether patients feel paradoxically stronger after climbing stairs. Enquire about autonomic features (especially dry mouth, impotence and constipation), smoking history and symptoms suggesting lung cancer.

Note that in LEMS:

- Ptosis occurs but diplopia is rare.
- 'Myopathy' with dry mouth is characteristic.

Examination

External ocular muscle fatigue is assessed by looking upwards or sideways for 1 min.

Cogan's twitch sign. Ask patient to look down for 15 sec then rapidly re-fixate to primary position. Note overshoot of upper eyelid.

Ventilatory muscle function assessment is important, using vital capacity.

Swallowing. Dysphagia is assessed by observing swallowing (Box 11.2). There may be tongue wasting (triple furrowing).

Limbs. Repeated strength testing of one muscle group (e.g. shoulder abduction) identifies decrement in MG but increment in LEMS. Note that limb fatigue also accompanies other neurological conditions (e.g. MND). MG and LEMS usually have no limb muscle wasting or sensory loss. Reflexes are normal or brisk in MG; LEMS reflexes are initially absent but can be potentiated (post-tetanic facilitation), e.g. by exercising one arm or leg whilst resting the other.

Differential diagnosis

Other neuromuscular junction disorders:

- Drug induced (penicillamine: seen in rheumatoid patients and associated with HLA DR1).
- LEMS.
- Botulism.
- Hypermagnesaemia.

Eye movement disorders:

- **Dysthyroid eye disease** (may co-exist). Consider forced duction test (performed by ophthalmologists – corneal forceps are used to pull eye in various directions – limitation suggests fibrosis of ocular muscles (rarely done now), imaging the orbits for muscle enlargement, thyroid function and antibodies.
- **Chronic external ophthalmoplegia.** Includes mitochondrial cytopathy (look for other features) and oculopharyngeal muscular dystrophy. Patients experience little diplopia despite the profound ophthalmoplegia, because the brain accommodates for decreased eye movement.
- **Brainstem** (especially midbrain) lesion can mimic fatiguable external ophthalmoplegia. Consider brain imaging in antibody-negative ocular MG.
- **Blepharospasm** patients have no diplopia; eye closure is forced with lower lid elevation.

Natural history

Ocular MG. 15% remain as ocular MG. However, 50% of initially ocular MG become generalized within 2 years.

Remission. MG rarely now runs its natural course; 10–20% achieve spontaneous remission for >1 year in older series. The clinical course broadly divides into 3 stages:

1. Active 1st stage (0–7 years). The extent of weakness is usually apparent in the first 3–7 years; there may be considerable lability.
2. Inactive 2nd stage (10 years). Late exacerbations are possible.
3. Burnt out 3rd stage.

Crisis. Respiratory crisis occurs in 15–20%.

Mortality has fallen from 80% in the 1950s to 4% by the 1990s.

Exacerbating factors include surgery, radiotherapy, stress, intercurrent illness, temperature extremes and several drugs, e.g. anti-arrhythmics, some antibiotics, neuromuscular blocking agents, thyroid, cimetidine and lithium.

Pregnancy. 20% improve, 20% worsen and 60% are unchanged; 30% worsen after delivery. The uterus (smooth muscle) is unaffected, but skeletal muscles are used during delivery. Steroids and anticholinesterase medications are safe in pregnancy; plasma exchange and intravenous immunoglobulin (IVIg) are sometimes used.

Investigations

- Immune features:
  - **Acetylcholine receptor (AChR) antibodies** occur in 85% of patients overall, but only 50% of ocular MG. The titre does not correlate with disease severity.
  - **Striated muscle antibodies** strongly predict thymoma in those aged <50 years (99% of thymoma patients have these antibodies, but also 30% of those without).
  - **Anti-titin antibodies and anti-ryanodine antibodies** also accompany thymoma. Anti-ryanodine titres correlate with MG severity.
  - **AChR antibody-negative MG.** 70% of seronegative generalized MG patients have a muscle-specific receptor tyrosine kinase (MuSK). Antibody-negative patients have more bulbar and respiratory problems than antibody-positive MG.
- Imaging:
  - Anterior mediastinum for thymoma.
- Associated conditions:
  - Check thyroid, B_{12} etc.
- Electrophysiological confirmation:
  - Increased jitter on single fibre EMG and decrement on repetitive stimulation.
- Pharmacological confirmation.

A positive Tensilon® test (edrophonium chloride) is dramatic. First, identify a reliable measure, e.g. ptosis. Perform the test on a ward with cardiac monitor and resuscitation equipment available in case of bradycardia or asystole. Atropine is given first (500 µg); then Tensilon® 2 mg and finally the remaining 8 mg.

Management

Anticholinesterases

Pyridostigmine 30 mg q.d.s. initially, maximum 360 mg/day. The effect peaks after 1 h and wears off 2–3 h later. Liquid pyridostigmine is useful, via nasogastric tube if unable to swallow. Intramuscular neostigmine can be used for myasthenic crisis. Propantheline 15 mg t.d.s. may prevent unwanted muscarinic effects, e.g. abdominal cramps and diarrhoea.

Intravenous immunoglobulin and plasma exchange

Plasma exchange (5 daily exchanges) or IVIg (0.4 g/kg for 5 days, start 25 ml/h, maximum 150 ml/h) give useful short-term benefit, particularly in myasthenic crisis, or pre-operatively for thymectomy in those with VC <2 L. Treatment works within 4–5 days and lasts for 5–6 weeks. IVIg and plasma exchange give similar benefit, although IVIg is more easily administered. If IVIg fails to improve, consider plasma exchange.

Corticosteroids

Benefit usually appears by 2–4 weeks, but beware of initial worsening within the first 10 days. If time allows, start a low dose (5 mg alternate days, increased in 10 mg steps every 5–10 days) to avoid worsening and to identify the lowest beneficial dose. Many neurologists admit patients with generalized myasthenia for initiation of steroids (steroids deplete ACh levels). Some 30% have a drug-dependent, symptom-free remission; a further 50% have significant improvement. Some surgeons avoid corticosteroids before thymectomy because of thymus involution and poor wound healing. Tapering should be slow; when symptom free for 1 month, reduce by 5 mg on alternate days each month, until on 20 mg alternate days. Review and further reduce by 2.5 mg monthly until on 10 mg alternate days. Most patients need a maintenance dose, but consider further reductions by 1 mg/month. Monitor the serum glucose and give bone protection prophylaxis.

Azathioprine

This takes >3 months for benefit to begin, maximal at 1–3 years. It is best avoided in women wanting pregnancy (fetal skeletal teratogenicity) or those with a malignancy history. 10–20% patients develop severe 'flu-like symptoms (so test thiopurine methyl transferase levels prior to introduction). Baseline bloods include full blood count, liver function, serum amylase and are repeated weekly during dose escalation. Start 50 mg daily, increased by 50 mg weekly to 2–3 mg/kg. Bone marrow depression, liver abnormalities and pancreatitis are dose-related side-effects. If liver enzyme levels double or a lymphopenia of $<2.8 \times 10^9$ develops, lower the dose. A raised MCV is normal with compliance.

Other immunosuppression

These include mycophenolate, methotrexate, cyclophosphamide and cyclosporin.

Thymectomy

This should be considered in MG patients with either:

- **Thymoma.** This accompanies 10% of MG. Surgery is essential but will not improve the MG.
- **All three of:**
  1. **Generalized MG.**
  2. **Anti-AChR antibodies** (thymectomy in anti-MuSK patients awaits assessment).
  3. **Aged <45 years:** with age the thymus involutes and surgical complications rise.

Patients may deteriorate immediately following thymectomy, so pre-operative FVC is essential. Improvement peaks after months or years (even 20 years). Some 25% remit within 3 years and a further 50% significantly improve.

Lambert–Eaton myasthenic syndrome

Causes: One-third are auto-immune but two-thirds are paraneoplastic (especially small cell lung carcinoma). Most precede tumour identification by a median of 1 year (can be up to 5 years).

Prevalence: One-tenth as common as MG.

Clinical features: Proximal lower limb weakness with reduced reflexes (80% show reflex potentiation). Autonomic symptoms include dry mouth (75%), impotence and constipation. Cranial nerves are much less prominently involved than MG.

Diagnosis: >90% of LEMS have anti-voltage-gated calcium channel antibodies. Electrophysiology findings are characteristic (Fig. 11.2d).

Management: 3,4-diaminopyridine (10 mg b.d., increased as tolerated to 20 mg q.d.s.); adverse effects include pins and needles and seizures. If control is incomplete in autoimmune LEMS, consider steroids and azathioprine.

Botulism

Botulism (*botulus*: sausage), named following a Southern Germany outbreak from tainted sausages in the 1700s. The toxin produced by the Gram-positive rod impairs acetylcholine release.

Common sources are wounds (i.v. drug users) or toxin ingestion in food. Symptoms appear after 1–3 days.

Clinical features: The most important distinction is from GBS.

- **Weakness pattern.** Botulism is 'top down': diplopia, ptosis, blurred vision, dysarthria and dysphagia precede limb weakness. GBS is often 'bottom up': only 10% of GBS have ophthalmoplegia although >50% have facial weakness. However, some GBS variants, particularly with GT1a antibodies, mimic top down spread and may have normal CSF protein.
- **Internal ophthalmoplegia** (fixed dilated pupils) may not be present in up to 50% of botulism cases.

- **Sensory problems.** None in botulism, but may be prominent in GBS.
- **Gag reflex** may be preserved in botulism despite the weakness.
- **Respiratory involvement** may not correlate with limb weakness in botulism, whereas most GBS patients needing ventilation have marked limb weakness.

Diagnostic tests include electrophysiology, biological assay (mouse neutralization test) with samples from serum, stool or food injected intraperitoneally (with and without anti-toxin or boiling inoculate as controls). Toxin is found in the serum in 30% of patients and culture is often undertaken with the supernatant from broth culture tested for toxin.

MOTOR NEURONE DISEASE

Motor neurone disease (MND) or amyotrophic lateral sclerosis (ALS) has a variable clinical presentation. The core features are a progressive motor problem with both upper and lower motor neurone features. There are no significant sensory symptoms, although some patients describe pain. Sphincter and extra-ocular muscles are generally unaffected. Some 10% are familial (usually autosomal dominant) but with a poor genotype–phenotype relationship and incomplete penetrance; prospective genetic testing is rarely possible.

Clinical subtypes

Onset may be bulbar (20%), upper limb (40%) or lower limb (40%).

- **Progressive muscular atrophy** accounts for 10%, although most eventually develop upper motor neurone signs. Survival is usually longer than in ALS.
- **Primary lateral sclerosis** is a pure upper motor neurone syndrome. Lower motor neurone signs (if they appear) do so by 5 years after onset. Bladder involvement may occur. Survival may be up to 20 years.

The relationship of MND to malignancy is controversial. There probably are rare associations between rapidly progressive MND with anti-*Hu* antibodies and primary lateral sclerosis with breast cancer.

History

Enquire about cramps, fasciculations, foot drop, breathlessness and pointers to frontal lobe dysfunction (behaviour change, etc). Ask for a family history.

Examination

Lower motor neurone (LMN): Fasciculations (including tongue), wasting in groups outside a single myotome. Facial fasciculations characterize Kennedy's syndrome.

Upper motor neurone (UMN): increased tone, clonus, loss of dexterity, brisk tendon reflexes (or preserved reflexes in wasted and/or fasciculating muscle), loss of superficial abdominal reflexes (may be retained), Babinski sign.

Frontal lobe dementia features (see Ch. 6).

The El Escorial criteria are principally for research purposes (see below). There is nothing to be gained in practice by labelling patients as 'probable' or 'possible', but the criteria do encourage a systematic clinical analysis. MND often (50%) has mild (sub-clinical) cognitive problems; 5% develop a significant frontotemporal dementia (see Ch. 6).

El escorial criteria for MND

- Definite:
  - UMN and LMN signs in three regions (from bulbar, cervical, thoracic, lumbosacral).
- Probable:
  - UMN signs and LMN signs in two regions, with some UMN signs rostral to LMN signs.
  - UMN signs in 1 region, with LMN signs (or EMG features) in at least 2 regions.
- Possible:
  - UMN together with LMN signs in one region.
  - UMN signs in two or more regions.
  - UMN and LMN signs in two regions, with no UMN signs rostral to LMN signs.

Differential diagnosis

Some 10% of patients are misdiagnosed in neurological practice.

Major

- **Cervical spondylotic myelopathy** and other degenerative vertebral disease (but the signs are confined to one myotome and with sensory features).
- **Foramen magnum/high cervical cord lesions**: pyramidal problems and sometimes wasted tongue and wasted hands. Joint position sense may be reduced in the fingers much more than the toes.
- **Chronic inflammatory demyelinating polyneuropathy (CIDP) and multi-focal motor neuropathy with conduction block** (2% of 'MND' cases in specialist centres): a rare but treatable cause that must not be missed.
- **Inclusion body myositis** (with an odd pattern of distal wasting and weakness in an elderly person).
- **Myasthenia gravis** because MND also has variability and fatigue at its onset; fasciculations may complicate anticholinesterase treatment.
- **Kennedy's disease** (X-linked bulbo-spinal neuronopathy) is caused by a CAG repeat on the androgen receptor. Clinical features include facial fasciculations, gynaecomastia and sensory symptoms. Electrophysiology shows denervation with small sensory potentials.

Less common

- Benign fasciculation syndrome. EMG shows no denervation and the condition does not progress.
- LEMS.

- Spinal muscular atrophy.
- Sjögren's syndrome.
- Hyperparathyroidism.
- Hyperthyroidism (Basedow's disease).
- Insulinoma (wasted hands).
- Fungal meningitis.
- Carcinomatous meningitis.
- Poliomyelitis.
- Hexosaminidase deficiency (Sandhoff's disease) may resemble MND or Friedreich's ataxia.
- Brown–Vialetto–van Laere (bulbar problems with deafness).

Investigations

Bloods. Full blood count, ESR, thyroid function, calcium, glucose, liver and renal function, CK, autoantibody screen. In MND with a serum paraprotein (up to 9% of cases) re-examine the nerve conduction: is there a hint of neuropathy?

MRI brain or cervical spine should be considered if there is any diagnostic doubt (e.g. degenerative back disease, foramen magnum lesion). Sometimes MRI shows pre-central gyrus atrophy (especially primary lateral sclerosis) or corticospinal tract signal change.

Chest radiograph for underlying malignancy.

Nerve conduction and EMG. Small amplitude and duration with excess of phases owing to decreased muscle fibre density. A similar pattern occurs with neuromuscular block or early re-innervation. Fibrillation and positive sharp waves are spontaneously firing motor units present whenever motor fibres lose contact with axons (e.g. in denervation) or are disconnected by segmental muscle necrosis (e.g. in inflammatory myopathies).

CSF. The protein is sometimes raised but if significantly raised, consider CIDP. The cell count should be normal; excess cells suggest malignant infiltration (lymphoma).

Management

Care is multidisciplinary; good communication between health care professionals and with the patient is essential. MND specialist nurses play a pivotal role. The neurologists' role is to make the diagnosis, communicate this to the patient, to prescribe appropriate medication and to decide with the patient on interventions such as gastrostomy or non-invasive ventilation (see below).

Giving the diagnosis

These are broad guidelines to help the process. Each consultation will differ and it is important to be sensitive to react appropriately to the patient.

- The diagnosis should be certain with investigations complete.
- The doctor giving the news should know the patient.

- Arrange a quiet, private room with enough time set aside for the discussion; everyone should be at the same level, usually seated.
- People usually present are the doctor, the patient, a nurse (MND nurse) and a close family member (usually partner), with the patient's agreement.
- Review the symptoms and investigations with the patient.
- State the diagnosis clearly; a diagram may help. Emphasize that although there is no cure, the disease may be inactive for some time, there are treatments for many symptoms and that riluzole can slow the disease.
- A range of survival estimates (2–5 years) can be given if the patient asks.
- Arrange for further discussion and follow-up.
- Give written information and advise about patient associations (e.g. website: http.www. mndassociation.org).
- Inform the general practitioner.

Riluzole

Riluzole, a benzothiazole derivative that inhibits glutamate release, is the only approved disease-modifying medication for MND. A Cochrane review reported that riluzole 100 mg daily modestly increased survival (median 2 months). Side-effects are uncommon but can include liver abnormalities: check liver function at 1, 2, 3, 6 and 9 months and then annually. There are no data that riluzole improves quality of life.

Gastrostomy

Percutaneous endoscopic gastrostomy (PEG) can prolong life in MND by up to 8 months. **Consider if:**

- Poor oral intake with significant bulbar problems.
- Failed swallowing assessment.
- Weight loss (>10% body weight) despite supplements.

Contraindications:

- Patient declines intervention.
- Survival >3 months is unlikely.
- Cannot manage feeds (e.g. no carer).

Assess respiratory function before deciding upon gastrostomy. A radiologically inserted gastrostomy (RIG) is preferable with FVC <50% normal. Non-invasive ventilation may be introduced before RIG if there is respiratory insufficiency. A nasogastric tube is a useful temporary solution (maximum for 6–8 weeks).

Other palliative aspects

Involve the palliative care team early.

Communication aids. It is important to involve speech and language therapy specialists. Writing, communication boards, Lightwriters, voice amplifiers may be useful.

Emotional lability with pseudobulbar palsy: consider amitriptyline or citalopram.

Pain may result from immobility, spasticity, or cramps. Re-take the history and treat appropriately.

Sialorrhoea. Hyoscine patches or glycopyrrolate (injected if necessary) are useful. Salivary gland irradiation or botulinum toxin injections are alternatives. Thick sputum sometimes responds to β-blockers.

Respiratory distress. Oral morphine or benzodiazepines are useful and used at the minimum effective dose.

Case history outcome

The diagnosis was MG (which often mimics 3rd nerve palsies and internuclear ophthalmoplegias). On Tensilon® testing the ptosis improved dramatically; anti-AChR antibody was positive, CT thorax excluded thymoma and electrophysiology showed a decrement in the weak deltoid muscle (normal in hand muscles). MR brain scan was not indicated. She responded well to pyridostigmine (with propantheline) without steroids.

KEY POINTS

- Do not rely solely on CK to diagnose a muscle condition; CK is often moderately raised in neurogenic disease.
- Check for fatiguable weakness; remember myasthenia mimics many eye movement disorders.
- Check respiratory function in all neuromuscular disease; patients will not always look in distress.
- Do not do a Tensilon® test if there is doubt about the patient's fitness; do the test on the ward and have a clear objective measure, e.g. improvement in ptosis.
- Investigate myopathy thoroughly before committing to treatment; biopsy, electrophysiology, bloods and (if appropriate) exclude underlying neoplasm or connective tissue disease.
- Consider cardiac and ventilatory muscle involvement, especially with inflammatory myopathies.
- Giving MND diagnosis: be certain of the diagnosis, set time aside, ensure you know the patient, results are available and complete and the appropriate people are with you.
- Question MND diagnosis (up to 10% are wrongly diagnosed); particularly consider multi-focal motor neuropathy with block.
- Consider cerebral imaging for isolated ocular and antibody-negative MG.
- Remember potential anaesthetic risks with some muscle conditions.

Further Reading

Polkey M, Lyall R, Moxam J, Leigh PN. Respiratory aspects of neurological disease. J Neurol Neurosurg Psychiatry 1999; 66: 5–15.

Neuropathy and radiculopathy

Case history

A 24-year-old woman presented with a 1-week history of progressive quadriparesis and distal sensory disturbance. She had been on a diet and had lost 15 kg in the previous 6 weeks. Four years earlier, during her first pregnancy, she had developed very similar symptoms complicated by type 2 respiratory failure necessitating admission to the intensive care unit (ICU). She was treated with plasma exchange and made a partial recovery although she had a residual foot drop. There was no family history of neurological illness. On examination, she had anosmia, pes cavus and optic disc pallor. She had bilateral sensory neural deafness. There was evidence of a severe quadriplegia with absence of deep tendon reflexes. Plantar responses were flexor. Sensory examination revealed loss of pinprick and light touch sensation in the hands and feet with more modest impairment of distal vibration sensation and proprioception.

INTRODUCTION

Peripheral neuropathies affect 2–8% of the population, the higher prevalence being among older age groups. Although there are many causes of neuropathy and many with unknown causes, most are distal sensorimotor axonal neuropathies from metabolic or toxic causes. The extent of necessary investigation depends upon the clinical presentation and likely cause.

CLINICAL ASSESSMENT

A thorough history and examination remain essential to establishing the cause and in tailoring investigations logically. Sensorimotor axonal neuropathies present with:

- Distal sensory symptoms often confined to the feet.
- Distal weakness and wasting, often confined to toes or feet.
- Loss of ankle reflexes.

Symptoms

Sensory and motor neuropathic symptoms may be positive or negative. Positive symptoms suggest an acquired rather than a symptomatic cause.

- **Positive** sensory features include pins and needles; positive motor features include fasciculations.
- **Negative** symptoms are characterized by loss of function, e.g. numbness or weakness.

Signs

Lower motor neurone features dominate the examination: wasting, no increase in tone, absent reflexes and flexor plantar responses. It is important to spot atypical neuropathies, e.g. chronic inflammatory demyelinating polyneuropathy (CIDP) in diabetic patients. The clinician should therefore address several questions when suspecting a neuropathy.

Is this a neuropathy?

This is not always a simple question. Myelopathy symptoms superficially resemble neuropathy, both presenting with distal sensory disturbance. Distinguishing acute myelopathy from acute neuropathy (particularly Guillain–Barré syndrome (GBS)) may be difficult:

Back pain occurs in both myelopathy and GBS.

- **Limb examination.** Tone, reflexes and plantar responses usually give the correct answer. However, note that acute myelopathy with spinal shock may not show increased tone and reflexes that develop later.
- **Cranial nerve signs.** Facial weakness, neck flexion weakness (particularly useful) and even ophthalmoplegia (10% of GBS) are against myelopathy.
- **Normal bladder function.** If there is sphincter involvement, myelopathy is much more likely.
- **Distal-only sensory features.** Mild distal sensory features are typical of GBS (though not of all acute neuropathies). There is no sensory level or significant proximal sensory symptoms, other than back pain.

What was the speed of onset?

This helps with differential diagnosis and in directing investigations.

- **Acute:** <4 weeks. Box 12.1 lists the main causes of acute neuropathy. In acute weakness, it is important to exclude potassium, magnesium and phosphate abnormalities. Note that vasculitis may give a hyper-acute presentation.
- **Sub-acute:** 1–3 months. The main cause is CIDP and its variants (see below).
- **Chronic:** >3 months. This is the most common onset and has a very broad differential diagnosis.

Box 12.1: Causes of acute neuropathy

- Guillain–Barré syndrome.
- Porphyria.
- Vasculitis.
- Diphtheria.
- Critical illness neuropathy.
- Infections, e.g. HIV, Lyme disease.
- Toxins, e.g. amiodarone, nitrofurantoin.
- Alcohol.

What is the pattern?

The main distinction is between:

- **Symmetrical and distal.** The most common pattern with a very large differential diagnosis.
- **Multifocal.** Box 12.2 lists the common causes of multiple mononeuropathy (mononeuritis multiplex).

Unusual distributions may also give clues, e.g. radiculopathies are associated with diabetes mellitus and facial sensory loss is associated with Sjögren's syndrome.

Sensory, motor or both?

Note that loss of reflexes generally implies a sensory component unless the patient is very weak with only a flicker of movement. Box 12.3 lists the causes of predominantly motor neuropathies.

Which sensory fibres are affected?

Small fibre neuropathies

These patients report burning discomfort rather than pins and needles. Sensory loss is to pin-prick rather than to joint position or vibration. Box 12.4 lists the common causes of small fibre neuropathy. Small unmyelinated axons outnumber large fibres four-fold, warm perception is mediated by type C unmyelinated fibres (conduction velocity 2 m/s); Aδ are small myelinated fibres that are the main afferents for cold perception (velocity about 20 m/s).

Note: Small fibre peripheral neuropathy is difficult to diagnose with certainty because the reflexes may be preserved and nerve conduction studies may be normal.

Box 12.2: *Multifocal mononeuropathies (mononeuritis multiplex)*

1. Vasculitis.
2. Infections, e.g. leprosy, HIV, Lyme disease.
3. Diabetes mellitus.
4. Hereditary liability to pressure palsies.
5. Some forms of CIDP.
6. Amyloidosis.
7. Sarcoidosis.

Box 12.3: *Motor neuropathies*

- Lead poisoning.
- Diabetes (diabetic amyotrophy).
- Multi-focal motor neuropathy with conduction block.
- Charcot–Marie–Tooth disease.
- Drugs, e.g. dapsone.

Box 12.4: Small fibre peripheral neuropathies

- **Idiopathic.** Some have an inflammatory autoimmune basis.
- **Diabetes mellitus.**
- **Erythromelalgia.** Episodic limb burning when standing, walking or with heat. It may be inherited or associated with connective tissue disease, essential thrombocythaemia and diabetes mellitus. The disorder might reflect C fibre sensitization to a lower temperature than normal.
- **Tangier disease.**
- **Fabry's disease.**
- **Sjögren's disease.** The neuropathy may precede sicca symptoms: check SS-A, SS-B, Schirmer test and consider lip (minor salivary gland) biopsy.
- **Amyloidosis** is suspected if the neuropathy starts as small fibre and progresses to large fibre with autonomic dysfunction.
- **HIV disease.**
- **Drugs,** particularly metronidazole.
- **Alcohol.**
- **Hereditary sensory and autonomic neuropathy** (types 1 to 5):
  1. Autosomal dominant disorder of serine palmitoyltransferase is rare.
  2. Autosomal recessive, childhood onset.
  3. Riley–Day syndrome is more common in Ashkenazi Jews and is characterized by postural hypotension, lack of tears but not sweat and impaired pain and temperature sensation.
  4. Congenital insensitivity to pain and anhidrosis, fever, autosomal recessive.
  5. Infantile onset, papillary involvement, nociceptive failure, autosomal recessive.

Large fibre neuropathies

These patients present with sensory ataxia, from loss of normal position sense (see below). The lesion is either in the large sensory fibres (e.g. in GBS) or in the dorsal root ganglion cells through immune or paraneoplastic phenomenon (neuronopathy). Box 12.5 lists the main causes of sensory ataxia.

Axonal or demyelinating?

Box 12.6 gives the common causes of demyelinating neuropathy. There are several clinical pointers to a demyelinating neuropathy including:

Box 12.5: Sensory ataxia causes

- CIDP.
- Paraneoplastic.
- Sjögren's syndrome.
- Pyridoxine (large amounts).
- Chemotherapy agents.

Box 12.6: Demyelinating neuropathies

- Genetic, e.g. CMT type 1, Refsum's disease.
- Guillain–Barré syndrome.
- CIDP (remember to check for paraproteins).
- Drugs, e.g. amiodarone.
- Some mitochondrial cytopathies (SANDO).

- Weakness without wasting, though many chronic demyelinating neuropathies also have wasting due to associated axonal damage.
- Weakness is both distal and proximal.
- Widespread loss of reflexes.
- Early loss of vibration sense, although other sensory modalities may also be affected.

Note: Electrophysiology is needed if demyelinating neuropathy is likely.

Is there an obvious cause?

- **The history** should include general medical points and particularly previous drug and toxin exposure.
- **The general examination** should include a search for alcoholic liver disease, diabetic retinopathy or ulcer, rash from vasculitis. More subtle signs are the rash of Fabry's disease, or the enlarged orange tonsils of Tangier disease.
- **Neurological examination** should include olfactory testing (reduced in B_{12} deficiency or Refsum's (Fig. 12.1) disease), nerve palpation (thickened in amyloidosis, Charcot–Marie–Tooth disease, neurofibromatosis and leprosy) and looking for pes cavus (implies a longstanding, often hereditary problem, from aged <14 years, when the feet were still growing (Fig. 12.2)).

Box 12.7 lists the common genetic neuropathies.

Is there autonomic involvement?

Perform a lying and standing blood pressure and pulse rate, looking for evidence of orthostatic hypotension.

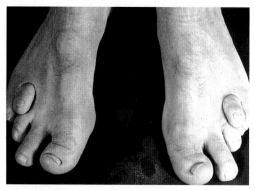

Figure 12.1
Syndactyly in Refsum's disease.

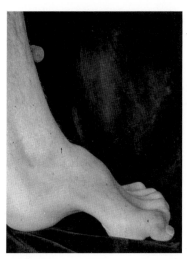

Figure 12.2
Pes cavus.

Box 12.7: *Common hereditary neuropathies*

- **Type 1 demyelinating**. 70% are caused by duplication of the peripheral myelin protein 22 (PMP-22) on chromosome 17 (17 p11.2).
- **Hereditary neuropathy with liability to pressure palsy** is caused by the deletion of the same portion of chromosome 17 and presents with recurrent mononeuropathy episodes that tend to recover quickly.
- **X-linked Charcot–Marie–Tooth disease (CMT-X)** is caused by a connexin-32 gene mutation. Affected males may have a demyelinating neuropathy, whereas females tend to have a milder axonal pattern. Sometimes it may be patchy and even mimic CIDP.

INVESTIGATIONS

With so many causes of neuropathy, there are many potential investigations. These should be guided by the clinical findings. Many patients require only simple blood tests, with more detailed tests reserved for particular clinical situations. Figure 12.3 summarizes the approach to investigating neuropathy.

Simple tests

Simple blood tests and urine dipstick assessment may be all that is required for patients with typical clinical presentations of distal sensory or sensorimotor neuropathy who are diabetic, or who have a history of alcoholism or drugs exposure. Electrophysiology may be unnecessary. More tests are needed when the pattern is not a standard distal sensorimotor neuropathy. Blood tests should include full blood count, ESR, serum B_{12}, random glucose, thyroid, liver and renal function tests, anti-nuclear antibody and serum protein electrophoresis. All

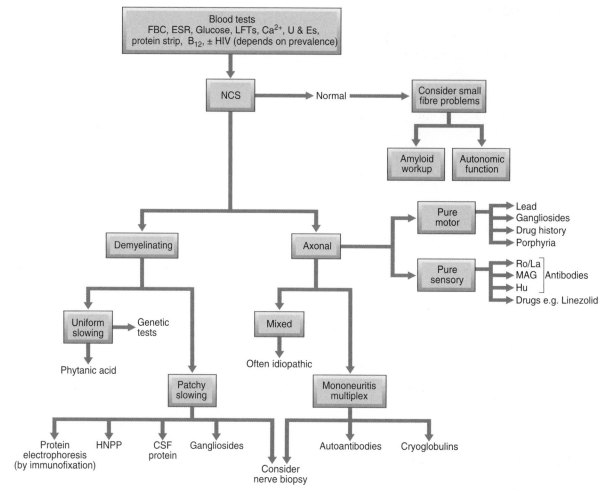

Figure 12.3
Investigating a peripheral neuropathy.

patients with 'cryptogenic' axonal neuropathies should have a glucose tolerance test and protein electrophoresis performed on an annual basis.

Detailed tests

These are best undertaken after consultation with a physician or neurologist with an interest in peripheral neuropathy.

Electrophysiology

This is important in atypical cases to confirm the diagnosis, severity, diffuse or multifocal nature of the neuropathy and to determine whether the neuropathy is demyelinating or axonal.

Cerebrospinal fluid

This may be useful in diagnosing CIDP or GBS. A CSF pleocytosis raises the possibility of infection, including HIV neuropathy or Lyme disease.

Nerve biopsy

This requires careful patient selection. It is most often undertaken to confirm or exclude vasculitis. A prospective study reported that the sural nerve biopsy changed the diagnosis in 7/50 patients; in 35 the suspected diagnosis was confirmed; in eight, the result was non-contributory. Overall, the biopsy helped the management in 60%. However, one-third of patients had persistent sensory problems at the biopsy site.

MANAGEMENT (GENERAL)

General measures. Physiotherapy may benefit patients by preventing contractures and helping to maintain independence. Foot care is essential particularly specialist fitting of shoes and orthoses. Patient organizations can help, support and advise:

- The Neuropathy Association (http://www.neuropathy.org).
- Guillain–Barré Syndrome Foundation International (http://guillain-barre.com).
- Charcot Marie–Tooth Association (http://www.charcot-marie-tooth.org).

Neuropathic pain remains a challenge; drugs can reduce the pain intensity by 30–40%. Table 12.1 shows several useful medications for neuropathic pain.

THE PATIENT WITH ACUTE ONSET WEAKNESS

Clinicians are commonly confronted by a patient with weak arms and legs, perhaps with facial or other cranial nerve weakness, with an onset over hours to days. There are various causes listed below, to consider before jumping to a diagnosis of GBS.

Table 12.1: Medications for neuropathic pain

Medication	Example	Dose	Side-effects	Number needed to treat
Anticonvulsants	Gabapentin	300–3600 mg	Drowsiness, dizziness, caution with renal failure	4.1
Antidepressants	Amitriptyline	10–100 mg	Anticholinergic effects, cardiac arrhythmias, orthostatic hypotension, weight gain	2.6
Opiates	Tramadol		Constipation, confusion, nausea, seizures	3.4
Topical agents	Capsaicin (0.075%)	Topically 3–4 times daily	Often limited by pain on application	5.9

Myopathy

- Inflammatory causes may have surprisingly abrupt onset.
- Toxins, e.g. colchicine in renal failure.
- Metabolic, e.g. potassium, phosphate, calcium, (selenium): check these serum concentrations in weak patients.

Neuromuscular junction disorder

- Myasthenia gravis gives a facio-bulbar weakness with ophthalmoplegia.
- Botulism: consider in 'top down' Guillain–Barré. Botulism may have autonomic features including internal ophthalmoplegia.
- Lambert–Eaton myasthenic syndrome more often presents as proximal limb weakness and resembles myopathy.
- Magnesium may disrupt the neuromuscular junction.

Neuropathy

- Guillain–Barré syndrome. Note that with lymphocyte pleocytosis, consider infection e.g. HIV.
- Diphtheria.
- Vasculitis.
- Drugs, e.g. amiodarone, nitrofurantoin.
- Porphyria.

Myelopathy and motor neurone disease

- **Back pain and areflexia** do not reliably distinguish GBS from acute myelopathy (Box 12.8).
- **Flaccid paraplegia** may characterize many acute myelopathies at their onset, e.g. acute transverse myelopathy.
- **Sensory symptoms** make myopathy and neuromuscular disease less likely, but note that acute neuromyopathy is still possible, e.g. sarcoidosis, colchicine toxicity.

Clinical evaluation of acute weakness

It can be deceptively difficult to recognize early weakness. GBS is often mistaken in casualty for hyperventilation or hysteria if there are only early distal sensory symptoms.

Box 12.8: Distinguishing GBS from myelopathy

Both may have back pain and reduced reflexes.
- Facial weakness favours GBS.
- Neck flexion weakness favours GBS.
- Sphincter involvement favours a myelopathy.
- Proximal sensory loss favours myelopathy.
- Upper motor neurone signs obviously favour myelopathy.
If there is doubt, image the cord.

- **Functional assessment.** Can the patient walk on their heels, toes or up a flight of stairs?
- **Review after a short interval** is useful, especially to reassess the reflexes: in GBS they quickly disappear.
- **Blood tests.** Check the serum potassium, phosphate and magnesium.
- **Consider early myelopathy** (Box 12.8). It is better to do an unnecessary scan than to miss early cord compression.
- **Beware top-down GBS.** Early facial weakness, bulbar weakness, dilated fixed pupils (blurred vision), minimal limb weakness but significant respiratory weakness might suggest botulism, particularly with a history of intravenous drug use.
- **Acute intermittent porphyria** has CSF changes similar to GBS (see below). Consider this especially if GBS ever seems to recur.

SPECIFIC NEUROPATHIES

No cause found

Despite all efforts, 20% of neuropathies remain undiagnosed. Some are later found to have impaired glucose tolerance or diabetes mellitus. Patients with painful sensory neuropathies should have repeat glucose sampling and even an oral glucose tolerance test. The management of these patients is uncertain and is the subject of ongoing trials. Some patients with chronic idiopathic axonal neuropathies have higher serum triglycerides and more environmental toxin exposure than controls, but it is unclear currently whether this finding will help in treatment. Those without a clear diagnosis generally have a benign prognosis, but clinicians must nevertheless remain vigilant about progression. Paraneoplastic neuropathy and vasculitic neuropathy in particular are potentially treatable and although presenting indolently, tend to progress.

Diabetic neuropathy

Diabetes is the most common cause of neuropathy; there are several types:

- **Diabetic symmetric distal polyneuropathy** is the most common. It is usually associated with a retinopathy or nephropathy and dominated by sensory symptoms, e.g. feelings of heat (worse at night), 'feet wrapped in cotton wool', or tingling. Detailed investigation is unnecessary.
- **Diabetic lumbosacral radiculoplexus neuropathy** (diabetic amyotrophy, Bruns–Garland syndrome) is a nerve microvasculitis. It typically presents in males with type 2 diabetes, giving severe pain, worse at night, followed by asymmetric and predominantly proximal weakness and progressing over several weeks. It does recover slowly although not fully. Investigations should include serum creatine kinase and electrophysiology. Malignant infiltration of the lumbo-sacral plexus presents in a similar way, so consider CT pelvic imaging in atypical cases.
- **Multiple mononeuropathy.** Diabetic damage renders nerves vulnerable to injury. Diabetes itself may involve the vasa nervorum. Management is to control the underlying condition, protect pressure areas from further trauma and await improvement.

- **Autonomic neuropathy**. Mild degrees are common in diabetes; severe forms are troublesome with nocturnal diarrhoea, postural hypotension and syncope.

Guillain–Barré syndrome

Guillain–Barré syndrome, or acute demyelinating polyradiculoneuropathy, is the most common cause of acute generalized paralysis. The annual incidence is 1–2 cases per 100 000 per year.

Clinical features

The classical presentation is with an ascending paralysis with positive sensory symptoms and facial and bulbar involvement. Low back pain is very common and can be severe. Examination shows a symmetrical flaccid tetraparesis, often with bilateral facial and neck flexion weakness, reduced or absent deep tendon reflexes but only minimal sensory loss. In severe cases, there may be weakness of the ventilatory muscles, external ocular muscles and dysphagia. Autonomic dysfunction may occur with sphincter involvement and propensity to brady- and tachy-arrhythmias. Typically, the illness progresses over 1–3 weeks before plateauing and gradually improving. Complete recovery is usual but residual deficit and even death may occur.

Management

Careful clinical monitoring is absolutely essential, if necessary in an intensive care setting.

- **Specific treatments** include plasma exchange or immunoglobulin (IVIg). These reduce median time to walking unaided from 100 to 50 days and improve long-term disability at one year. It is uncertain whether treatment helps to treat mild cases or those presenting after two weeks. Treatment can be repeated after two weeks if there has been no improvement.
- **Respiratory muscle strength**. Vital capacity (VC) should be measured (normal 70 ml/kg body weight); consult ITU urgently if VC deteriorates quickly, or reaches <20 ml/kg, or if there is significant bulbar weakness. Ventilatory muscle strength usually reflects limb weakness in GBS: if the limbs are strong, respiratory function is usually good. Note that this is not true of other conditions, e.g. myasthenia gravis or botulism. GBS patients needing ventilation may require this for 1–3 months (mean 49 days).
- **Autonomic function**. Arrhythmic complications can occur in patients without severe weakness or respiratory muscle involvement. The ECG must be continuously monitored until there is clinical improvement or removal of tracheostomy. Sinus tachycardia is common but about 1 in 40 patients develop significant brady-arrhythmia or complete heart block, requiring pacing.
- **Physiotherapy**. Prevention of pressure sores and contractures is essential and too often overlooked; splinting is often needed. Fixed contractures appear quickly and may defeat an otherwise good functional outcome.

- **Antibiotics.** Over half of GBS patients develop chest infections. Antibiotics are indicated for purulent sputum, radiographic changes or significant sputum bacterial growth.
- **Anticoagulation.** Heparin is indicated as prophylaxis against deep venous thrombosis.
- **Bulbar function** is disturbed in 25–50%, especially in those with facial or neck flexion weakness. A preserved gag reflex is no guarantee against aspiration. A speech and language therapist should assess patients with suspected bulbar dysfunction.
- **Enteral nutrition.** Patients may require PEG feeding. It is also important to monitor their weight.
- **Neuropathic pain** may respond to gabapentin or to small doses of opiates, e.g. MST 10 mg once or twice daily.
- **Other complications** will be identified by meticulous daily review: hyponatraemia (common in ventilated patients) is best treated with fluid restriction; papilloedema reflecting high CSF protein may lead to visual loss and is best treated by repeat lumbar punctures.

Chronic inflammatory demyelinating neuropathy (CIDP)

CIDP is an acquired demyelinating neuropathy (or polyradiculoneuropathy). It is important because it is treatable yet potentially disabling. The incidence is 1–2 per 100 000 per year, with age of onset 40–60 years. CIDP presents as a chronic sensorimotor neuropathy, with onset over >2 months.

- **Motor features** are typically proximal and distal with widespread reflex loss. Motor problems predominate (20% are almost purely motor).
- **Sensory features** are less prominent (although 6% are purely sensory) and may need to be specifically sought. Sensory involvement is large fibre, causing paraesthesiae, which are sometimes painful.
- **Respiratory involvement** occurs in 15%, faciobulbar and even extraocular muscles are affected in 5–10%.

The diagnosis is confirmed electrophysiologically and with CSF.

- **Neurophysiology** reveals demyelination: look for any hint of this, as only 70% have 'barn-door' demyelination.
- **CSF** shows albuminocytological dissociation (high protein in 90% but <10 white cells per mm^3).
- **Nerve biopsy** is rarely needed: demyelination is found in only half and the biopsy is normal in 20%.

Chronic inflammatory demyelinating polyneuropathy (CIDP) variants

These are defined largely on clinical features.

- **CIDP with paraprotein.** Serum paraproteins should be checked in any neuropathy. Box 12.9 lists the common paraprotein-associated neuropathies. All patients with paraprotein-associated CIDP require specialist haematology review, screening for osteosclerotic bone lesions, urinary Bence-Jones protein, serum calcium and renal function.

> **Box 12.9: Neuropathies associated with a paraprotein**
>
> - Cryoglobulin neuropathy.
> - Amyloidosis. This typically gives a small fibre neuropathy with autonomic dysfunction.
> - Monoclonal gammopathy of uncertain significance (MGUS)-associated CIDP.
> - POEMS (polyneuropathy, organomegaly, endocrinopathy, M-proteins and skin changes) often has a low serum titre of lambda paraprotein and high CSF protein.
> - CIDP. 10–20% have a paraprotein:
>   - Those with IgA or IgG paraprotein-associated CIDP usually respond to immunomodulation.
>   - Those with IgM paraprotein-associated CIDP often have predominately distal demyelination and are unresponsive to immunomodulation.

- **CIDP with diabetes.** CIDP is more common in diabetes than in the general population. CIDP in diabetics should be suspected if there is significant weakness in proximal legs or arms, or sensory loss in the hands before sensory loss has reached the mid-thigh. Management is with immunoglobulins rather than steroids.
- **CIDP with other illness.** Several other conditions may have superimposed CIDP, e.g. chronic active hepatitis, inflammatory bowel disease, HIV, hereditary neuropathies.
- **Distal acquired demyelinating symmetric neuropathy (DADS):**
  - Paraprotein-associated DADS (DADS-M). Two-thirds of DADS patients have an IgM kappa paraprotein (anti-MAG). They are mostly male, in their sixth decade, with tremor and prominent sensory findings.
  - Idiopathic DADS (DADS-I). One-third of DADS patients have no paraprotein and no age or sex preponderance.
- **Multifocal motor neuropathy with block.** This important treatable imitator of motor neurone disease (MND) presents asymmetrically with focal weakness, often in the arm with localized fasciculations (not generalized like MND). Occasionally sensory symptoms occur without signs. The reflexes are preserved but not brisk. It is diagnosed electrophysiologically with motor block at sites not subject to compression and with normal sensory conduction through the same length of nerve. The CSF protein is normal. Patients may deteriorate on corticosteroids and so IVIg is used.
- **Multifocal acquired demyelinating sensory and motor neuropathy (MADSAM).** This condition, also known as the Lewis–Sumner syndrome, presents asymmetrically, again often with upper limb involvement and both sensory and motor problems. The CSF protein is raised in 80%. Most respond to either corticosteroids or IVIg.

Differential diagnosis

- **Guillain–Barré syndrome.** CIDP progresses for >2 months, whereas GBS reaches a nadir in <4 weeks.
- **X-linked Charcot–Marie–Tooth disease (CMT-X)** can resemble CIDP clinically, but without pain and paraesthesiae (rare symptoms in genetic motor neuropathies).

Management

- **Corticosteroids.** In classical CIDP, start prednisolone 1.5 mg/kg on alternate days, with appropriate bone protection. With high doses early on, watch for diabetes, hypertension and low potassium. Motor predominant CIDP may deteriorate. Steroids may be reduced after a month according to response, aiming for a maintenance of 10–20 mg on alternate days. Steroids do have some relative contraindications, e.g. diabetics with CIDP.

- **Intravenous immunoglobulin (IVIg).** There is clear evidence for benefit of IVIg compared to placebo in CIDP. In motor CIDP and multifocal motor neuropathy with block IVIg is better than corticosteroids. The treatment often requires repeating every 2–3 months.
- **Azathioprine** or **cyclophosphamide** may be added to corticosteroids (see Ch. 11).

Neuropathies with sensory ataxia

Sensory ataxia results from loss of proprioceptive information (including muscle spindle afferents) and is caused either by a dorsal root ganglionopathy, large fibre peripheral neuropathy or spinal cord lesion affecting the dorsal columns. Distinguishing cerebellar from sensory ataxia may be difficult. The following features favour sensory rather than cerebellar ataxia:

- Abnormal joint position sense and positive Romberg's sign.
- Normal eye movements: accurate saccades and smooth pursuit movements.
- Normal speech.

Sensory ganglionopathy

This represents a specific subset of neuropathies, with degeneration of the central and peripheral connections of the dorsal root ganglion. Patients present with sub-acute pain (sometimes severe) and paraesthesiae, often beginning in the upper limbs, with sensory ataxia and pseudoathetosis of the hands (and feet). Autonomic dysfunction is common, especially bowel pseudo-obstruction.

- **Paraneoplastic.** The ganglionopathy precedes carcinoma diagnosis by a mean of 4.5 months, sometimes considerably longer. The underlying tumour is usually small cell lung carcinoma, often with only mediastinal lymph nodes visible at diagnosis. Consider [18]FDG-PET scanning to detect malignancy. Features suggesting paraneoplasia are additional CNS abnormalities, e.g. encephalomyelitis, or finding anti-*Hu* antibody (specificity 99%: sensitivity 82%). Note that absence of anti-*Hu* is still consistent with a paraneoplastic cause.
- **Sjögren's syndrome** is the most common disimmune cause. Box 12.10 shows the neuropathies associated with Sjögren's syndrome. Only half of all patients report sicca symptoms and antibody tests have a low sensitivity. Labial salivary gland biopsy is often needed for diagnosis. Immunosuppression is needed to treat extraglandular Sjögren's syndrome.

Box 12.10: Neuropathies with Sjögren's syndrome

- Sensory neuronopathy (20%).
- Trigeminal neuropathy.
- Small fibre peripheral neuropathy.
- Polyradiculopathy.
- Motor neurone syndrome.
- Sensorimotor peripheral neuropathy.
- Multiple mononeuropathy.

Other causes of sensory ataxia

- **Chemotherapy**, particularly platinum agents (cisplatin, oxaliplatin). The symptoms may appear long after treatment is stopped (coasting).
- **Pyridoxine toxicity.** Occasionally even 200 mg/day can cause a large fibre neuropathy.
- **Syphilis.** (See Ch. 13).
- **Diphtheria.** Some cases may resemble tabes dorsalis.
- **HIV myelopathy** clinically resembles B_{12} deficiency.
- **Tropical sensory ataxia.** Strachan's syndrome may cause a sensory ataxia, as well as optic neuropathy and painful small fibre neuropathy.
- **CANOMAD:** chronic ataxic neuropathy, ophthalmoplegia, IgM paraprotein cold agglutinins and disialosyl antibodies. Disialosyl antibodies react against GQ1b and other gangliosides (95% of Miller Fisher syndrome cases have GQ1b antibodies) causing ataxia. There may be demyelinating and axonal features and a partial response to IVIG.

Porphyria

Porphyrias are rare autosomal dominant metabolic disorders characterized by defects in porphyrinogen biosynthesis or transformation of porphyrinogens to haem. Haem is an oxygen carrier in haemoglobin or myoglobin. Haem precursors are overproduced; in excess some are neurotoxic. They are excreted in urine which turns dark red when left to stand (Greek: *porphuros*: purple). The defective metabolic step in acute hepatic porphyrias, including acute intermittent porphyria, is in the liver.

Clinical features

Neurological involvement is peripheral or central. The classic triad is psychosis, abdominal pain and neuropathy. Additional problems are cortical blindness (clinically resembling posterior leucoencephalopathy), seizures and neuropathy. The neuropathy often starts in the arms, typically motor although sometimes with sensory features, e.g. 'bathing suit' sensory loss and autonomic problems.

Investigations

CSF protein is raised without excess white cells. The first episode is therefore often misdiagnosed as GBS.

Management

- **Remove identifiable precipitants**, e.g. porphyrinogenic drugs including alcohol, carbamazepine, valproic acid, phenytoin, contraceptive pill, ergots, calcium channel blockers.
- **Medications.** Consider propranolol for dysautonomia.
- **General measures.** Hydration, increase carbohydrate intake (2500 kcal/day = 300–400 g carbohydrates).

- **Specific measures.** If the above is ineffective, consider intravenous haem (haematin 4 mg/kg per day for 4–14 days according to response).

Amyloid neuropathy

This is an uncommon but important cause of a predominantly small fibre neuropathy. Autonomic features are very prominent, e.g. severe symptomatic postural hypotension. Consider sural nerve biopsy and protein electrophoresis.

MONONEUROPATHIES

Foot drop

This is a challenging clinical condition with many possible causes.

Common causes

- Common peroneal nerve (CPN) or deep PN palsy.
- Sciatic nerve palsy.
- Lumbar plexopathy.
- L5 radiculopathy, including cauda equina lesion.
- Upper motor neurone lesion: motor neurone disease is a relatively common cause of painless foot drop in people aged >50 years.
- Distal myopathies, e.g. inclusion body myositis.

History

Common peroneal nerve palsy is the most common cause of foot drop and usually occurs within days. The clinician should directly seek several points in the history.

- **Trauma to the CPN** includes long flights, habitual leg crossing, recent operations, plaster of Paris application, or yoga.
- **Predisposing factors.** Mononeuropathies are more likely with underlying diabetes mellitus, alcoholism, recent significant weight loss, malignancy or radiotherapy. With a previous or family history, consider hereditary liability to pressure palsies.
- **Back pain** favours an L5 root lesion rather than CPN palsy.
- **Nerve pain.** Vasculitic foot drop is often preceded by pain from nerve infarction.
- **Sphincter or sexual dysfunction** suggest an intraspinal lesion, i.e. conus or cauda equina.

Examination

A careful examination will often localize the lesion.

- **General examination** should include palpation of pulses and feeling for a large vessel aneurysm.
- **Wasting** suggests a more longstanding or pre-existing lesion.
- **Spina bifida.** Pointers include a hairy lower lumbar patch, as in spina bifida cystica or occulta.

- **Straight leg raising tests.** Lasègue's sign (flex the hip, knee straight with patient supine and then dorsiflex foot) can reproduce L5 or S1 root pain and so helps to distinguish an L5 root problem from CPN palsy. The femoral stretch test (extending the hip with the patient facing downwards) can reproduce L4 (or higher) root pain, but is also positive in femoral neuropathy, pelvic haematoma and abscess.
- **Patterns of weakness and sensory loss** are really helpful (see Fig. 12.4 and Fig. 12.5).
- **Reflexes.** The ankle jerk (tibial nerve) is preserved in a CPN palsy. Hamstring reflexes (L5) are tested in same position as knee reflexes.
- **An extensor plantar** (or spasticity) clearly suggests an UMN problem.

Common syndromes

Common peroneal nerve palsy

- **Causes:** There may be a history of trauma to the fibular head region (see above).
- **Clinical picture:** There is weakness of eversion and foot dorsiflexion, but normal inversion. The ankle jerk is retained.

A   B   C

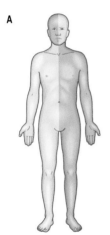 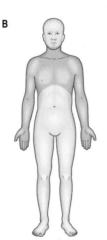 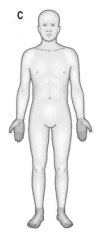

'Crossed' sensory loss
Lesion midpons down to C2

Cape distribution
Central cord (often dissociated pain and temperature loss but not vibration or joint position). Conversely loss proprioception only– dorsal column– consider syphilis, Friedreich's ataxia or paraneoplastic neuropathy, Sjögren's, CIDP or chemotherapy agents

Distal extremities
Neuropathy (patchy loss may indicate mononeuritis multiplex e.g. vasculitis, leprosy)
If only face bilaterally consider Sjögren's syndrome

Figure 12.4
Sensory patterns of weakness. (a) 'Crossed' sensory loss. Lesion mid pons down to C2. (b) Cape distribution: central cord (often dissociated pain and temperature but not vibration or joint position). Conversely, loss of proprioception only – dorsal column – consider syphilis, Friedreich's ataxia or paraneoplastic neuropathy, Sjögren's, CIDP or chemotherapy agents. (c) Distal extremities: neuropathy (patchy loss may indicate mononeuritis multiplex, e.g. vasculitis, leprosy). If only face bilaterally, consider Sjögren's syndrome.

A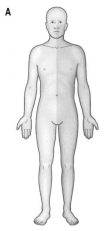

B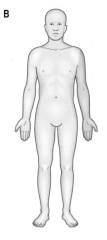

C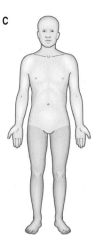

Hemiplegia
Face (lower half), leg and arm
– cortical
– capsule
– brainstem
So– look for the company they keep, e.g. dysphasia, neglect– more likely cortical

Monoplegia
Think cortex. Cord possible if ipsilateral limb and other limbs follow 'round the clock' pattern i.e.
R arm →**R** leg →**L** leg →**L** arm

Legs
– cord
– remember parasagittal lesions
– sometimes basilar vascular events

D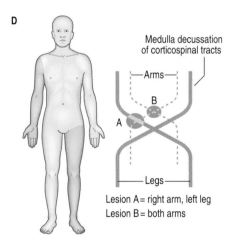

Medulla decussation of corticospinal tracts

—Arms—

B

A

—Legs—

Lesion A= right arm, left leg
Lesion B= both arms

Crossed weakness
e.g. **R** arm; **L** leg are possible reflecting decussation of fibres destined for arm and leg in medulla

E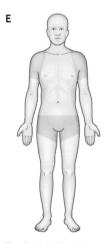

Proximal weakness
Think – myopathy
– demyelinating neuropathies (may be distal also)
– Lambert-Eaton myasthenic syndrome
Fasciobulbar and eye
– myasthenia gravis

Figure 12.5
Motor patterns of weakness. (a) hemiplegia – face (lower half); leg and arm – cortical, capsule, brainstem. Look for company they keep, e.g. dysphasia, neglect – more likely cortical. (b) Monoplegia – think cortex (cord possible if ipsilateral limb and other limbs follow 'round the clock' pattern, i.e. right arm → right leg → left leg → left arm). (c) Legs – cord; remember parasagittal lesions; sometimes also basilar vascular events. (d) Crossed weaknesses, e.g. right arm, left leg are possible, reflecting decussation in medulla of fibres destined for arm and leg. Lesion A, right arm, left leg; lesion B, both arms. (e) Proximal weakness, think – myopathy; demyelinating neuropathies (may be distal also); Lambert–Eaton myasthenic syndrome. Fasciobulbar and eye – myasthenia gravis.

Sciatic nerve palsy

- **Causes:** Most follow hip surgery. The common peroneal nerve component of the sciatic nerve is much more vulnerable to damage than the tibial, because it is anchored at the hip and knee more than the tibial and also the peri-neural connective tissue properties differ. Vasculitis may also cause sciatic nerve mononeuropathy.
- **Clinical picture:** Sciatic nerve foot drop is strongly suggested by additional tibial nerve involvement: hamstring and toe plantar flexion weakness and loss of the ankle reflex (all tibial nerve).

Piriformis syndrome

This is a controversial entity localizing to the piriformis muscle. The inferior gluteal nerve passes with the sciatic nerve beneath the piriformis muscle. An inferior gluteal nerve palsy gives weakness of hip extension (gluteus maximus) but sparing of hipabduction (gluteus medius and minimus).

L5 root lesion

An L5 root lesion presents as a foot drop with dorsal foot sensory loss, but is distinguished from CPN palsy by:

- Back and leg pain.
- Weakness of hip extension and abduction (superior and inferior gluteal nerves).
- Weakness of ankle inversion (tibial nerve).
- With associated S1 compression, there may be a reduced ankle jerk.

Distinguishing conus from cauda equina lesions

Features favouring a conus lesion:

- Early loss of sphincters or sexual dysfunction.
- Spontaneous sweating over sacral dermatomes.
- Perianal numbness early with loss of anal 'wink' reflex.
- Loss of ankle reflexes, but retained knee jerks.

Features favouring a cauda equina lesion:

- Widespread weakness of the legs.
- Asymmetric weakness.
- Loss of both knee and ankle reflexes.

Cauda equina lesions

The cauda equina lies in the spinal canal between T12 and S5. The filum terminale is a fibrous band from tip of cord to sacrum. There are many possible causes of a cauda equina lesion.

Benign tumours:

- Chordoma. 80% are sacrococcygeal, presenting with bone pain and destruction.
- Ependymoma. These present in filum terminale of middle-aged adults: the associated high CSF protein may cause papilloedema.
- Dermoid tumours are associated with spina bifida.
- Neurofibromas. One-third are below L1, two-thirds are above L1.
- Meningioma.

Malignant tumours:

- Secondaries from myeloma, prostate, breast or lung.
- Malignant meningitis: cells settle where there is little flow, e.g. in the basal meninges or around the cauda equina. Examine for confusion, papilloedema and cranial nerve function (including hearing).

Arteriovenous malformation (AVM):

- Cauda equina AVM is often initially overlooked on imaging. Typically, there is a raised CSF cell count and protein (Foix–Alajouanine syndrome).

Arachnoiditis:

- Infective causes, e.g. syphilis.
- Following contrast, e.g. myelography (oil-based contrast agents).
- Connective tissue disease, e.g. ankylosing spondylitis.

Viral infection:

- The main viral causes are HIV, CMV, or HZV.

Trauma.

Radial nerve palsy

There are four main compression sites:

1. **Axilla.** This is rare. It causes weakness of triceps and other extensors and minor sensory involvement. Consider trauma and long crutches.
2. **Upper arm.** This is often encountered as 'Saturday night palsy': the patient passes out with an arm draped over a chair compressing the radial nerve. It may also follow a general anaesthetic, a supracondylar fracture, or occur in HNPP. It causes inability to extend the wrist, fingers and thumb (triceps spared).
3. **Forearm.** Involvement of the posterior interosseous nerve causes 'supinator syndrome' with dropped fingers without wrist drop. Causes include tendinous stricture of the arcade of Frohse, lipoma and rheumatoid arthritis.
4. **Wrist.** Involvement of the superficial radial nerve causes shooting pain in wrist, without motor involvement. Causes include handcuffs, direct trauma, neuromas and shunt operations for haemodialysis.

Ulnar nerve palsy

This commonly occurs at the elbow ('tardy ulnar palsy'). Ulnar clawing (hyperextension of fingers 4 and 5 at metacarpophalangeal joints and flexion of interphalangeals) occurs through weakness of 3rd and 4th lumbricals allowing EDC to exert unopposed pull and tension in flexor digitorum superficialis and profundus because of hyperextension. Froment's sign (Figs 12.6, 12.7) results from using FPL instead of adductor pollicis.

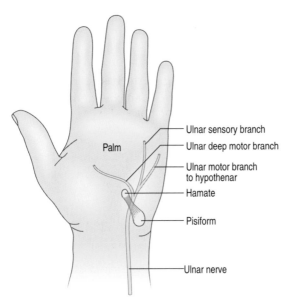

Figure 12.6
Canal of Guyon.

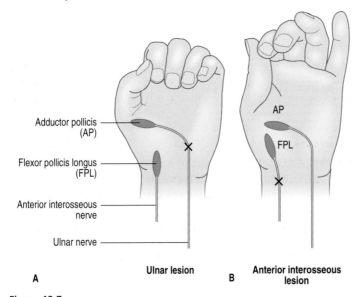

Figure 12.7
Comparison of thumb pinch manoeuvre in ulnar and anterior interosseous nerves. (a) Froment's sign. Ulnar lesion. (b) Anterior interosseous lesion.

A deep ulnar nerve palsy is an important cause of a wasted hand (see below).

The wasted hand

There are several causes of wasted hand. Clinical examination must include testing for numbness (would exclude MND) and examining the feet (wasted in hereditary neuropathy).

- Ulnar neuropathy (with or without carpal tunnel syndrome).
- Motor neurone disease.
- Radiculopathy (C8/T1).
- Syrinx.
- Charcot–Marie–Tooth disease.
- High cervical cord lesion (brisk reflexes but normal or depressed jaw jerk).
- Disuse or rheumatological conditions.
- Thoracic outlet syndrome.
- Brachial plexus lesion.

RADICULOPATHIES

Lumbar radiculopathies

Posterior thigh/leg pain

Lumbar radiculopathies are a common cause of posterior leg pain, sometimes with discrete myotomal weakness. They almost exclusively involve the L5 or S1 roots (95%); other roots should be accepted with caution.

Which disc, which root?

Since the cord finishes adjacent to the T12-L1 vertebral bodies, the lower roots travel long distances before exiting at their respective foramina. Each root branches from the cauda equina to pass inferolaterally and emerge at its respective foramen. Each lumbar root relates to two intervertebral discs.

- The L5 root branches from the cauda equina at the L4/5 disc level and exits via the L5/S1 foramen. It is compressed shortly after its origin by a L4/5 disc postero-lateral protrusion and only rarely by a large lateral L5/S1 protrusion.
- The S1 root (origin at L5/S1 disc level; exit via S1/2 foramen) is compressed by a L5/S1 postero-lateral protrusion.
- Large L5/S1 fragments may compress both the S1 root posteriorly and the L5 root laterally.

Thus, a disc prolapse at one spinal level can cause different syndromes according to the direction of herniation. For example, at the L4/5 level:

- A postero-lateral disc prolapse irritates the L5 root.
- A central prolapse damages the cauda equina: asymmetric bilateral symptoms follow.

- A lateral prolapse may damage the L4 root.

MRI is the investigation of choice. Surgery is considered if:

- There is pain that does not respond to conservative management (usually at least 6–8 weeks of conservative measures – 85% will resolve by this time).
- There are bilateral symptoms or signs (suggesting a cauda equina lesion).
- There is a significant motor problem.

Anterior thigh pain

This is due to an L4 root lesion (rare), plexopathy (see below), diabetic amyotrophy or femoral neuropathy. Femoral neuropathy may follow pelvic surgery through the lithotomy position, through haematoma (e.g. from anticoagulation), or through retraction and pressure on the nerve. A pure femoral neuropathy spares the obturator nerve, i.e. hip adduction and adductor reflex are preserved. Note a femoral neuropathy may cause sensory loss below the knee (saphenous nerve may be damaged during varicose vein surgery).

Exercise induced symptoms

Lumbar canal stenosis may present with symptoms similar to vascular claudication, but with important differences (Table 12.2).

PLEXOPATHIES

Supraclavicular

Upper plexus

- **Burner (or stinger)** usually follows a contact sports injury. Separation of the shoulder and head causes traction on the upper brachial plexus. Pain is felt in the shoulder radiating to the lateral border of arm, often to the thumb; permanent problems are rare.
- **Rucksack or cadet palsy** follows pressure on the upper trunk of the brachial plexus (often demyelinating). There is usually pain in the upper trunk and involvement of the suprascapular nerve.

Table 12.2: Differences between symptoms of vascular claudication and lumbar canal stenosis

Vascular	Neurogenic
Peripheral pulses reduced	Pulses present
Walking provoked	Walking or standing provoked
Constant claudication distance	Variable distance
Brief rest relieves symptoms	Prolonged rest relieves symptoms
No differences in posture	Better if leaning forward, e.g. shopping trolley, bicycle
Reflexes present	Reflexes may disappear after walking

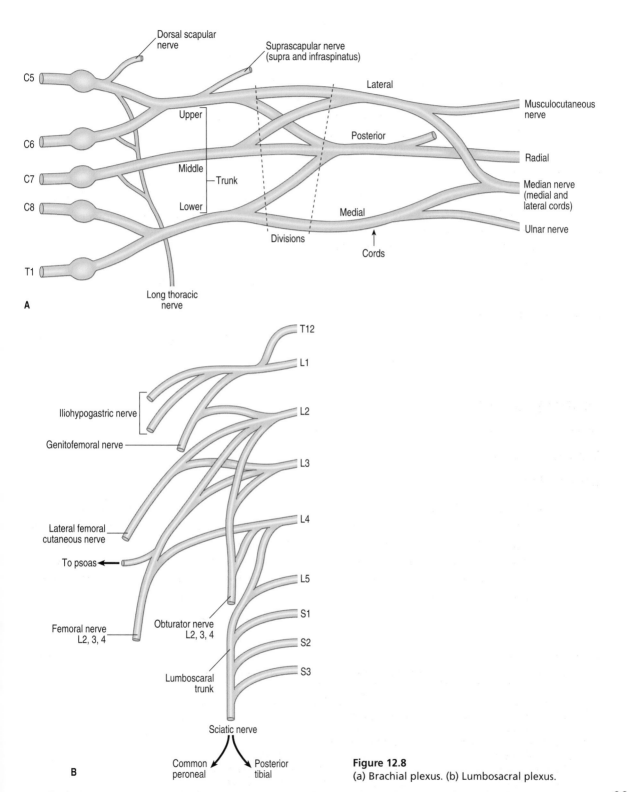

Figure 12.8
(a) Brachial plexus. (b) Lumbosacral plexus.

- **Postoperative**. This reflects stretching of the upper trunk typically in a patient under anaesthesia, with the shoulder abducted, the head turned away from abducted shoulder and in the Trendelenburg position. Presents with parasthesiae and weakness, e.g. of brachioradialis or biceps.

Lower plexus

- **True neurogenic thoracic outlet syndrome** is a rare condition (1 in 1 000 000) usually affecting young women. There is pressure from a cervical rib or fibrous band with pressure especially on T1 motor fibres causing APB wasting and C8/T1 sensory loss (medial forearm and finger).
- **Post-median sternotomy** results from pressure from retracted ribs on the lower plexus. Patients present with pins and needles in the ulnar fingers but with weakness in other C8 muscles, e.g. flexor pollicis longus.
- **Pancoast syndrome** (described 1924) from a lower plexus lesion is the presenting feature of 3% of lung cancers. Patients describe a burning, boring pain, worse at night, down the medial forearm (less often the medial fingers) and have a Horner's syndrome. If cancer invades the posterior rami, then patients may have midscapular pain.

Lumbosacral

Structural

- **Pregnancy**. This usually follows a large baby causing pressure on the lumbosacral trunk. Clinically it resembles an L5 radiculopathy (Note NCS showing normal sensory action potentials and paraspinal denervation favours L5 root involvement). Weakness of ankle inversion and toe flexion should distinguish a common peroneal nerve lesion from an L5 or lumbosacral trunk lesion.
- **Haematoma** (often on warfarin).
- **Malignant**. Upper plexus involvement suggests rectal carcinoma; lower plexus involvement suggests sarcoma; whole plexus involvement (panplexopathy) suggests urological malignancy. The presentation may be with a warm, dry (non-sweating) foot, or with the classic pentad of oedema, rectal mass, hydronephrosis, pain and weakness. Another manifestation is inguinal pain from L1 root or genitofemoral nerve involvement. Box 12.11 shows the features distinguishing malignant plexopathies from radiation causes.
- **Trauma**.

Non-structural

- **Diabetes mellitus**. A common cause of plexopathy.
- **Vasculitis**. Beware as this can resemble malignancy.
- **Radiation** plexopathy typically develops after a latency of 1–35 years (median 5 years). It typically involves L5 and S1 and is usually progressive (Box 12.11).
- **Idiopathic**.

Other conditions

Malignant plexopathy

Breast and lung cancer may involve brachial plexus by extrinsic compression or infiltration – it often spreads from an axillary lymph node and therefore affects the medial cord. Pain in shoulder and pain in medial forearm are the earliest features (loss of SAP from medial cutaneous nerve of forearm). As in lumbosacral plexopathies, loss of sympathetic activity can be a presentation – a dry warm hand with Horner's sign.

Radiation plexopathy

These may be observed following radiotherapy for breast cancer. The damage may reflect fibrotic radiation induced damage, disrupting the microcirculation. There is often early lateral cord involvement – parasthesiae in lateral three fingers, no pain (although there may be later) and no Horner's – all different from malignant plexopathies. The condition can be progressive. Electrophysiologically there may be myokymic discharges and denervation in paraspinal muscles (more often than in malignant plexopathies). Investigations to help distinguish malignant and radiation plexopathies include MRI, PET, EMG and cerebrospinal fluid examination for cytology. Occasionally radiation can induce malignant nerve sheath tumours – presenting with pain and suitable motor deficits according to lesion location.

Neuralgic amyotrophy

The usual pattern is:

- Preceding immunization or infection (recalled in about half).
- Pain can be very severe in the shoulder, enough to require opiates and take patients to hospital, lasts about 1 week to 10 days.
- Weakness, particularly picks off motor nerves, presenting as a mononeuropathy or multiple mononeuropathies, particularly long thoracic nerve (winging scapula when stopping traffic), or suprascapular nerve, anterior interosseus nerve (test by doing the OK sign, Fig. 12.7).

Box 12.11: Radiation vs malignant plexopathy

Features favouring malignancy
- Unilateral.
- Pain first symptom (may be severe).
- Unilateral loss of knee reflex.
- Varied weakness pattern, including proximal weakness or panplexopathy weakness.

Features favouring radiation
- Bilateral although asymmetric.
- Pain occurs in half (usually not severe).
- Bilateral loss ankle and knee reflexes.
- Predominantly distal weakness.
- EMG commonly shows paraspinal involvement and myokymic discharges (60%).

Features of both malignant and radiation
- Sphincter symptoms occur in both, with involvement of the lower plexus or lower cord.

- Phrenic nerve involvement presenting with orthopnoea (estimated to be 7% unilateral or bilateral diaphragm involvement).
- 90% do improve – but takes up to 3 years.
- Steroids not shown to influence course of disease.

Cervical spondylosis

Cervical spondylosis describes a degenerative condition causing stenosis of both cervical canal and emerging nerve roots. The degenerative processes include disc disease, thickened ligamentum flavum, osteophytes (oncovertebral and facet joints). Cervical spondylosis may cause nerve root compression from disc or osteophytes. The characteristics of cervical root pain include:

- Exacerbation with coughing or straining (10%).
- Relief by arm elevation.
- Occasional worsening by using the arm.
- Pain reproduced by axial compression with the head laterally tilted (rarely done).

Despite major sensory symptoms, there are few signs reflecting the overlapping dermatomes and nerve territories.

C5 radiculopathy

- **Pain** in the shoulder and upper arm and does not radiate below the elbow.
- **Weakness** in shoulder abduction, elbow flexion and internal and shoulder external rotation. Axillary nerve involvement may cause weakness in the second 90° of abduction and may cause shoulder pain.
- **Reflexes.** Reduced or absent biceps reflex (musculocutaneous nerve).

C6 radiculopathy

- **Pain** from biceps into the lateral forearm and thumb.
- **Weakness** in biceps (musculocutaneous), brachioradialis (radial) and forearm supinator (radial).
- **Reflexes.** Reduced or absent supinator reflex (radial nerve).
- **Sensory** symptoms superficially resemble carpal tunnel syndrome (the motor features differ).

C7 radiculopathy

- **Pain** radiates to the middle finger, with aching in the medial and lateral forearm.
- **Weakness** in shoulder adduction, elbow extension, wrist extension and flexion.
- **Reflexes.** Reduced or absent triceps and pectoral jerks (C7/8).

Radial nerve palsy can look very similar.

Motor: Radial nerve palsy involves brachioradialis (C6) (easy to see) but spares shoulder adduction and wrist flexion.

Reflexes: The triceps jerk is involved in both C7 radiculopathy and radial nerve palsy. However, radial nerve palsy involves the supinator reflex (C6) but spares the pectoral jerk (C7/8, lateral medial anterior thoracic nerves).

C2 or C3 radiculopathy

These are unusual, so consider causes other than cervical spondylosis, e.g. meningioma, Chiari malformation, or rheumatoid disease. 25% of rheumatoid patients have atlantoaxial subluxation (anterior subluxation of C1 on C2). Often there are other features of foramen magnum disease.

- C2 pain radiates over occipital region.
- C3 pain may radiate to behind the ear. Remember the angle of the jaw is innervated by C3.

Cervical spondylotic myelopathy

Cervical spondylosis is the most common cause of cord compression in patients aged >55 years.

Clinical features

This presents with various combinations of radicular and myelopathic symptoms:

- **Numb and clumsy hands**, e.g. difficulty with buttons (also seen in many other neurological conditions, particularly parkinsonism).
- **Sensory symptoms** in the hands, which can be very unpleasant, but with few sensory signs.
- **Bladder involvement** is only a late feature.
- **Upper motor neurone symptoms** in the legs are frequent: ask specifically about legs jumping in bed (clonus).
- **Impaired joint position sense**: in high cervical spine lesions, this is more marked in the fingers than the toes.
- **Hand muscle wasting** is due to radicular or high cord involvement.

Investigation

MR scanning is the investigation of choice. A rule of thumb is that compression is significant if the cord diameter is reduced to <50% and there is signal change in cord (T1 signal change carries a poor prognosis, most experts regard signal change on T2 as significant).

Plain cervical radiograph (flexion and extension) is helpful in excluding atlantoaxial subluxation.

Blood tests should include serum B_{12} and syphilis serology.

Incidental compression

Ten percent of apparent cervical spondylotic myelopathy has another cause, e.g. ALS or multiple sclerosis (MS). Cord imaging may reveal intrinsic cord lesions in MS (and sometimes incidental compression). Intrinsic cord signal change in inflammatory conditions is often above the level of compression, whereas signal change at the level of compression suggests a mechanical cause.

Management

An operation is often indicated for myelopathy. The aim of surgery is to arrest decline. The earlier the operation is performed, the better: 50% improve if operated upon within 1 year of symptom onset, whereas only 15% do if operated upon after 1 year. A repeat MRI cervical spine is indicated if the patient has worsened at follow-up.

KEY POINTS

- Break down the problem: symmetrical vs multifocal, axonal vs demyelinating.
- Look for paraproteins (10–20% CIDP, 10% neuropathies).
- Do a glucose tolerance test and remember diabetics develop superadded inflammatory neuropathies.
- Genetic causes rarely have positive sensory features: pes cavus suggests the problem has existed since childhood.
- Look for vasculitis: do a biopsy and use EMG to select a nerve.
- If the reflexes are present, consider a myelopathy, e.g. in rheumatoid disease.
- Do BP lying and standing.

Further Reading

Willison HJ, Winer JB. Clinical evaluation and investigation of neuropathy. J Neurol Neurosurg Psychiatry 2003; 74 (Suppl II): ii3–ii8.

Neurological infections 13

Case history

A 60-year-old man was admitted with a 3-day history of agitation, confusion and headache. He had developed diabetes 6 years earlier necessitating treatment with oral hypoglycaemics. His alcohol consumption was excessive. On examination he was pyrexial (39°C) with neck stiffness and a positive Kernig's sign. He had bilateral 6th nerve palsies and bilateral extensor plantar responses. Fundoscopy revealed no evidence of papilloedema. CT brain scan was normal. Cerebrospinal fluid (CSF) opening pressure was 30 cm water. CSF white count was elevated (150 cells: 60% polymorphs, 40% lymphocytes), CSF protein 2 g/l, CSF glucose 3 mmol/l (serum 18).

BACTERIAL MENINGITIS

The three common bacteria causing meningitis are *Streptococcus pneumoniae* (pneumococcus), *Neisseria meningitidis* (meningococcus) and *Haemophilus influenzae*. Each colonizes the nasopharynx and secretes IgA protease, which breaks down the mucous lining, allowing bacterial attachment and subsequent cell entry. Their polysaccharide capsules protect them from neutrophil phagocytosis. The subarachnoid space has few complement components or immunoglobulins to hinder rapid bacteria multiplication.

Meningeal inflammation is triggered by the bacteria and their cell wall components (lipo-oligosaccharide of *H. influenzae* type b, or lipoteichoic acid of pneumococcus). It is mediated by cytokines, e.g. tumour necrosis factor and interleukin-1. Bactericidal antibiotics cause cytokine release, potentially worsening inflammation. Thus inflammation has several consequences:

- Polymorphs increase blood–brain permeability and cause vasogenic oedema.
- Proteinaceous inflammation may obstruct CSF flow and cause interstitial oedema.
- Cytotoxic oedema increases blood flow.
- Intracranial pressure rises in response to the above.
- Cerebral autoregulation is disturbed.
- Inflammation in arterial and venous systems may cause infarction and venous thrombosis.

Clinical presentation

The classical triad is fever, headache and neck stiffness, often with photophobia, confusion, drowsiness or even coma. About 20% (particularly the elderly) present more subtly, e.g. with fever and confusion without neck stiffness.

History and examination

There are several specific points relevant to possible meningitis:

- Search for a history of preceding upper respiratory tract infection.
- Ask about any antibiotics already received, as these change the CSF polymorph to lymphocytic ratio (see below).
- Has the patient had a brain operation or head injury either recently or remotely (look for a cranial scar); these provide a bacterial route of entry and change the antibiotic choice.
- Look for evidence of immunocompromise e.g. malignancy history, sickle cell anaemia, splenectomy scar, lymphadenopathy or Kaposi sarcoma.
- Look for petechiae (hands, feet and conjunctivae).
- Examine the ears: has the infection spread from otitis media?
- Chest examination and radiograph are important (25–50% of pneumococcal meningitis have pneumonia).
- Neck stiffness: test by flexing (not by rotating) the head.
- Brudzinski and Kernig's signs (Fig. 13.1).
- Seizures are uncommon in adults with acute pyogenic meningitis and suggest cortical infarction (arterial and venous), subdural empyema or electrolyte abnormality.

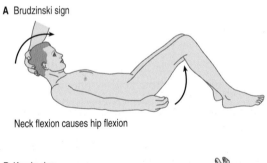

A Brudzinski sign

Neck flexion causes hip flexion

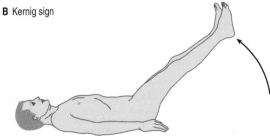

B Kernig sign

Neck pain on hip flexion
N.B. neck stiffness in meningitis is more apparent
on flexion/extension than rotation

Figure 13.1
Brudzinski and Kernig signs. (a) Brudzinski sign. Neck flexion causes hip flexion. (b) Kernig sign. Neck pain on hip flexion. *Note*: Neck stiffness in meningitis is more apparent on flexion/extension than rotation.

Investigations

- **CT head scan must be done before lumbar puncture (LP)**, if:
  - Reduced level of consciousness (GCS <13).
  - Papilloedema.
  - Focal neurological signs.
  - Immunocompromise (even if only suspected) because of the risk of a space-occupying lesion.
  - A recent seizure (within 2 weeks).
  - Age >65 years.
- **CSF examination** is essential to confirm the diagnosis and to identify the organism and its sensitivities:
  - CSF should have <5 WBC/mm^3. With a traumatic CSF tap, calculate the white cell to red cell ratio in CSF and blood. A CSF to blood ratio of >1 indicates that CSF pleocytosis was present before the LP.
  - The white cells in bacterial meningitis are polymorphs, typically >1000 cells/mm^3. However, lymphocytes may predominate both early on and in partially treated cases. Some viral meningitides, e.g. enteroviral, also show polymorphs. If in doubt, treat as bacterial.
  - CSF glucose is considered abnormal if <60% of the blood glucose level.
  - CSF protein is increased, but remember a traumatic LP also raises it.
  - Bacterial CSF antigen tests may help in diagnosis where patients have a negative Gram stain and culture, or have received antibiotics.

Pneumococcal meningitis: special features

- There often is preceding upper respiratory tract involvement.
- Pneumococcal meningitis may present fulminantly or subacutely.
- Search for a predisposing cause: examine the ears.
- Conscious level: patients are more obtunded than in meningococcal meningitis and most have impaired consciousness at presentation.
- Focal signs and seizures may occur; cranial nerve palsies (3, 4, 6, 7, 8) reflect inflammation, vasculitis or thrombosis, e.g. cavernous sinus. Hemiparesis suggests infarction, oedema, abscess, or post-ictal Todd's paresis.

Meningococcal meningitis

This is more common in children and young adults, sometimes occurring in epidemics (types A and C). The petechial rash is important for diagnosis, but some rash also accompanies haemophilus and pneumococcal meningitis. Look in the conjunctivae and mucous membranes as well as the skin. Blood cultures as well as CSF are important. Blood from the cutaneous purpuric lesions may reveal the organism. Meningococcal septicaemia may present with the Waterhouse–Friderichsen syndrome: a sudden onset, large haemorrhagic rash, disseminated intravascular coagulation and septic shock (caused by massive bilateral adrenal haemorrhages): lumbar puncture is contraindicated in these circumstances.

Differential diagnosis of bacterial meningitis

- Other infections. Herpes simplex encephalitis, fungal, tuberculous, spirochaetal (syphilis and Lyme disease), protozoal (malaria).
- Neuroleptic malignant syndrome (rigidity and fever).
- Acute disseminated encephalomyelitis (see Ch. 10).
- Subarachnoid haemorrhage.
- Cerebral abscess.
- Bacterial endocarditis.
- Parameningeal infection.

Meningitis in the immunocompromised

Immunocompromise increases the likelihood of meningitis, but the organism may be atypical and the signs more subtle. There are four main immunocompromised groups:

1. **Defective polymorph function.** Consider Gram-negative bacilli (*E. coli*, klebsiella, pseudomonas), candida, aspergillus and abscess.
2. **Defective antibody**, e.g. leukaemia or lymphoma. Consider pneumococcus and haemophilus.
3. **Impaired cell-mediated immunity**, e.g. HIV and iatrogenic immunosuppression. Consider listeria, cryptococcus, nocardia, aspergillus, toxoplasma, varicella, cytomegalovirus and tuberculosis.
4. **Splenic abnormality**, including sickle cell disease. Consider pneumococcus and haemophilus.

Fungi

Several conditions increase vulnerability to fungal infections:

- AIDS.
- Transplantation.
- Immunosuppressive chemotherapy.
- Lymphoreticular malignancy.

Fungal meningitis may present as typical meningitis, but also as a stroke syndrome, a rhinocerebral syndrome (often with carotid artery involvement), or as a space-occupying lesion. Skin cryptococcal lesions may resemble molluscum contagiosum.

Cryptococcus

Cryptococcus is a yeast-like fungus found in pigeon droppings and soil. It can spread haematogenously from a primary lung infection to the CNS.

Cryptococcal meningitis presents as indolent headache with fever, rather than as acute meningitis. Cranial nerve palsies may occur if the basal meninges are affected.

Beware of AIDS patients with cryptococcal meningitis: 25% have normal CSF or show isolated high CSF pressure. A cryptococcal antigen test is therefore essential in immunocompromised patients.

Candida

Candida meningoencephalitis presents either subacutely or as chronic meningitis. Typically it follows disseminated candidal infection, the fungaemia seeding the meninges. Consider candida in ITU patients with central line infections who have received antibiotics. Candida cultures grow quickly (positive within 2–4 days).

Aspergillus

Aspergillus and zygomycetes may invade blood vessels giving stroke-like presentations. The CSF shows either polymorphs or lymphocytes and a normal glucose. Aspergillus may also cause abscesses. On MR scanning, aspergillus often has both parenchymal lesions and ependymal lesions. Zygomycetes (mucor) often present in diabetic patients (acidosis and hyperglycaemia), with infection originating in the palate or paranasal sinuses. There may be a black eschar that can be biopsied or blackish purulent nasal discharge.

Investigating the immunocompromised

CSF examination
This is essential but beware:

- Patients are often ill: check the platelet count before undertaking lumbar puncture (should be $>50 \times 10^9$/L).
- CT must precede lumbar puncture in immunocompromised patients because of the high incidence of space-occupying lesions.

Usually the CSF shows elevated pressure, high protein, low glucose and a lymphocytic pleocytosis. Note however that these CSF markers are sometimes normal in AIDS patients with meningitis. A CSF India ink test is positive in 50% of cryptococcal cases and 75–88% of HIV-positive patients. A CSF cryptococcal antigen is highly sensitive and specific (95% in AIDS). For fungi other than cryptococcus, then take a large CSF volume for culture on at least three occasions. If these are normal but fungal meningitis remains possible, consider a cisternal puncture before either empiric therapy or meningeal biopsy.

Ancillary tests

Several other tests can help the diagnosis in immunocompromised patients.

- **Cryptococcus** requires cultures of blood, urine, sputum and even bone marrow. Consider biopsying any skin lesions.
- **Candida** diagnosis requires biopsy of skin lesions and culture of catheters.
- **Aspergillus** requires blood culture, chest radiograph and biopsy of skin lesions, e.g. the black eschar for mucormycetes.

Management

Specific medications. Intravenous amphotericin-B should be given for 2 weeks; nephrotoxicity is the main side-effect. Flucytosine (2 weeks) may be synergistic, the main side-effects being marrow toxicity and hepatitis. Chronic fluconazole therapy (400 mg/day for 8 weeks, then 200 mg/day) should be considered in AIDS patients, because they risk relapse with clinically silent, persistent or recurrent urinary cryptococcus.

Treating complications. Raised CSF pressure (from impaired CSF drainage) occurs in 50% of HIV cases with cryptococcus. Corticosteroids must be avoided: treat with several daily lumbar punctures until the pressure improves.

Prognosis

Features suggesting a poor prognosis include high CSF pressure, abnormal mental status and high cryptococcal antigen titres.

Tuberculous meningitis

During either primary tuberculous infection or reactivations, tubercles may be deposited in the brain substance or meninges. These caseous (soft and exudative) lesions discharge bacilli into the subarachnoid space. An inflammatory reaction follows, particularly around the basal cisterns, as a reaction both to the bacilli and associated antigenic material.

Clinical presentation

Tuberculous meningitis presents in several ways:

- As an acute meningitis (relatively rare).
- As a subacute meningitis (most common):
  - Prodromal illness, e.g. headache, weight loss or night sweats.
  - Fever, meningism, long tract signs and cranial nerve palsies appear within 2–3 weeks. Cognition is often affected in adults before meningism appears. Sometimes dementia is prominent.
  - The illness may then accelerate, with convulsions and coma; death becomes almost inevitable within 5–8 weeks.
- As an indolent illness, developing over weeks or months, sometimes with prominent cognitive features.

Complications

The basal meningeal inflammatory exudate of tuberculous meningitis influences its presentation and complications.

- **Obstructive hydrocephalus** may result from inflammation around the 4th ventricle or aqueduct.
- **Blood vessel inflammation** causes infarctions either directly (thrombosis) or indirectly (vessel compression); this is a major determinant of prognosis and residual neurological deficits.
- **Systemic complications.** Patients with tuberculous meningitis must be examined in detail looking for fever (20% are said to be apyrexial, but fever sometimes appears only in the late afternoon), chest involvement, lymphadenopathy, joint disease and scrotal masses or draining fistulae. Fundoscopy may reveal choroidal tubercles and/or papilloedema.

- **Tuberculomas**, conglomerate caseous foci in the brain or cord parenchyma, occur in 10–30% patients.
- **Cranial nerve palsies** also result from the inflammation. The most common is a 6th nerve palsy, but 3rd or 4th also occur.
- **Spinal complications.** The inflammatory reaction may encase the cord in a gelatinous exudate. Alternatively, tuberculomas may mimic tumours (extradural, intradural or intramedullary). Furthermore, a vasculitis may involve the cord. Most spinal TB presents as an acute or subacute radiculomyelopathy. The term arachnoiditis is often used, although this actually means arachnoid inflammation whereas it actually involves all three meningeal layers. Chronic spinal arachnoiditis more usually implies meningeal scarring following trauma (e.g. surgery), foreign material, tumour or infection. A syrinx may follow arachnoiditis, including as a complication of spinal TB. CSF shows abnormalities similar to those above, including the potential for spinal block.

Investigations

- **Chest radiograph** is often helpful, but tuberculous meningitis can occur without pulmonary disease: only 50% have chest radiograph changes of active or previous tuberculosis. Chest films may reveal the 'Ghon complex' (primary lung lesion); the associated secondary infection manifests as tracheobronchial lymphadenopathy, upper lobe infiltrate, or as miliary spread.
- **CT brain imaging** is important, to demonstrate either hydrocephalus or basal meningeal contrast enhancement.
- **CSF** is the key to diagnosis. The typical findings are a high protein, low glucose and a lymphocyte pleocytosis (usually >100 cells/mm^3, range 50–500). Polymorphs are found early in the illness but sometimes only on starting treatment (a therapeutic paradox which, when seen, strongly suggests TB). Very high CSF protein (2–20+ g/L) suggests spinal block (Froin's syndrome) and implies a poor prognosis. Involve the microbiology or TB laboratory. Collect 10–20 ml of CSF, using the last sample for an acid-alcohol fast bacilli (AAFB) smear. If the CSF clots send this. Culture is definitely required but takes 6 weeks (it is positive in 75%). Polymerase chain reaction (PCR) analysis lacks sensitivity and specificity.

Management

TB meningitis was invariably fatal before streptomycin (the 1948 MRC trial reduced mortality by 30%). If you suspect the diagnosis, do not delay treatment.

Antituberculous treatment

Start with:

- Isoniazid (bactericidal with good CSF penetration).
- Rifampicin.
- Pyrazinamide.
- Either streptomycin or ethambutol.
- Remember to prescribe pyridoxine.

Beware of multi-drug resistance and discuss with an infectious diseases expert. Continue treatment for 1 year minimum (4 drugs 2 months, 2 drugs thereafter).

Corticosteroids

Steroid treatment for tuberculous meningitis remains controversial. It appears to reduce mortality but not morbidity. Consider dexamethasone (12 mg/day for 3 weeks, tapering to 0 over a further 3 weeks) if there are the following features:

- Altered consciousness.
- Papilloedema.
- High CSF opening pressure (>30 cm H_2O).
- Focal deficit.

Prognosis

The prognosis remains grave (mortality 20% overall). With altered consciousness (the most important prognostic feature) the mortality is 50–70%. The early phase is critical: 90% of deaths occur during the first month. Improvement should not be expected early on and CSF variables take months to normalize (glucose, cell counts abnormal for 1–2 months; protein for longer).

Cranial nerve palsies mostly resolve, although deafness persists (caused by damage to the internal auditory artery, acoustic nerve or cochlear involvement from drugs).

Meningitis in older adults (>50 years)

Organisms

- Pneumococcus is a common cause at this age.
- Gram-negative bacilli are more common if there are chronic respiratory problems or urinary tract infection (organisms include *E. Coli*, klebsiella and pseudomonas).
- *Listeria monocytogenes* is an important and increasingly recognized cause of meningitis. It presents either subacutely with a lymphocytic or neutrophilic CSF, or with small abscess cavities in the brainstem parenchyma. Ampicillin or gentamicin is the best treatment.

Prognosis. The mortality is higher in older persons (30–40% if aged >60 years with pneumococcal meningitis).

Neurosurgical patients

Shunts. *Staphylococcus aureus* or coagulase-negative staphylococci may complicate shunts early on, presenting often non-specifically, without classical meningitis features.

Head injury. Pneumococcal infection is common in the week following a head injury; beyond that, staphylococcus or *H. Influenzae* predominates.

MANAGEMENT OF MENINGITIS

Treatment must begin before knowing the organism sensitivities; remember blood cultures as well as CSF can help. Liaise with the medical microbiologists.

Antibiotics

- Pneumococcus can be penicillin resistant (some outside the UK are cephalosporin resistant). Treatment of bacterial meningitis usually involves a third generation cephalosporin, e.g. intravenous ceftriaxone 2–4 g/day. Ceftriaxone also covers Gram-negative bacilli (except pseudomonas which requires ceftazidime). Pneumococcal meningitis is treated for 2 weeks. Gram-negative meningitis is treated for 3 weeks.
- In those aged >50 years, add ampicillin (12 g/day i.v., 4-hourly for 2 weeks) to cover *Listeria*.
- In those with a neurosurgery history, either recent or remote, add vancomycin to cover staphylococcus.
- In immunocompromised patients, consider medications to cover likely organisms in individual patients.

Corticosteroids

The role of corticosteroids for bacterial meningitis remains controversial.
- Dexamethasone for the first 2–4 days reduces mortality and morbidity without increasing the risk of gastrointestinal haemorrhage. The patient requires a repeat CSF examination after 48 h, since corticosteroids can mask treatment failure.

Prophylaxis

The household contacts of a patient with meningococcal meningitis (particularly children) are at increased infection risk (500–1000 times the general population): they require chemoprophylaxis to prevent secondary cases.

- Adults: Rifampicin 600 mg 12-hourly for 2 days. Rifampicin should not be used in pregnancy.
- Children aged >1 year: 10 mg/kg 12-hourly for 2 days.

ASEPTIC MENINGITIS

Meningitis with predominately mononuclear cells in the CSF and no bacteria on culture or smear and no parameningeal infection is termed aseptic meningitis and generally has a benign course.

Cause. Viral infection causes most cases (70%); others include intravenous immunoglobulin therapy.

Clinical features. Consciousness is almost never disturbed in viral meningitis.

Differential diagnosis. The causes of aseptic meningitis are listed in Box 13.1.

Prognosis. The symptoms rarely persist beyond 10 days: a repeat lumbar puncture should be considered if they do. However, note that CSF abnormalities may lag a few weeks behind clinical improvement. A few patients have recurrent aseptic meningitis, described by Mollaret; sometimes this is caused by recurrent Herpes simplex type 2 reactivation.

LYME DISEASE

An Ixodes tick transmits the organism, *Borrelia burgdorferi*, which disseminates widely, including the CNS. The first manifestation is often the rash, erythema chronicum migrans (ECM). In the UK the New Forest has Lyme disease; most people are bitten in their gardens since deer carrying the tick come and go from such areas. The classic neurological characteristics may appear within 4 weeks:

- Meningism.
- Cranial neuropathies (particularly unilateral or bilateral 7th nerve palsies).
- Painful radiculopathy.
- Features consistent with Bannwarth syndrome (lymphocytic meningoradiculitis).

CSF results include near normal glucose, mildly elevated protein and lymphocytes generally $<200/mm^3$.

Box 13.1: *Causes of aseptic meningitis*

Viral
- Enterovirus (the vast majority), includes echovirus and coxsackie.
- Mumps.
- Lymphocytic choriomeningitis.
- Herpes simplex type 2 (type 1 causes encephalitis and less commonly meningitis).
- HIV.

Non-viral
- Mycobacteria.
- Spirochaetes: syphilis and Lyme.
- Listeria.
- Parameningeal infections.
- Bacterial endocarditis.
- Mycoplasma (consider assessing cold agglutinins).
- Fungi.
- Malaria.

Non-infective
- Vasculitis.
- Uveo-meningitis, e.g. sarcoidosis, Vogt–Koyanagi–Harada disease.
- Malignant meningitis.
- Drugs, e.g. immunoglobulins, co-trimoxazole, naproxen and other NSAIDs.

ENCEPHALITIS

Encephalitis implies brain inflammation. Thus, patients with meningism, fever, photophobia and CSF findings similar to those in viral meningitis, but also with focal signs, seizures or reduced level of consciousness, have encephalitis (or meningoencephalitis). MRI may show signal change in the brain parenchyma (often temporal lobe in H. simplex type 1); EEG may show slow waves or periodic complexes (the latter again with H. simplex 1).

Herpes simplex encephalitis (HSE)

Herpes (Greek: 'to creep'). Herpes simplex type 1 virus is a common cause of encephalitis (annual frequency 1 in 300 000) with no season or gender predilection; two-thirds of cases are caused by endogenous reactivation; one-third represent new infection.

Clinical features

HSE often starts with a prodrome of fever and headache, later progressing to seizures, confusion, aphasia or hemiparesis. Psychosis and behavioural change may be prominent. 'Cold sores' are not more common in these patients.

Investigations

- MRI abnormalities occur in 60% (Fig. 13.2), particularly the temporal and inferior frontal brain regions; frequently brain swelling can result in uncal herniation.
- EEG abnormalities occur in 80%.
- CSF lymphocytosis (10–500 cells/mm^3) is common; CSF protein may be surprisingly raised, e.g. 5–6 g/L. CSF PCR for herpes virus is positive in 95% and remains positive for 5 days after starting treatment; note that blood-stained CSF can give falsely negative PCR.

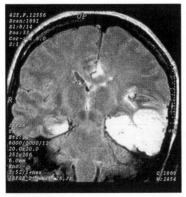

Figure 13.2
MRI showing asymmetrical signal change in herpes simplex encephalitis.

Management

- Intravenous aciclovir must be given promptly (10 mg/kg TDS for 14 days), while maintaining good hydration and monitoring renal function. Aciclovir is phosphorylated by viral thymidine kinase; aciclovir triphosphate inhibits viral DNA polymerase. Its use has reduced HSE mortality from 70% to 30%.
- Foscarnet may be added if the diagnosis is established but the patient still deteriorates.
- Corticosteroids may be required for cerebral oedema.
- Deteriorating conscious level suggests either raised intracranial pressure (may require discussion of ventilation or even decompressive craniectomy) or on-going seizure activity (may require EEG monitoring).

Prognosis

The two main prognostic determinants are:

1. Level of consciousness at presentation.
2. Time from illness onset to starting treatment.

Other viral encephalitides

- Herpes zoster.
  - Peripheral complications, especially radiculopathy, commonly follow shingles, particularly in the elderly. Motor radiculopathy occurs in 5%. Post-herpetic neuralgia is diagnosed if pain persists for >4 weeks after resolution of shingles.
  - CNS complications occur in up to 5% (more common than generally thought) and include cerebellitis but also myelitis, meningitis and encephalitis. These complications sometimes appear days or weeks following zoster infection.
  - *H. zoster* encephalitis may be severe and haemorrhagic, particularly in the immunocompromised; the leucoencephalitis and vasculopathy (with necrotizing cerebral vasculitis causing infarction and haemorrhage) is due either to direct viral invasion of vessel walls or to a delayed immunopathological or allergic reaction during convalescence. PCR in CSF is very helpful in diagnosis; CSF for IgG specific for *H. zoster* is useful later in the disease.
- Japanese B encephalitis.
  - This is spread by the Culicine mosquito. The virus affects the basal ganglia and thalamus, causing tremor, parkinsonism and extrapyramidal features in the acute and recovery stages.
- Western Nile virus.
  - This has gained some notoriety; the Culex mosquito spreads the flavivirus. It may manifest with typical encephalitic features (severe in only 1% of infected persons) but may cause additional lower motor neurone problems in the limbs and cranial nerves.
- Cytomegalovirus.
- HIV encephalitis (see below).

Infections resembling viral encephalitis

- **Cerebral malaria.** Patients with suspected encephalitis must always be asked about foreign travel. The female Anopheline mosquito spreads this protozoal infection. Falciparum infection causes neurological involvement, with reduced consciousness level, meningism, fever and oculogyric crisis. Hypoglycaemia can result either directly from infection or from intravenous quinine. Cerebral malaria is diagnosed using thick and thin blood films and with CSF (raised opening pressure and mild lymphocytosis). Lumbar puncture also helps to exclude other causes.
- **Endocarditis,** especially from fungal and mycobacterial causes may present with an encephalitis-like picture.
- **Atypical pneumonia,** e.g. mycoplasma or legionella.
- **Pneumococcal meningitis** presenting with reduced level of consciousness is easily mistaken for encephalitis.

Other conditions mimicking encephalitis

- **Space occupying lesions,** e.g. subdural haematoma, can cause fluctuating consciousness and often fever without long tract signs (especially in the elderly).
- **Vascular causes.** There are four main groups to consider:
  1. **Vasculitis,** either from systemic disease or isolated cerebral angiitis.
  2. **Vasculitic mimics,** including haemolytic uraemic syndrome, thrombotic thrombocytopenic purpura, lupus anti-coagulant syndrome, endocarditis, cholesterol embolization.
  3. **'Funny strokes'** (see Ch. 7). Thalamic strokes may present with confusion, drowsiness and eye movement disorder.
  4. **Cerebral venous thrombosis.** This is an important mimic. Patients present with headache and reduced level of consciousness. Cerebral imaging shows oedema and so LP is not usually undertaken. CT or MR venogram often give the diagnosis.
- **Metabolic causes,** e.g. renal failure, liver failure, diabetic coma. These are sometimes difficult to diagnose because often there is no fever (except with neuroleptic malignant or serotonin syndrome), no focal signs and seizures are generalized.
- **Others:**
  - Hashimoto's encephalopathy.
  - Wernicke's encephalopathy.
  - Neuroleptic malignant syndrome.
  - Toxins, e.g. carbon monoxide poisoning.
  - Demyelination, particularly acute disseminated encephalitis (ADEM). This usually affects children and is often associated with myelopathy or optic neuritis, but sometimes also fever.

Whipple's disease

This infection, although extremely rare, commonly crops up at clinicopathological conferences. The organism is *Tropheryma whipplei*. It causes gastrointestinal symptoms in 45%

of patients (malabsorption, diarrhoea and abdominal pain); 10–20% have neurological complications:

- Cognitive problems.
- Supranuclear gaze problems.
- Movement disorders, including one peculiar to Whipple's: oculomasticatory myorhythmia (pendular vergence oscillations synchronized to rhythmic mouth or palate movements).
- Hypothalamic problems, e.g. sleep abnormalities.

The diagnosis requires intestinal biopsy (PAS-positive macrophages) and CSF (PCR for *T. whippelii*).

Treatment is with a 3rd generation cephalosporin and trimethoprim/sulfamethoxazole, given for 1–2 years.

Subacute sclerosing panencephalitis (SSPE)

Pathogenesis: This is a subacute inflammatory and neurodegenerative encephalitis related to measles virus. It is thought to arise through defective virus maturation in neural cells containing aberrant M (matrix) protein.

Clinical features: The symptoms appear after a latent period, e.g. in teenagers who had measles aged <2 years (M:F ratio = 3:1). It begins with personality change or deterioration in school performance, but later with movement disorders and odd periodic stereotyped movements (corresponding EEG complexes) and ultimately akinetic mutism and death. Some have prominent visual symptoms, e.g. cortical blindness, chorioretinitis.

Investigations include CSF with high measles titres and oligoclonal bands (hence SSPE may be mistaken for MS, particularly if the visual symptoms are prominent). EEG is useful in diagnosis, showing long, repetitive complexes.

Prognosis: The mean survival is 18 months; 20% survive beyond 4 years.

Human immunodeficiency virus (HIV)

HIV affects the entire neuraxis. Highly active anti-retroviral therapy (HAART) increases CD4+ counts and has drastically changed mortality and morbidity in the developed world.

Seroconversion

Some 10% of patients have neurological problems during the seroconversion illness, e.g. meningitis, encephalitis, myelitis, myositis or cauda equina syndrome. Note that Guillain–Barré syndrome with a raised CSF cell count is highly suspicious of HIV seroconversion.

Peripheral nerve complications

There are three main causes of peripheral nerve involvement in HIV patients:

1. **HIV itself** is a common cause of distal sensorimotor neuropathy, often with pain and burning (small fibre involvement, which may be an isolated symptom).
2. **HAART** may cause a painful neuropathy: withdrawal of neurotoxic drugs (ddI, ddC, d4T) should be discussed with HIV physicians and the patient.
3. **Other explanations** should not be overlooked, e.g. alcohol or diabetes mellitus.

Treatment of HIV neuropathy is considered elsewhere (see Ch. 12).

HIV dementia

Consider HIV in young dementia patients. Before HAART was introduced, 20% of AIDS patients developed significant dementia. HIV dementia is typically associated with vacuolar myelopathy. There is usually a subcortical pattern of dementia with behavioural and psychiatric features.

Opportunistic infections

Relationship to CD4+ count. The CD4+ T lymphocyte count provides a guide to the level of immunosuppression and determines the type of opportunistic infection:

- With CD4+ counts <200/mm^3, toxoplasmosis is seen.
- At <100/mm^3, cryptococcal meningitis can develop.
- At <50/mm^3, CMV infections develop.

Mass lesions

- **Toxoplasmosis.** This often manifests as multifocal or basal ganglia lesions. The management is based on clinical and radiology findings, regardless of toxoplasma serology. Repeat MR scanning after 2 weeks of therapy: if responding, continue; if not responding, consider a biopsy.
- **Primary CNS lymphoma.** This often manifests as a single lesion next to ventricles, with considerable oedema. If CSF is taken, request EBV titres (causally related to lymphoma).
- **Tuberculoma.** Consider the patient's country of origin and check the chest radiograph.

Progressive multifocal leucoencephalopathy (PML)

- **Pathogenesis.** PML is caused by reactivation of the (confusingly named) JC virus, which is normally dormant within the kidney and reticuloendothelial system. It affects mainly the occipito-parietal white matter. Microscopically, there is demyelination with enlarged oligodendrocyte nuclei and bizarrely shaped astrocytes.
- **Clinical features.** PML presents with weakness, speech and language disturbance, often with cortical visual problems or other cortical problems, e.g. dyspraxia.
- **Diagnosis** is by imaging and CSF PCR for JC virus; CSF often contains a few lymphocytes (usually <20).
- **Treatment** aims to reverse the predisposing immunocompromise, e.g. with antiretrovirals. Note however, that HAART may be associated with the immune reconstitution syndrome: a deterioration, clinically, in PML and other infections.

Neurosyphilis

Neurosyphilis (*Treponema pallidum*) is now uncommon.

Clinical features

- **The primary infection** causes a chancre, usually on the genitals and self-limiting.
- **Secondary syphilis** may follow, characterized by a rash, condyloma lata (warty lesions in moist areas, e.g. perianal), lymphadenopathy and sometimes uveitis.
- **Neurosyphilis** may follow, often following a latent interval, relating mainly to chronic meningitis and comprising four overlapping entities:
    - Syphilitic meningitis, manifests as a leptomeningitis, vasculitis (Heubner's arteritis) and cord arachnoiditis. There may be meningitic symptoms and sometimes cranial nerve palsies.
    - Meningovascular syphilis. The chronic meningitis may cause a large vessel stroke, e.g. middle cerebral artery. However, a raised CSF protein and cell count after a stroke is non-specific and may follow a large non-infectious stroke.
    - Tabes dorsalis. Here the chronic meningitis affects the spinal cord causing the classical quartet of loss of deep tendon reflexes, ataxia, lightning pains and Argyll Robertson pupils; but also sometimes causing myelopathy or lower motor neurone bladder.
    - General paresis of the insane. This manifests as neuropsychiatric problems: hallucinations, frontal lobe deficits and sometimes Argyll Robertson pupils (see Ch. 14).

Antibody testing

There are two main antibody types in blood and CSF:
1. **Blood**
    - Non-specific. VDRL (venereal disease research laboratory), which often becomes negative with age and in chronic syphilis; RPR (rapid plasma reagin).
    - Specific. FTA-ABS (fluorescent treponemal antibody absorption), which is highly sensitive; TPHA (*T. pallidum* haemagglutination).
2. **CSF**
    - A positive VDRL is very specific, but not sensitive.
    - A positive FTA-ABS is very sensitive but not specific. A negative CSF FTA makes neurosyphilis very unlikely.

Note: Involve microbiologist, as diagnostic certainty may be elusive.

Management

- **Antibiotics.** Aqueous crystalline penicillin G 18–24 million units daily for 10–14 days, *or* procaine penicillin 2.4 million units i.m. once daily, with probenecid orally 500 mg four times per day for 10–14 days.
- **Repeat CSF** at 6, 12 and 24 weeks. If the cell count does not fall after 6 months, or if the CSF is abnormal after 2 years, repeat the treatment.

Treatment note
- Clinicians must have a low threshold to treat neurosyphilis.

- CSF cell count may be very low with indolent chronic meningitis.
- FTA and TPHA remain positive for a long time after treatment.

PRION DISEASE

(See Ch. 6)

Case history outcome

The patient had listeria meningitis. He made a good recovery following treatment with intravenous ampicillin and gentamicin.

KEY POINTS

- Guillain–Barré syndrome with a raised CSF cell count is suspicious of HIV seroconversion.
- All three common organisms causing meningitis in adults (pneumococcus, meningococcus and haemophilus) usually respond to an intravenous cephalosporin.
- In older patients with meningitis, consider listeria and Gram-negative organisms.
- HIV patients are susceptible to a wide range of opportunistic infections including toxoplasmosis, TB, PML and fungi.
- Herpes simplex encephalitis has a poor prognosis if treatment is delayed; where clinical suspicion is high start i.v. aciclovir immediately.
- VDRL is very specific for syphilis, but not sensitive; FTA-ABS is very sensitive but not specific. A negative CSF FTA makes neurosyphilis very unlikely.
- Suspected MS in a teenager may sometimes be SSPE, particularly with prominent visual symptoms and oligoclonal bands.
- Consider HIV in young dementia patients, particularly if there is associated myelopathy.

Further Reading

Roos KR. Meningitis 100 maxims. London: Edward Arnold; 1996.

Ophthalmic neurology 14

Case history

A 28-year-old female social worker of Afro-Caribbean ethnicity presented with a gradual onset of visual loss in her right eye. Her first symptoms were blurring and greying of vision, improving on covering the right eye. Her right eye vision had diminished over 2 days to the extent that she was blind in that eye. The eye was uncomfortable and she had mild photophobia. There was no eye trauma or other antecedent illness apart from a single episode of vertigo 1 year previously. On examination her visual acuity was 6/60 (right) and 6/6 (left). She had a right-sided relative afferent pupillary defect. Visual field examination revealed a large right-sided centrocaecal scotoma. Ishihara plate testing showed colour desaturation in the right eye. The remaining neurological examination was normal.

NEURO-OPHTHALMOLOGY

Visual loss or impairment is a common problem in neurological practice: occasionally ocular emergencies also present to neurologists, needing urgent identification and treatment. There is a broad spectrum of ophthalmological symptoms, with many potential causes: several symptoms are 'red flags' and must not be missed (Box 14.1). Fortunately, the constancy of the anatomical visual pathway allows reliable clinical localization. This, taken together with the chronology and context of the problem, usually facilitates a clinical diagnosis. This chapter provides a pragmatic framework to help to avoid pitfalls.

THE CONSULTATION

The nature of the visual disturbance determines the focus of history taking. Visual loss and diplopia are the common symptoms but others include positive visual phenomena and unusual visual alteration (occipital cortex) syndromes.

Box 14.1: When to call the ophthalmologist (URGENTLY)

Visual loss with:
- Painful, red eye.
- History of trauma.
- Previous severe ophthalmological disease in the affected eye.
- History (previous or current) of severe ophthalmological disease in the fellow eye.

VISUAL LOSS

This is the most common ophthalmic complaint. The pattern of visual loss gives the biggest clue to its cause. A working knowledge of the visual system anatomy is essential to undertaking and interpreting the necessary detailed examination (see Fig. 4.1).

Pattern

The pattern of visual loss, together with symptom chronology and context, should provide the diagnosis.

- **One or both eyes?** It is essential first to distinguish whether the visual loss is monocular or binocular. A patient may describe blindness in the right eye when in fact there is a right homonymous hemianopia. Does the symptom improve with covering either eye? Monocular visual loss implies damage in the eye or optic nerve. However, the clinician should search for visual loss in the other eye, as it is easy to miss a junctional scotoma from chiasmal compression. Binocular visual loss implies damage further back, anywhere from the optic chiasm through the optic tracts and optic radiation, to the visual cortex.
- **Persistent monocular blindness** is a neuro-ophthalmological emergency and requires immediate referral. Within 90 min of suspected central retinal artery thrombosis, consider ocular massage and oculocentesis (in collaboration with on call ophthalmologist). If blindness persists after 90 min of ischaemia, it is very likely to persist: the emergency is then to save the sight in the other eye, usually with high dose steroids (for suspected temporal arteritis).
- **An altitudinal defect** 'like a curtain coming down' if monocular, suggests retinal ischaemia (carotid origin); if binocular, suggests posterior cerebral circulation ischaemia.
- **An enlarging blind spot:** if monocular, points to papillitis; if binocular, suggests papilloedema.

Progression

The speed of progression is diagnostically helpful (Table 14.1).

- **Acute or instantaneous** monocular blindness (especially if altitudinal) is usually ischaemic, even if the cause of the ischaemia is actually compression. Note also that there may be apparently sudden onset if patients notice a pre-existing visual loss for the first time, e.g. when closing one eye, looking at a clock face, or driving at night.
- **Sub-acute visual loss** usually has an inflammatory or compressive cause. The exception is Leber's hereditary optic neuropathy, which is degenerative but presents sub-acutely.
- **Chronic visual loss** usually has a degenerative or compressive cause.
- **Transient symptoms** may be trivial and harmless (see below), or may be ominous, as with amaurosis fugax heralding a possible stroke.

Drugs and toxins affect vision both acutely and chronically and so should be considered in any pattern of visual loss.

Table 14.1: Neurological visual loss

Presentation	Mechanism of insult	Diagnosis
Acute	Ischaemia	Central retinal artery occlusion, branch retinal artery occlusion, anterior ischaemic optic neuropathy (e.g. giant cell arteritis), pituitary apoplexy (usually bilateral)
Sub-acute	Inflammation	Optic neuritis (e.g. multiple sclerosis, sarcoidosis), chronic relapsing inflammatory optic neuropathy (CRION)
	Compression/raised ICP	Idiopathic intracranial hypertension, tumours (metastases)
	Infection and neoplasm	Chronic meningitis (tuberculous, syphilis, neoplastic, fungal)
	Toxic and nutritional	Tobacco-alcohol syndrome, B_{12} deficiency
Chronic	Compression	Tumours (gliomas (e.g. neurofibromatosis type 1), craniopharyngiomas, meningiomas, metastases), thyroid ophthalmopathy, Wegener's granulomatosis
	Degenerative	Leber's hereditary optic neuropathy, retinitis pigmentosa, Refsum's disease

Associated features

Additional features may give the clue to the diagnosis.

- **Headache** is common in giant cell arteritis and migraine; masticatory claudication should be specifically asked about, as it is sufficiently uncommon to be highly suggestive of arteritis. Remember to palpate the temporal arteries (are they non-pulsatile and tender?) and the occipital arteries.
- **Pain on eye movement** suggests optic neuritis or other optic nerve inflammation; it is unusual following ischaemia.
- **Persistent eye pain,** particularly with conjunctival suffusion, strongly suggests ocular causes including glaucoma and uveitis; ophthalmological review is essential.
- **Ocular trauma** requires ophthalmological assessment, usually involving pupil dilatation, so complete the neurological examination first.

Clinical context

- **Age** influences the order of differential diagnosis. Among patients with monocular blindness, those aged <45 years are likely to have migraine, idiopathic intracranial hypertension or optic neuritis; those aged >45 years are likely to have anterior ischaemic optic neuropathy or central retinal artery occlusion.
- **Previous symptoms** may be diagnostically helpful. Visual loss may be associated with vertigo, ataxia and dysarthria (suggesting posterior fossa pathology), disseminated central nervous symptoms (suggesting multiple sclerosis), or systemic complaints such as myalgia and arthralgia (suggesting a connective tissue disease or giant cell arteritis).
- **Drugs and toxins** are particularly important. The history should include specific questioning about herbal drugs, as the patient may not consider these to be 'medications' (Table 14.2).

Table 14.2: Drugs causing eye disease

Condition	Drug
Scleritis	Bisphosphonates
Keratopathy	Amiodarone, chloroquine, clofazimine
Posterior cataracts	Glucocorticoids
Maculopathy	Tamoxifen, hydroxychloroquine, chloroquine
Retinopathy	Tamoxifen, thioridazine, vigabatrin, Talc (in i.v. drug abuse)
Open angle glaucoma	Glucocorticoids
Closed angle glaucoma	Topiramate, tricyclic antidepressants, tetracyclic antidepressants
Optic neuropathy	Amiodarone, ethambutol, chloramphenicol
Nystagmus, diplopia and extra-ocular muscle palsies	CNS depressants, antihistamines, antiepileptic drugs
Idiopathic intracranial hypertension	Glucocorticoids, tetracyclines, sodium valproate

- **Nutritional status** is important. A careful dietary history may unearth a restricted or limited diet, requiring vitamin supplementation. 'Alcohol-tobacco amblyopia' is now considered to be a nutritional condition exacerbated by toxins. It is potentially treatable: parenteral thiamine can prevent further visual loss.
- **Family history** of visual and neurological disorders is sometimes revealing; familial visual loss occurs in Leber's disease (especially males), mitochondrial cytopathy (retinopathy, ptosis, ophthalmoparesis or strokes), or CADASIL (cerebral autosomal dominant arteriopathy with subcortical ischaemic leucoencephalopathy) where there are associated migraine and strokes (see Fig. 10.4).

DIPLOPIA

Double or blurred?

Patients often report seeing double, but actually mean something else. The distinction is clearly essential.

Which muscle(s)?

Having established that the patient is seeing double, there are two main localizing questions:

- Are the images side by side or one on top of the other (i.e. horizontal, vertical or oblique)?
- In which direction is the double vision worst (i.e. widest separation of the images)?

One or both eyes?

Clarify whether the diplopia is binocular. Diplopia that persists when one eye is covered suggests an ocular abnormality (retinal detachment, dislocated lens or keratoconus), an occipital lesion (causing the phenomena of monocular polyopia or palinopsia), or a non-organic disorder.

Variability

Myasthenia gravis can initially mimic single cranial nerve lesions or posterior strokes through eye muscle fatiguability and patients may not volunteer fluctuating symptoms. Rarer reasons for variability are dysthyroid eye disease and progressive extra-ocular ophthalmoplegias, as in mitochondrial disease.

Chronology

All diplopia starts suddenly (the patient either has double vision or not); gradual onset therefore refers to the diplopia becoming more persistent and the images more widely separated. As a general rule:

- **Acute onset** suggests an ischaemic insult.
- **Subacute onset** suggests a compressive lesion.

The cover test

On testing pursuit eye movements, identify where the double vision is worst. The outer image (furthest away from the patient either horizontally or vertically) is the 'false' image from the eye that is not moving fully. Cover either eye to confirm the eye responsible for this false image.

Upper or lower motor neurone?

This distinction is important in localizing the cause.

- Lower motor neurone ophthalmoparesis refers to pathology of the cranial nerves (3, 4, or 6), extra-ocular muscles, or neuromuscular junction.
- Upper motor neurone (supra-nuclear) ophthalmoparesis refers to pathology of the centres controlling conjugate gaze, disrupting either horizontal or vertical gaze.

Simple eye movement disorders

Cranial nerve palsies

The 3rd, 4th or 6th nerve palsies have specific patterns and are considered in Chapter 1. Note that the 6th nerve may be damaged anywhere along its long and tortuous path; a 6th nerve palsy is usually due to a microvascular lesion but a false localizing 6th may occur with raised intracranial pressure and need emergency management.

Gaze palsies

An isolated conjugate gaze palsy should not give diplopia, though the patient may report being 'unable to see' on the affected side.

- **Supranuclear vertical gaze disorders** may manifest first as slowing of vertical saccades and only later as limitation and subsequent loss. The vertical gaze centre is in the floor of the third ventricle at the superior colliculus level.

- **Supranuclear horizontal gaze disorders** are caused by contralateral frontal lobe damage (usually stroke): the patient cannot look towards the hemiparetic side. Passive involuntary eye movements are preserved on the doll's eye manoeuvre, confirming the upper motor neurone nature.

Complex eye movement disorders

Where movement is abnormal bilaterally and complex, pure cranial nerve or nuclear pathologies are less likely.

- **Anterior internuclear ophthalmoplegia (INO) and 'one and a half' syndrome** are more complex and unusual conditions that commonly present with diplopia (see Fig. 2.12). They usually occur in multiple sclerosis, although sometimes with brainstem strokes. The medial longitudinal fasciculus is disrupted in both disorders, but in the 'one and a half' syndrome there is also conjugate gaze palsy.
- **Nuclear ophthalmoplegia** giving horizontal gaze palsy is caused by ipsilateral brain stem pathology, usually pontine stroke, where the patient involuntarily gazes towards the hemiparetic side. The eyes remain fixed during the doll's eye manoeuvre, confirming the lower motor neurone nature. There may be co-existing nystagmus or vertical gaze disruption including skew deviation.

Finding no clear pattern does not necessarily imply a brain stem lesion, even with apparent nystagmus at extremes of gaze. Dysthyroid eye disease and myasthenia gravis are possible diagnoses (Table 14.3).

Table 14.3: Causes of diplopia

Site	Timing	Mechanism	Diagnosis
Brainstem	Acute or stuttering	Ischaemia	Stroke
	Subacute	Inflammation	Multiple sclerosis
	Chronic	Tumours	Glioma
		Inflammation	Progressive multifocal leucoencephalopathy
Cranial nerves			
3	Acute	Infarction	Diabetes mellitus, hypertension
		Mechanical	Posterior communicating artery aneurysm
	Chronic	Tumour	Cavernous sinus, glioma or metastases
		Infection	Chronic meningitis
4	Acute	Infarction	Diabetes mellitus, hypertension
6	Acute	Raised ICP	False localizing sign due to tortuous path of 6th cranial nerve (unilateral or bilateral).
		Infarction	Diabetes mellitus, hypertension
3, 4 and 6	Sub-acute	Inflammation	Miller Fisher syndrome
3, 4 and 6	Chronic	Inflammation	Cavernous sinus syndrome or orbital apex syndrome
Neuromuscular junction	Chronic	Autoimmune	Myasthenia gravis, rarely Lambert–Eaton myasthenic syndrome
Muscle paresis	Chronic	Inflammation	Dysthyroid eye disease
		Degenerative	Progressive external ophthalmoplegia (mitochondrial cytopathy)

Patient context

This can provide useful diagnostic clues.

- **Cranial nerve palsies** are the most common with diabetes mellitus and hypertension, but remember syphilis is historically the most common cause and is re-emerging.
- **Gaze palsies** (particularly with internuclear ophthalmoplegia) in young people are usually due to multiple sclerosis.

POSITIVE VISUAL PHENOMENA

Benign

- **Fortification spectra (teichopsia)** are characteristic of migraine with aura, but can occur in isolation (migraine equivalent). They are named after the zigzag outline of medieval forts (*teichopsia*: town wall vision). Aspirin is usually effective.
- **Phosphenes** (intermittent flashes) are common benign phenomena in older people which are alarming to the patient but do not require detailed investigation. However, phosphenes can be seen in impending retinal detachment.
- **Floaters** are common in health, but severe persistent unilateral floaters suggest retinal detachment or vitreous haemorrhage.

Serious

Spectra (rainbows) or haloes surrounding objects in the vision, especially when monocular, suggest glaucoma and require urgent ophthalmological referral.

VISUAL ALTERATION (OCCIPITAL CORTEX) SYNDROMES

Several syndromes listed in Table 14.4 cause sometimes bizarre-sounding symptoms that are easily misdiagnosed or dismissed.

Table 14.4: Occipital cortex syndromes

Syndrome	Localization within occipital lobe	Clinical features
Anton's syndrome	Bilateral calcarine	Bilateral loss of vision with patient denial
Balint's syndrome	Bilateral occipito-parietal	Simultagnosia, optic ataxia and ocular apraxia
Bonnet's syndrome	Unilateral or bilateral	Lilliputian visual hallucinations
Palinopsia	Calcarine	Afterimage persistence
Prosopagnosia	Right or bilateral inferior calcarine	Inability to recognize faces
Occipital lobe epilepsy	Any	Lateralized unformed visual hallucinations culminating in convulsion

EXAMINATION POINTS

General examination

The examination should include:

- Weight and body mass index (BMI): typically raised in idiopathic intracranial hypertension.
- Temperature: fever may suggest giant cell arteritis or infective endocarditis.
- Head position: a head tilt is often seen in diplopia.
- Evidence of trauma may suggest eye injury including retinal detachment.
- Cardiovascular examination is important if there is a suspected retinal ischaemic insult and should include blood pressure measurement (hypertension) and cardiac rhythm (atrial fibrillation).
- Skin examination may identify rashes of suspected varicella zoster infection, vasculitis or HIV.

Neurological examination

This should include:

- Cognitive and alertness assessment (reduced with raised intracranial pressure).
- Detailed neurological examination to identify clues to more generalized conditions, e.g. myasthenia gravis (evidence of fatiguability) and multiple sclerosis (pyramidal, cerebellar or sensory signs).
- Temporal artery palpation is important.
- Listen for bruits over the orbit (cavernous sinus) and carotid areas.

General ocular examination

This should include:

- Inspection of the eyes and periorbital areas.
- Eye position at rest may show skew deviations and strabismus.
- Orbital symmetry, assessed from above, may show proptosis (retrobulbar mass) or dysthyroid eye disease.
- Orbital or periorbital swelling suggests either orbital cellulitis or cavernous sinus pathology.
- Chemosis or inflammation of the corneas and conjunctivae must prompt urgent ophthalmological referral.

Practice note: Red, inflamed eyes require urgent ophthalmological review.

Visual acuity

This should be quantified in each eye. It is important to have optimal refractive correction, using the patient's (cleaned) spectacles. Alternatively, pinhole acuity assessments are useful and certainly better than uncorrected acuities. Where corrected vision improves with a pinhole, this clearly implies an uncorrected refractive error. Where there is very severely reduced visual acuity (worse than 6/60), the next three measures are the patient's ability to count fingers, detect hand movements and finally, to perceive light. In optic neuritis, the centrocaecal scotoma can be so large that hand movements are not seen: it is therefore important that in apparent monocular blindness, hand movements are tested in the far periphery of vision. In people who cannot use a Snellen chart, e.g. preverbal children or adults who do not read or speak English, alternatives include assessing the patient negotiating obstacles or by preferentially looking towards objects of interest. For example, one might offer two objects, one plain and one coloured, then move their position and observe whether the patient registers this.

Pupil examination

This includes assessing the pupil's regularity and shape. A painful red eye with an oval pupil suggests acute glaucoma requiring urgent referral and treatment. There is often a previous history of trauma or previous surgery. Anisocoria (unequally sized pupils) is often longstanding but previously unnoticed; ask to see old photographs and remember to enquire about topical agents. Establish which pupil is abnormal and check the light and accommodation responses. *A relative afferent pupillary defect* (RAPD) is identified by a direct search, *'the swinging flashlight test'*. Shine the light directly into one eye and then the other at several second intervals. It is not necessary to dip the light source under the nose or to place a barrier between the two eyes. If the pupil dilates upon shining the light directly into it, it means the consensual response is preserved and the direct response is impaired, i.e. there is ipsilateral optic nerve damage.

Fundoscopy

This is important in patients with visual symptoms, in particular to examine the optic disc, the macula and the retinal periphery.

Optic disc abnormalities

The disc may be pink in acute haemorrhage or inflammation or pale following optic nerve damage. In general, ask an ophthalmologist to photograph abnormal fundi and to chart the visual fields. A fluorescein angiogram can help to demonstrate papilloedema in equivocal cases, but surprisingly often is equivocal.

Papilloedema

Papilloedema (Fig. 14.1) is almost always bilateral but beware of Foster–Kennedy syndrome and occasional asymmetrical presentations. Spontaneous venous pulsations are absent in papilloedema, owing to elevated intracranial hypertension, but note that up to 10% of the normal population have absent venous pulsations. Visual acuity is usually preserved. There are many causes:

- Space occupying lesion.
- Idiopathic intracranial hypertension:

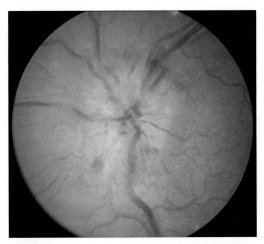

Figure 14.1
Papilloedema.

- Venous sinus thrombosis.
- Drugs, e.g. tetracycline.
- SLE and other connective tissue disorders.
- Endocrinopathies e.g. Cushing's disease.
- **Carbon dioxide retention.**
- **Hypertension.**
- **Hypocalcaemia.**
- **Chronic meningitis (meningitis present for >4 weeks):**
  - **Infections** including spirochaetal, mycobacterial, fungal (particularly cryptococcus: note that 25% have otherwise normal CSF so a cryptococcal antigen test is important if there is diagnostic doubt).
  - **Malignant meningitis** patients are less obtunded than with chronic infection and often have lower cranial nerve involvement (unusual with chronic infections). Remember to look for cauda equina problems and myeloradiculopathy: absent reflexes are common.
  - **Vasculitis**, e.g. Wegener's granulomatosis, has frequently been present for several months before diagnosis.
  - **Uveo-meningitic conditions,** especially sarcoidosis.
- **Diabetic papillopathy.**

Papillitis

- **Papillitis** is almost invariably unilateral and often accompanied by discomfort and impaired visual acuity. There are four main conditions to consider:
  1. **Optic neuropathy** may result from demyelination (optic neuritis) or a vascular cause. Typically, there is reduced visual acuity and a visual field defect (altitudinal defect with vascular causes, central scotoma with optic neuritis).

2. **Optic nerve tumour** (compression or infiltration). An optic nerve sheath meningioma may give ipsilateral visual loss when looking to the side (a form of claudication); field testing may show both a scotoma and peripheral loss and fundoscopy may show cilio-retinal shunt vessels.
3. **Central retinal vein occlusion** gives haemorrhages all over retina, not just at the disc margins.
4. **Drusen** is often mistaken for papillitis or papilloedema. If doubt exists, an ophthalmological opinion is essential. Signs favouring drusen include preserved spontaneous venous pulsations and a heaped appearance to the disc, especially of blood vessels. Drusen sometimes runs in families (autosomal dominant).

Optic disc cupping

This suggests glaucoma, something to consider with all visual loss.

Macular abnormalities

Macular disease that presents acutely is either ischaemic or haemorrhagic.

- **Ischaemia** presents with macular pallor, sometimes with secondary vasospasm (occurs within 90 min) or visible cholesterol emboli (requiring careful and experienced fundoscopy).
- **Haemorrhage.** Large macular haemorrhages are easily visible but it may be difficult to decide if it is of arterial or venous origin. Micro-haemorrhagic areas are harder to see, but usually suggest vasculitis. The diagnosis may need an expert ophthalmology assessment.

Visual field assessment

This should be attempted for each eye, even with an apparently clear monocular deficit. See Figure 4.1 for the anatomy of the anterior visual pathway including the tracts, chiasm and radiation. Clinically important anatomical points are:

- The representation of superior images by inferior parts of the optic tract.
- The involvement of the chiasm by crossed and uncrossed fibres (junctional lesions affect both eyes).
- By convention, field diagrams are drawn as though one is looking through them, i.e. the right eye is situated on the right of the paper.

The initial visual field screening is done by confrontation with both eyes open. This should identify homonymous deficits (by definition retro-chiasmal) but may not pick up incongruent deficits.

- **Unilateral altitudinal defects** are typical of anterior ischaemic optic neuropathy.
- **Centrocaecal scotomas** are typical of optic neuritis.
- **Blind spot enlargement** supports a diagnosis of papilloedema, e.g. in idiopathic intracranial hypertension.

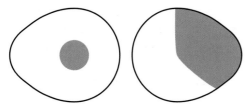

Figure 14.2
Junctional scotoma of Traquair. Scotoma plus contralateral temporal hemianopia caused by involvement of the optic nerve near the chiasm, which impairs conduction in the ipsilateral crossing fibres but too anterior to affect nasal retinal fibres crossing from the fellow eye.

- **Junctional lesions** at the chiasm have a central scotoma in one eye, a temporal cut in the other eye. This is because of involvement of the forward sweeping lower nasal fibres (giving vision to the upper outer quadrant) (Fig. 14.2).

Visual field testing tips

Vertical field loss suggests a 'neurological' cause, whereas horizontal suggests retinal pathology. A stationary target is more sensitive than a moving one when testing congruent field deficits; thus asking for a finger count in varying quadrants is better than asking for identification of a moving finger. Always test all four quadrants and remember that a red pin is a useful way of testing colour desaturation (which may occur without frank blindness) and is a sensitive test of field loss. Remember to test the central 6° of vision served by the macula. Colour vision testing with Ishihara plates is particularly useful in probable optic neuritis. Figure 14.3a–f illustrates several typical field deficits.

Extra-ocular movements

These must be examined in each eye separately and then together. Cranial nerve palsies should be readily identifiable on individual eye assessment (Fig. 14.4), while disruption of the medial longitudinal fasciculus is best appreciated when examining both eyes together.

INVESTIGATIONS AND MANAGEMENT (Table 14.5)

Blood tests

The targeting of investigations depends upon the clinical context.

- **Probable ischaemic episodes** should be investigated for diabetes mellitus, raised ESR, anaemia and hypercoagulable states.
- **Cranial nerve palsies** should be investigated for diabetes mellitus and syphilis.
- **Optic neuritis** symptoms should be investigated for multiple sclerosis, sarcoidosis and lupus.

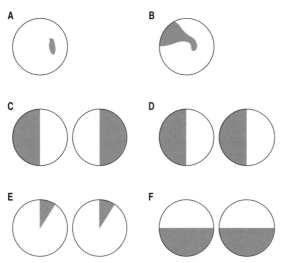

Figure 14.3
Patterns of visual field loss. (a) Seidel scotoma: early optic nerve damage. (b) Arcuate nerve fibre defect due to optic nerve lesion. (c) Bitemporal hemianopia due to chiasmal compression. (d) Homonymous hemianopia; congruous, thereby implying posterior lesion (parietal or occipital). (e) 'Pie in the sky' field loss implying a temporal lesion. (f) Bilateral inferior altitudinal defects caused by bilateral parieto-occipital lesions (usually infarctions).

Table 14.5: Common diagnoses requiring immediate management

Condition	Clinical features	Management
Central retinal artery occlusion	Often associated with hypertension or arrhythmia	Consider ocular massage and oculocentesis in presentations within 90 min, in association with ophthalmology (cherry-red spot consistent with infarction excludes these manoeuvres). Search for an embolic source, (carotid Doppler, and echocardiogram) and heparinize until definitive treatment is complete
Arteritic ischaemic optic neuropathy	Visual loss and headache in aged >65 years, with anorexia, fever, myalgia and jaw claudication	Prevent contralateral visual loss (occurs in up to 40%). Start prednisolone 100 mg daily (or 1–1.5 mg/kg) and monitor ESR. Arrange temporal artery biopsy within 1 week. Prepare patient for long-term treatment of 1–2 years
Transient monocular blindness	Vascular risk factors	Search for stroke risk factors. Treat with anti-platelet regimen as a minimum and heparinize if awaiting endarterectomy
Retrobulbar mass lesion	Proptosis, visual loss and ophthalmoplegia	Expert neuroradiology advice for best mode of imaging: may need both MRI and CT thin orbital cuts (for bony erosion).
Inflammatory optic neuritis	Presenting symptom in 15% of MS. Also consider vasculitis. If relapsing and steroid-responsive, consider CRION	i.v. methylprednisolone 1 g for 3 days if no contraindication. Search for disseminated demyelination (brain MRI); exclude vasculitis. CRION requires oral prednisolone in slowly tapering dose with acuity and fields monitoring
Idiopathic intracranial hypertension	Papilloedema and enlarged blind spots. Worsening acuity requires urgent intervention	Exclude intracranial mass lesions and venous sinus thrombosis. Lumbar puncture for both diagnostic and (short-term) treatment. Stop potential causative agents. Prescribe acetazolamide. Advise weight loss. Monitor with perimetry and frequent review. If medical treatment fails, consider optic nerve fenestration or lumboperitoneal shunt

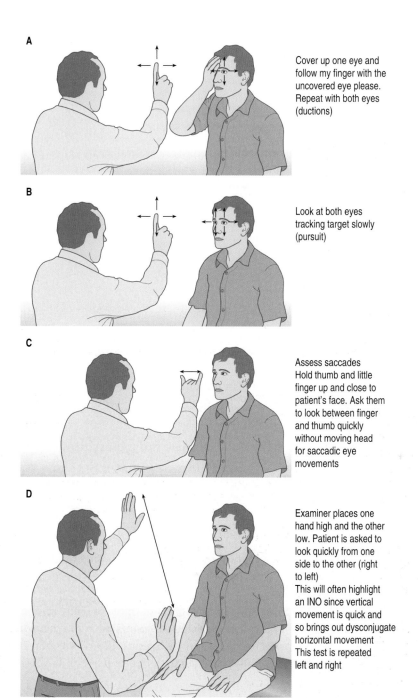

A

Cover up one eye and follow my finger with the uncovered eye please. Repeat with both eyes (ductions)

B

Look at both eyes tracking target slowly (pursuit)

C

Assess saccades
Hold thumb and little finger up and close to patient's face. Ask them to look between finger and thumb quickly without moving head for saccadic eye movements

D

Examiner places one hand high and the other low. Patient is asked to look quickly from one side to the other (right to left)
This will often highlight an INO since vertical movement is quick and so brings out dysconjugate horizontal movement
This test is repeated left and right

Figure 14.4
Extra-ocular movements. (a) Test eye movements with ductions and versions. Examiner: 'Cover one eye and follow my finger with the uncovered eye please'. Repeat with both eyes (ductions); then (b) Look at both eyes tracking the target slowly (pursuit); then (c) Assess saccades: examiner holds thumb and little finger up and close to the patient's face. Ask the patient to look between finger and thumb quickly without moving his head for saccadic eye movement; then (d) Patient looks quickly from right to left. This will often highlight internuclear ophthalmoplegia (INO), since vertical movement is quick and tends to highlight horizontal dysconjugate movement. This test is repeated left to right.

- **A chronic meningitis** clinical picture should be investigated for neoplasm, tuberculosis, HIV, fungal and other opportunistic infections.

Imaging

This is indicated for patients whose visual symptoms occur with:

- **Suspected raised intracranial pressure** clearly requires cerebral imaging, to exclude mass lesions but also venous sinus thrombosis.
- **Focal ocular or CNS neurology** requires imaging targeted according to whether the pathology is more likely in the orbit or brain.
- **Probable optic neuritis.** Here, although the optic nerve is affected, imaging aims to identify previous or disseminated pathology.

Lumbar puncture

This is usually performed for visual symptoms when there is a suspicion of an inflammatory cause.

- **Routine tests.** The CSF opening pressure should always be recorded, along with the cell count, protein and paired glucose.
- **Paired oligoclonal bands** must be sought in patients with probable inflammatory causes.
- **Other tests** might include tuberculosis PCR and culture, CSF syphilis serology, fungal staining, cytology and immunophenotyping.

Traditional advice always to save a CSF sample is currently difficult to justify, so aim to request all your tests the first time.

Static perimetry

Formal perimetry is useful in several situations.

- **Localization.** Perimetry is at its most helpful in characterizing unilateral defects or incongruent non-homonymous defects (usually pre-chiasmal) or incongruent homonymous defects (optic tract).
- **Monitoring.** Perimetry is useful in monitoring progress in optic neuritis, idiopathic intracranial hypertension and CRION (chronic relapsing inflammatory optic neuropathy).
- **Driving eligibility.** Legal requirements for driving in UK require 120° horizontal field of binocular vision and 70° vertically unilaterally; perimetry is often required in borderline cases.

Case history outcome

The patient was given methyl prednisolone i.v. (1 g daily for 3 days) and by day 3, her visual acuity was 6/18 (right) and 6/6 (left). Field-testing demonstrated a persistent but smaller centrocaecal scotoma in the right eye, including colour desaturation. Brain MRI revealed multiple periventricular lesions and two infratentorial lesions. CSF showed a normal cell count and protein, but positive unmatched oligoclonal bands. Serum angiotensin converting enzyme, antinuclear antibody, anti-double stranded DNA, anticardiolipin antibody, lupus anticoagulant tests and chest radiograph were all normal or negative. Multiple sclerosis was diagnosed.

KEY POINTS

- Clarify the nature of the visual problem in the history.
- Enquire about drugs and consider stopping potential causative agents.
- Family history may be illuminating.
- Examine both eyes carefully.
- In bilateral acute visual loss, consider raised ICP and pituitary apoplexy.
- Acute visual loss is an emergency.
- Acute glaucoma, uveitis and retinal detachment require urgent expert ophthalmology help: do not delay.
- In ischaemic optic neuropathy, attempt to preserve sight in the symptomatic eye (by involving the on-call ophthalmologist) and if impossible, prevent blindness in the fellow eye.

Further Reading

Acheson J, Riordan-Eva P. Neuro-ophthalmology. London: BMJ Books; 1999.

General medicine and neurology

15

Case history

A 20-year-old man presented to the Accident and Emergency Department following a first generalized seizure earlier that day. His parents (who are first cousins) reported that over the last year, he had become rather apathetic and withdrawn and he had struggled at college, having previously been a very bright student. He had no siblings. A cousin (aged 28) was reported as having Parkinson's disease. He did not drink alcohol and was not on any medication. On examination, he was drowsy and confused (post-ictal). He had widespread, jerky, choreiform movements. The rest of the neurological examination was normal. He had a 3 cm smooth enlarged liver. There was no evidence of jaundice. He had no stigmata of liver failure.

HAEMATOLOGY

Anaemia

Symptoms include tiredness, fatigue, tinnitus, headache and occasionally pica. Reversible hemiparesis may occur from the combination of arteriosclerotic carotid vessels and severe anaemia (Hb <7.5 g/L). In severe anaemia, papilloedema may occur.

Vitamin B$_{12}$ deficiency (Fig. 15.1)

Vitamin B$_{12}$ is involved in forming methionine (promoting DNA synthesis) and succinyl CoA. Defective methylation results in altered sized fatty acids and an abnormal myelin sheath compact array, allowing myelin breakdown. The many causes of vitamin B$_{12}$ deficiency include pernicious anaemia, malabsorption and nitrous oxide exposure. It may be precipitated by folic acid supplements. B$_{12}$ deficiency causes sub-acute (over months) neuropathy, myelopathy and encephalopathy.

- **Anaemia.** Major blood film changes do not necessarily accompany the neurology. Painful glossitis is often recalled if specifically sought.
- **Neuropathy** is usually sensory (tingling or sensory loss), i.e. identical to the myelopathic symptoms. However, it often starts in the hands and reflexes are lost.
- **Myelopathy** involves the most myelinated fibres (posterior columns) causing striking joint position loss in the lower limbs. Lhermitte's phenomenon is characteristic. There is usually a spastic paraparesis with extensor plantars, but bladder involvement is typically late.

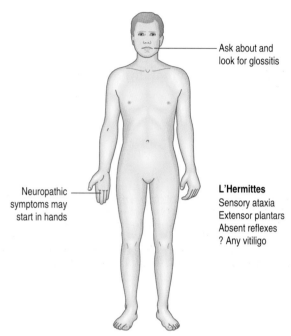

Ask about and
look for glossitis

Neuropathic
symptoms may
start in hands

L'Hermittes
Sensory ataxia
Extensor plantars
Absent reflexes
? Any vitiligo

Figure 15.1
The effects of B_{12} deficiency.

- **Encephalopathy** gives confusion, auditory and visual hallucinations and mood disturbance. The demyelination involves the corpus callosum, frontal and parietal cortex and sometimes the cord.
- **Optic neuropathy** is rare (bilateral centrocaecal scotomata).

Investigations include blood film and serum vitamin B_{12} assay. Methylmalonic acid and total homocysteine measurements may also help. High methylmalonic acid levels may be the only abnormality after nitrous oxide exposure.

Sickle cell disease and thalassemia

- **Sickling** occurs at low oxygen tensions, usually in veins. Stroke can result directly; myelopathy and radiculopathy usually result from bony vertebral infarcts.
- **Thalassemia** causes extramedullary haemopoiesis (e.g. liver and spleen). Myelopathy can result from bony enlargement secondary to compensatory haemopoiesis. Peripheral sensorimotor neuropathy also occurs.

Polycythaemia

- **Stroke** (thrombotic and haemorrhagic) becomes more likely.
- **Chorea** may develop, especially in women aged >50 years.

- **Hyperviscosity symptoms** (auditory and visual disturbances, headache, lethargy, somnolence and TIA-like events) accompany high blood cell counts, e.g. $>200 \times 10^9$/L.
- **Headache with a raised haemoglobin** may occur with chronic carbon monoxide poisoning, haemangioblastoma, renal cell cancer and chronic hypoventilation.

Thrombocytopenia

This complicates several neurological conditions.

SLE and lupus anticoagulant syndrome

The clinical associations of lupus anticoagulant syndrome are described in Chapter 7.

Thrombocytopenia is one of the 11 diagnostic criteria for systemic lupus erythematosus (SLE) (American Rheumatism Association). Lupus anticoagulant interferes with phospholipid binding to form prothrombin activator, a complex of calcium ions, Factors Xa and V and a phospholipid (platelet Factor III). Clinical features include:

- Valvular lesions (often ventricular, but marantic often atrial).
- Livedo reticularis (and stroke: Sneddon's).
- Migraine.
- Recurrent fetal loss.
- Arterial and venous thrombosis.

Thrombotic thrombocytopenic purpura

This comprises:

- Fever.
- Renal dysfunction.
- Neurological features (often fluctuating) including coma, headache and seizures.
- Microangiopathic haemolysis, with low platelets.

Gaucher's disease

This condition (glucocerebrosidase deficiency) comprises:

- Horizontal gaze palsy.
- Cognitive impairment (mild to severe).
- Ataxia.
- Thrombocytopenia.
- Dystonia and/or seizures.

Haemophilia

Severe Factor VIII deficiency (<1% activity) gives a high risk of haemorrhagic complications.

- **Peripheral nerve lesions** are the most common neurological complication, resulting mostly from intramuscular haematomas.
- **Intracranial haemorrhage** is a major cause of mortality (30% of deaths).

Paraproteins and neuropathy

Some 10% of neuropathy patients have a paraprotein. There are several causes:

- **Monoclonal gammopathy of uncertain significance (MGUS).** MGUS is a low-level paraprotein (<3 g/dL); patients with MGUS differ from those with myeloma in having less than 5% plasma cells in their marrow, no Bence–Jones protein, no anaemia, normal calcium and normal renal function. However, 30% of MGUS become malignant within 20 years. The associated neuropathy is usually demyelinating, but occasionally axonal. IgA- or IgG-associated demyelinating neuropathies respond to CIDP-like treatment. Those with IgM MGUS appear different, presenting as a DADS-M (see below); they respond less well, but sometimes improve with chlorambucil, cyclophosphamide, fludarabine or rituximab (anti-CD20).
- **Myeloma.** (See below).
- **Waldenström's macroglobulinaemia** causes a (usually demyelinating) neuropathy, affecting bulbar function as well as limbs.
- **Motor neurone disease.** 10% of MND patients have a paraprotein. Great care and meticulous neurophysiology are needed to avoid missing neuropathy presenting as MND.
- **Cryoglobulins.** 70% of patients with mixed cryoglobulins have hepatitis C.
- **Amyloid AL** causes a small fibre peripheral neuropathy with autonomic involvement, occasionally with myopathic features and systemic problems (heart and kidney).

Myeloma

This causes central and peripheral neurological problems.

- **Spinal metastases.** Myeloma is the second most common cause of spinal metastases leading to myelopathy or cauda equina syndrome.
- **Cerebral metastases** typically involve the sella or cavernous sinus.
- **Peripheral neuropathy** has four main causes:
  1. Amyloidosis causes nerve infiltration or ischaemia from vasa nervorum involvement.
  2. Paraneoplastic.
  3. Direct infiltration.
  4. Plasmacytoma (osteosclerotic myeloma: 3% of myeloma) commonly presents with a demyelinating neuropathy associated with a low level lambda paraprotein, high CSF protein and sometimes a normal ESR. There is a male predominance. It occurs with POEMS syndrome (Polyneuropathy, Organomegaly, Endocrinopathy, M-protein and Skin changes). The marrow may be normal as the plasmacytoma is localized. It can respond to radiotherapy.

Lymphoma

Hodgkin's (HL) and Non-Hodgkin's lymphoma (NHL)

CNS complications are far more common with NHL than HL. They are mainly caused by direct spread either from a primary node or an extranodal site. Some 25% of NHLs present extranodally, although only 1% present with CNS disease.

Lymphoma and neurological illness. In a patient neurologically ill with lymphoma (or other cancers), consider several disease mechanisms:

- **Direct effects.** Spinal cord and meningeal involvement are common in lymphoma. Extra-dural deposits arise from direct spread from the retroperitoneum or post-mediastinal space via the intervertebral foramina; or from the vertebral body itself. *Note therefore that most lymphomas with CNS involvement have abnormal bone marrow.* The spinal dura prevents cord invasion; however, the cord becomes damaged by secondary ischaemia from dural compression.
- **Paraneoplastic effects** are more common in HL than NHL.
- **Predisposition to infection.** These include viral (including PML), bacterial and fungal (particularly aspergillus).
- **Metabolic effects.**
- **Treatment effects** (radiotherapy and/or chemotherapy): there is a huge range, from ifosfamide encephalopathy to cisplatin neuropathy.

Other neurological lymphomas

- **Primary CNS lymphoma** typically presents with brain parenchymal lesions, usually single, near the ventricles and with mass effect. They present with focal symptoms and headache. Seizures are rare owing to their sub-cortical and periventricular distribution. They are high-grade B cell lymphomas, perhaps causally related to Epstein–Barr virus infection. Thallium SPECT is useful, especially in HIV-positive patients, in showing a hotspot in lymphoma, but not in tuberculoma or toxoplasma.
- **Neurolymphomatosis.** This is a rare lymphoma of the peripheral nerves and although half have systemic lymphoma at autopsy, only the nerve pathology is obvious clinically. The lymphoma may also infiltrate into perivascular spaces of the brain parenchyma. It presents as a sub-acute painful, asymmetric neuropathy with cranial nerve involvement (including prominent bulbar involvement).
- **Intravascular lymphoma (neoplastic angioendotheliomatosis).** This unusual lymphoma presents like a vasculitis (see below) with radicular symptoms, encephalopathy, stroke-like events and sometimes a skin rash. It is difficult to diagnose in life and usually fatal, so frequently appears as the diagnosis at clinicopathological conferences.

Leukaemia

The neurological complications of lymphoma patients overlap with those of leukaemia. CNS problems are caused mainly by acute rather than chronic leukaemias.

- **Meningeal leukaemia** occurs particularly with acute lymphoblastic and acute myelomono-cytic leukaemia. Headache, lethargy and drowsiness are the most common symptoms. Papilloedema is the most common sign; cranial nerves 2, 3, 6, 7, 8 may be affected but lower cranial nerve involvement is rare. Myelopathic symptoms are unusual.
- **Solid non-lymphatic leukaemia** (chloroma) may cause space occupying brainstem lesions, cord compression, or venous sinus thrombosis, e.g. cavernous sinus with proptosis.
- **Intrathecal chemotherapy.** Methotrexate, Ara-c (used for CNS lymphomas and leukae-mias) and thiopental cause many complications including encephalopathy (white matter)

and myelopathy. Complications are particularly likely if also given radiotherapy; thus chemotherapy is therefore usually administered before radiotherapy.

NEPHROLOGY

Neurological disease arises through complications of renal failure, dialysis, renal transplantation and immunosuppression.

Renal failure

Uraemic encephalopathy

This is characterized by fatigue, obtundation, seizures, dysarthria, occasional focal signs and 'uraemic twitching,' a combination of negative (asterixis) and positive myoclonus. Muscle tone may be increased with extensor plantars.

Drugs exacerbate several aspects of the encephalopathy:

- **Myoclonus**, e.g. with tranexamic acid.
- **Confusion**, e.g. with ciprofloxacin.
- **Impaired consciousness**, sometimes prolonged for days, e.g. with opiates.

Hyperkalaemia

Renal patients risk developing hyperkalaemia, presenting as:

- **Severe weakness**, mimicking Guillain–Barré syndrome.
- **Cardiac arrhythmia**, common and more serious, presenting with cardiogenic syncope or sudden death.

Dialysis

Dialysis dysequilibrium

Dialysis causes major changes in:

- Circulating volume.
- Osmotic gradients between the brain (where urea concentrations remain high) and the blood (where urea is rapidly removed).

Dialysis dysequilibrium probably results from the cerebral oedema. This condition varies in severity from mild headache (the most common symptom) to coma.

Dialysis dementia

This was previously a common cause of intermittent dysarthria and later myoclonus and dementia in dialysis patients. The incidence fell dramatically by removing aluminium from dialysate. Aluminium inhibits dihydropteridine reductase and hence leads to impaired tetra-hydrobiopterin synthesis, needed for neurotransmitter synthesis. Desferrioxamine chelates aluminium and helps the problem.

Dialysis neuropathy

- **Peripheral neuropathy.** 60% of patients develop neuropathic symptoms on starting dialysis. 40% of renal failure patients develop cramps and restless legs.
- **Carpal tunnel syndrome** arises first as a complication of an arteriovenous fistula with high venous pressures and second through β_2 microglobulin accumulation causing, after 5 years or so, nerve (or rarely spinal cord) compression.

Renal transplantation

The necessary long-term immunosuppression risks several neurological complications.

- **Primary cerebral lymphoma** may develop as quickly as 3–6 months after transplantation (see above).
- **Opportunistic infections.** Up to 50% patients with allografts at autopsy have disseminated fungal infection; 30% of these have brain abscess, often from the lung. The most common are aspergillus, candida and nocardia. Cryptococcal meningitis may present with stroke.

HEPATOLOGY

Hepatic encephalopathy

This has four stages:

- Stage 1: impaired concentration and dysphoria.
- Stage 2: lethargy and personality change.
- Stage 3: somnolent but rousable, dysarthria.
- Stage 4: coma.

Asterixis becomes more evident with progression from stages 2 to 4; this roughly correlates with arterial ammonia concentration (Stage 1: 150–200 μg/dL through to stage 4: >301 μg/dL).

Acute (fulminant) hepatic failure

Viruses or drugs, e.g. paracetamol, are the usual causes. The encephalopathy appears within eight weeks of the liver disease. Neurological manifestations are prominent and death is usually from cerebral oedema.

Chronic liver disease

Chronic liver disease, notably alcoholic liver disease, may lead to encephalopathy arising either spontaneously or following certain precipitants, e.g. diuretics, gastrointestinal bleeding, high oral protein intake, or sepsis.

Pathogenesis

There are several mechanisms:

- **Toxin accumulation.** Gut derived toxins (e.g. ammonia, mercaptans, phenol), derived from bacterial degradation of lipids and protein are usually hepatically metabolized and so accumulate in liver disease.
- **Blood–brain barrier breakdown.** Manganese accumulates in the pallidum (high T1 signal on MRI), accounting for extrapyramidal features.
- **Aromatic amino acid accumulation** alters the ratio of aromatic to branched chain amino acids; this inhibits dopamine and noradrenaline synthesis and favours formation of false neurotransmitters such as octopamine.

Management

Reduce gut-derived toxins by:

- **Reducing protein intake** (20–30 g/day: discuss with dietician).
- **Increasing gut acidity.** Lactulose, an acidic non-absorbable disaccharide, binds to and promotes ammonia excretion, so promoting intracolic acidosis.

Prognosis

The coma of chronic liver disease has a relatively good prognosis compared to other causes of coma (although the underlying disease has a high mortality) and may cause recurrent coma episodes.

ELECTROLYTES

Sodium

Sodium abnormalities cause predominantly central neurological complications.

Hyponatraemia

Understanding the mechanism of hyponatraemia helps to guide management.

- **Hypovolaemia**, e.g. renal or gut fluid loss.
- **Euvolaemia**, e.g. inappropriate ADH secretion, hypothyroidism, Addison's disease.
- **Hypervolaemia**, e.g. cirrhosis, heart failure.

A serum sodium of <125 mmol/L causes confusion; <120 mmol/L causes seizures. This partly depends upon the rate of change, acute changes being more likely symptomatic.

Osmotic demyelination follows rapid hyponatraemia correction (>10 mmol/L per 24 h). It develops where white and grey matter are adjacent. Grey matter is more vascular than white and so here oligodendroglia are more vulnerable to osmotic forces.

- **Central pontine myelinolysis** (90% of cases) causes tetraparesis, pseudobulbar palsy, or locked-in syndrome (Fig. 15.2).
- **Extrapontine demyelination** (10% of cases) causes ataxia or extrapyramidal features.

Hypernatraemia

High sodium causes obtundation. The osmotic forces tend to shrink brain parenchyma; this may cause subdurals from disruption of bridging veins.

Potassium

Potassium abnormalities cause predominantly peripheral neurological complications:

- **Weakness** from low potassium levels.
- **Rhabdomyolysis and cardiac arrhythmias** from either high or low potassium levels.

Calcium

- **High calcium** reduces neuromuscular excitability, causing weakness.
- **Low calcium** causes tingling, muscle twitching and positive Chvostek and Trousseau signs. Chronically low calcium, e.g. from hypoparathyroidism, may cause movement disorders (parkinsonism or chorea) with basal ganglia calcification, myelopathy (secondary to vertebral foramina overgrowth), raised intracranial pressure and seizures.

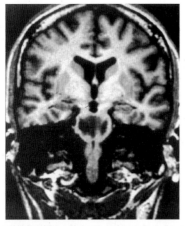

Figure 15.2
MRI showing central pontine myelinolysis.

Phosphate

Low phosphate is a commonly overlooked cause of weakness in sick patients.

Magnesium

- **Low magnesium levels** cause problems similar to low calcium levels.
- **High magnesium levels** (usually a renal or eclampsia patient) cause neuromuscular junction abnormalities and hence weakness and loss of reflexes (similar to LEMS).

ENDOCRINOLOGY

Diabetes mellitus

Neuropathy

Diabetes commonly causes neuropathy (see below).

Stroke

Stroke is twice as common in diabetics, even allowing for confounding risk factors, e.g. hypertension ($\approx$3 times more common among diabetics than the general population). Strokes affect both large and small vessels. Diabetes also increases the mortality and morbidity from stroke.

Acute complications

Diabetic ketoacidosis (DKA)

- **Coma** complicates 10% of DKA. Hyperosmolality forces water from brain cells. The hyperosmolality of DKA must be corrected only slowly, using normal saline to reduce the chance of cerebral oedema.
- **Mucor mycosis** (fungal rhinocerebral infection) may complicate the acidosis. It frequently involves the carotid artery causing stroke.
- **Thromboembolic events** may be precipitated by increased blood viscosity.

Hyperosmolar non-ketotic coma (HONK)

This manifests as very high glucose concentrations without acidosis (the small quantities of circulating insulin prevent hepatic ketogenesis).

- **Lethargy, obtundation and coma** occur in HONK more commonly than DKA. Seizures may occur and HONK is a cause of epilepsia partialis continua.
- **Transient focal features** have also been described, e.g. hemiparesis, hemianopia and hemichorea.
- **Cerebral oedema** is surprisingly rare, despite fluids and correction of the high serum glucose.

Hypoglycaemia

This may cause coma, focal problems and seizures. The symptoms are usually rapidly reversed, but repeated attacks can lead to cognitive decline.

Thyroid

Hyperthyroidism

Thyrotoxicosis presents to neurologists in various ways:

- **Mood and cognitive disturbance.** Irritability, emotional lability and sometimes confusion. Apathetic hyperthyroidism occurs in the elderly.
- **Worsening of pre-existing conditions,** e.g. epilepsy and migraine.
- **Cerebral venous thrombosis** from an increased thrombotic tendency (increased Factor VIII levels).
- **Dysthyroid orbitopathy** occurs with Graves' disease, unrelated to thyroid status. The oedema and lymphocytic infiltration of orbital tissues cause an external ophthalmoparesis and optic neuropathy. Early features of optic nerve involvement are colour vision disturbance and abnormal VEPs. Orbital imaging shows extra-ocular muscle enlargement. It is important to recognize and treat with steroids, surgery or radiotherapy. Note that diplopia in hyperthyroidism may be from myasthenia (5% of myasthenics are thyrotoxic). Imaging has largely supplanted the forced duction test.
- **Motor features.** Tremor, chorea, clonus and brisk reflexes are well-known features. Thyrotoxicosis enters the differential diagnosis of motor neurone disease.
- **Thyrotoxic myopathy** causes limb girdle weakness and sometimes wasting. The creatine kinase may be normal.
- **Thyrotoxic hypokalaemic periodic paralysis** occurs mainly in Orientals. It presents later than the familial periodic paralysis but has similar triggers (see Ch. 8).

Hypothyroidism

Hypothyroidism also presents to neurologists under various guises:

- **Mood and cognitive disturbance** occur in hypothyroidism. Occasionally a florid psychiatric picture may emerge ('myxoedema madness'), comprising delirium, hallucinations, abulia or irritability.
- **Hashimoto's encephalopathy** presents as cognitive problems and is unrelated to thyroid status. Patients develop confusion, seizures, myoclonus and catatonia. The EEG shows slow waves, CSF protein is raised and (although often euthyroid) there are high serum titres of thyroid microsomal or antithyroglobulin antibodies. The thyroiditis may be accompanied by a cerebral vasculitis or autoimmune encephalitis. It is among the differential diagnosis of CJD.
- **Motor features** are the most common hypothyroid neurological symptoms:
  - Proximal myopathy (with enlarged muscles: Hoffmann's syndrome).
  - Slow relaxing reflexes (Woltman's sign) are classical, best seen at the ankle.

- Electrically silent muscle depression on percussion (myoedema).
- Peripheral nerves features, e.g. carpal tunnel syndrome and polyneuropathy.
- Myasthenia gravis may co-exist.
- Ataxia (5–10% of cases).

PREGNANCY

Epilepsy

Epilepsy may become more difficult to control during pregnancy; it is the second most common cause of maternal death (after eclampsia). Seizure frequency increases through sleep deprivation, fatigue, reduced adherence to medications and altered pharmacokinetics, e.g. increased hepatic metabolism. A maternal convulsion risks direct fetal or placental trauma. However, the far greater fetal risk is teratogenicity from antiepileptic medication, especially in very early pregnancy. Advice on pre-conception counselling and epilepsy management in pregnancy are detailed in Chapter 3.

Migraine

Migraine typically improves during pregnancy. It is sensible to avoid medications in pregnancy if possible, although propranolol and amitriptyline prophylaxis are often used.

Idiopathic intracranial hypertension

This may present during (or be exacerbated by) pregnancy. Beware not to miss venous sinus thrombosis. It is generally managed by lumbar puncture during confinement, avoiding acetazolamide, which is potentially teratogenic.

Space occupying lesions

- **Tumours** sometimes enlarge during pregnancy, e.g. meningiomas and neurofibromas.
- **Arteriovenous malformations** may become symptomatic, particularly in the spinal cord. They typically cause both upper and lower motor neurone signs in the legs, sometimes with a spinal bruit.

Movement disorders

- **Chorea** may present in pregnancy: 70% have had rheumatic fever or previous chorea. The symptoms usually appear early in pregnancy. It is best to avoid medication if possible, using only small doses of benzodiazepine if needed. Those with previous possible rheumatic fever must undergo proper cardiac investigation.
- **Restless legs** are common (see Ch. 9).

Stroke

Stroke occurs for many reasons in pregnancy (1 in 3000 deliveries).

- **Dissection** of the carotid or vertebral arteries may occur during labour.
- **Venous thrombosis** (cerebral veins and sinuses) may result from the procoagulant state (decreased Protein S and C, increased procoagulants except Factors XI and XIII).
- **Embolic stroke** typically occurs post-partum and may be caused by lupus anticoagulant syndrome or cardiomyopathy developing following pregnancy, or by a paradoxical embolus (procoagulant state, Valsalva during delivery and patent foramen ovale). Choriocarcinoma embolus is rare.
- **Haemorrhage** may result from low platelets or hypertension in eclampsia. Aneurysm formation or rupture may also be more likely.

Multiple sclerosis

MS is unpredictable in pregnancy. The relapse rate appears lowered in late pregnancy and increased in the 3 months post-partum; overall, there is no adverse effect in the pregnancy year. Neither the pregnancy itself nor the number of pregnancies affects long-term disability.

Nerve lesions

Mononeuropathies. Carpal tunnel syndrome is more common during pregnancy. During labour, nerves become compressed, including the lumbosacral trunk (from the baby's head), obturator, femoral or common peroneal nerves from the lithotomy position.

Bell's palsy becomes more common in the third trimester. The decision to give medication in pregnancy needs to be taken individually. In non-gravid patients presenting within 72 h, consider corticosteroids and aciclovir (400 mg, 5 times daily), checking liver and renal profiles beforehand.

Myasthenia gravis (MG)

- **Clinical course.** MG may worsen with pregnancy (20%); one-third relapse after delivery. Corticosteroids and cholinesterases may be used; intravenous immunoglobulin and plasma exchange are also used.
- **Magnesium** (for eclampsia) may exacerbate the symptoms.
- **Transient neonatal myasthenia.** 10–15% of babies born to myasthenic mothers have transient MG, often not immediately but within 3 days; it usually resolves by 6 weeks. Note this is quite different from congenital myasthenia, a group of genetic conditions that persist.

FSH

For reasons that are unclear, FSH can deteriorate acutely in pregnancy and the resulting pelvic muscle weakness may make labour difficult (consider caesarean section).

Eclampsia

Clinical features. Hypertension, proteinuria and visual symptoms (eclampsia: Greek: 'to shine forth') herald eclampsia; seizures often follow. There may be low platelets and other organ dysfunction. MRI brain shows marked cortical and posterior white matter high signal abnormality (especially occipital).

Management is to deliver the baby and treat urgently with antihypertensives, anticonvulsants and steroids. Magnesium sulphate remains the best treatment for eclamptic seizures.

'Pre-eclampsia'. Note that thrombotic thrombocytopenic purpura (see above) affecting pregnant women before 24 weeks' gestation, causing headache, fluctuating consciousness and seizures, may be misdiagnosed as pre-eclampsia.

CARDIOLOGY

Infective endocarditis

This diagnosis is worth considering in many neurological situations. A total of 30% have neurological complications ranging from young stroke to elderly-onset confusion. Remember Osler's triad: fever, murmur and hemiparesis.

Embolic complications (infected or bland) are the most common cause of neurological complications:

- **Large emboli** often cause middle cerebral artery infarcts.
- **Micro-emboli** cause meningoencephalitis: the presentation includes psychiatric disorder, delirium, fluctuating consciousness and TIA-like events.
- **Immune complexes** settling on capillary walls contribute to the neurological manifestations. Elsewhere, these immune complexes cause glomerulonephritis, Janeway lesions, petechiae and Osler nodes.
- **Infected emboli** can cause cerebral abscess and meningitis (often sterile). Some 30% of staphylococcal meningitis, excluding trauma causes, originates from endocarditis. Infected emboli cause arteritis and mycotic aneurysms, with cerebral haemorrhage in up to 7% of endocarditis patients.

Cardiac surgery

Patients are commonly referred to neurologists after cardiac surgery.

Cognitive decline is the most common neurological problem after cardiac surgery, though most cases are not referred. It may be subtle and the reported incidence reflects the sensitivity of its measurement. The causes are multifactorial: drugs, micro-emboli (including cholesterol), hypoperfusion, metabolic complications, anaesthesia and infections.

Stroke is the most common referral (occurs in 2% of cardiac operations, of which 25% are fatal). Embolic causes are the most common, cerebral hypoperfusion less so. Severe aortic atherosclerosis and calcinosis usually pre-exist in those with stroke. The aortic cross-clamping time is often longer in those who develop strokes.

Prosthetic heart valves present challenging management dilemmas, e.g. how to treat intracerebral haemorrhage when a mechanical heart valve requires anticoagulation. Some statistics can help in managing this problem.

- The embolization risk from a prosthetic valve to the brain and other organs is 4% per patient year, reduced to 2.2% by anti-platelet drugs and to 1% with warfarin.
- The risk of prosthetic heart valve thrombosis without antiplatelet agents or anticoagulation is 1.8% per year. Thus, the risk of embolism from a prosthetic heart valve causing stroke is 4% per year plus 1.8% per year, i.e. 0.016% risk per day. Thus stopping anticoagulation for 6 weeks following an intracerebral haemorrhage carries a risk of stroke or valve thrombosis of 0.67%.
- The intracranial haemorrhage risk from anticoagulation increases 7–10-fold on warfarin (0.3–1% per year). The mortality from intracerebral haemorrhage in those on warfarin is 60%. Half of these continue to bleed beyond 24 h, compared with 10% of those with intracerebral haemorrhage who are not anticoagulated. There is therefore potential benefit to stopping anticoagulation early.
- The balance of risks may therefore favour reversing anticoagulation in prosthetic valve patients for 6 weeks.
- If anticoagulation is needed, heparin is recommended, being quickly reversible; however, its prolonged use is difficult owing to thrombocytopenia (>1%) and a paradoxical risk of thrombosis.

ALCOHOL

Alcohol affects all levels of the nervous system (Fig. 15.3); neurological referrals with alcohol-related neurological problems are common.

Seizures

Alcohol is often associated with seizures.

Epilepsy control is poorer with alcohol. Patients may avoid medication when they intend to drink, forget to take tablets if inebriated, vomit medication or become sleep deprived.

Withdrawal seizures ('rum fits') occur in patients with alcohol dependence, usually 7–48 h after stopping alcohol (95% within 12 h). Seizures affect 10% of alcoholics and are usually generalized tonic-clonic; focal seizures are unusual. Other withdrawal features include nervousness, tachycardia, tremor and hyperreflexia.

Hypoglycaemia must always be excluded in alcoholic patients presenting with seizures.

Delirium tremens

This occurs 2–5 days after stopping alcohol and affects 15–20% of alcoholics. It manifests as delirium, agitation, increased sympathetic activity, psychiatric problems (including visual

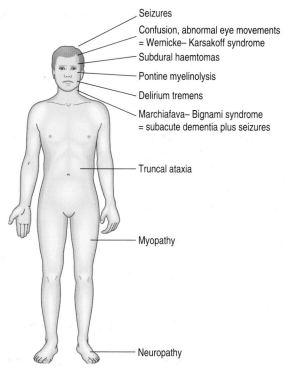

Seizures

Confusion, abnormal eye movements
= Wernicke– Karsakoff syndrome

Subdural haemtomas

Pontine myelinolysis

Delirium tremens

Marchiafava– Bignami syndrome
= subacute dementia plus seizures

Truncal ataxia

Myopathy

Neuropathy

Figure 15.3
The effects of alcohol on the nervous system. If co-existing nutritional problems consider Strachan's syndrome (optic nerve involvement and neuropathy) and pellagra.

hallucinations) and fever. Benzodiazepines are used; phenothiazines must be avoided as they lower the seizure threshold. General management includes correcting dehydration and low serum magnesium and potassium levels.

Dementia

Dementia and cognitive problems are common in alcohol abusers, with various causes.

- **Liver damage** (see above).
- **Wernicke's encephalopathy.** This is a common clinical problem which classically presents as ataxia, ophthalmoparesis and confusion. However, the 'full-house' is seen only in a minority. The ophthalmoparesis includes ptosis, extra-ocular muscle palsies and nystagmus, but seldom pupillary involvement. Blindness occurs rarely. There may be autonomic features, e.g. hypothermia. With thiamine treatment, the eye signs should resolve in hours to days. Thiamine pyrophosphate is a co-factor for many enzymes including pyruvate dehydrogenase: giving glucose can use up any last reserves and precipitate Wernicke's.

- **Korsakoff's psychosis.** This amnestic syndrome follows repeated Wernicke's episodes. Immediate recall (e.g. digit span) is unaffected but episodic memory is disrupted with confabulation. Other causes of the amnestic syndrome include hydrocephalus, tumours around the third ventricle, herpes simplex and human herpes virus 6, limbic encephalitis (paraneoplastic or potassium channelopathy: Morvan's fibrillary chorea), hypoxic-ischaemic encephalopathy and posterior circulation infarcts particularly to the dorsomedial or anterior thalamus.
- **Subdural haematoma** should be considered in alcoholics with confusion or dementia.
- **Pellagra** (nicotinic acid deficiency) causes diarrhoea, glossitis, anaemia and dermatitis (erythematous lesions in sun-exposed areas: Casal's necklace).
- **Porphyria cutanea tarda** may also cause a blistering rash in sun-exposed areas in alcoholics.
- **Marchiafava–Bignami disease** is corpus callosum demyelination presenting with frontal lobe dysfunction (e.g. abulia), pyramidal and extrapyramidal problems. Abstinence seldom completely reverses the symptoms.

Ataxia

The eye signs usually distinguish Wernicke's encephalopathy from alcoholic ataxia. Both predominantly affect axial coordination, giving gait ataxia rather than upper limb ataxia or dysarthria.

Central pontine myelinolysis

See above.

Infections

These are more common in alcoholics. It is important to consider bacterial infections including listeria (rhombo-encephalitis or micro-abscess formation) and tuberculosis.

Neuropathy

A distal sensorimotor neuropathy is common. It is unclear whether it is nutritional or the toxic effect of alcohol.

Myopathies

- **Acute painful myopathy** occurs 1–2 days after drinking, presenting as weakness with a high serum creatine kinase; rhabdomyolysis is a possibility.
- **Potassium or phosphate deficiency** may give acute but painless weakness.
- **Chronic myopathy,** typically painless and with a normal serum creatine kinase, progresses over weeks to months.

Stroke

- **Haemorrhagic stroke** is more common, due to abnormal clotting and higher blood pressure.

• **Ischaemic stroke** risk is reduced by moderate alcohol intake, but increased risk with heavier intake: this may relate to alcoholic cardiomyopathy or to thrombocytosis on alcohol withdrawal.

RHEUMATOLOGY

Vasculitis

These disorders often have neurological manifestations. Each causes dysfunction by ischaemia from increased vasomotor tone, activation of clotting cascades by endothelial dysfunction and vascular lumen narrowing by inflammation within vascular walls. The mechanism is either antibody-dependent (the most important) or cell-mediated.

Vasculitis can be classified according to the size of vessel involved.

Systemic necrotizing vasculitis

This comprises Churg–Strauss syndrome and polyarteritis nodosa (30% have hepatitis B).
Clinical features

• **Systemic manifestations** include fever, arthritis, weight loss and rash. It is important to check renal function and to test urine for protein and blood. Pulmonary features (asthma, lung infiltrates and eosinophilia) typify Churg–Strauss syndrome.
• **Peripheral manifestations** include:
  • Mononeuritis multiplex, hyperacute and often painful. Many have a sensory level at mid-extremity due to increased risk of nerve infarcts at watershed areas.
  • Diffuse polyneuropathy probably represents end-stage mononeuritis multiplex, unrecognizable due to multiple nerve involvement.
  • Cutaneous neuropathic symptoms include hyperaesthesia on soles or individual digits.
• **Central nervous system manifestations** are less common (see below).

Investigations. The diagnosis relies mainly upon the clinical features, but important investigations include nerve and muscle biopsy (or tissue obtained from another affected organ, e.g. skin or kidney) and c-ANCA.

Management. The following are used in severe vasculitis:

• Corticosteroid induction with methylprednisolone for 3 days, then high dose oral steroids (1 mg/kg per day).
• Cyclophosphamide (2.5 mg/kg per day) for 3 months. This may cause leucopenia (total white cells $<4 \times 10^9$, neutrophils $<2 \times 10^9$) and lung or heart toxicity, necessitating dose reduction. Transitional cell bladder cancer risk is increased (33 fold if >3 years treatment).
• Azathioprine helps to reduce the corticosteroid dose and is withdrawn slowly after 1 year of remission.

Prognosis. If untreated, the 5-year survival is only 10%. Immunosuppressive treatments improve survival.

Wegener's granulomatosis

Clinical features.

- Age of onset is 30–40 years.
- Upper and lower respiratory tract granulomas.
- Renal disease.
- Ear or nose discharge or sinus disease.
- Neurological manifestations (30%) including central and peripheral vasculitis and cavernous sinus disease.

Investigations. The diagnosis is clinical, but supportive investigations include biopsy, c-ANCA and chest X-ray.

Management is as for vasculitis.

Prognosis without treatment is poor (90% mortality after 2 years), but reasonably good with aggressive immunosuppression (90% remission).

Large vessel vasculitis

This comprises several conditions.

- **Giant cell arteritis.** (see Ch. 7).
- **Polymyalgia rheumatica** occurs mainly in women aged >55 years, presenting with limb muscle aching and stiffness. Investigation clues include elevated ESR and elevated platelet count. The symptoms melt away with steroids.
- **Takayasu's (pulseless) arteritis** affects young (often Asian) females (aged 11–30 years) with aortic and proximal vessel arteritis (98% have a major arterial pulse missing) and systemic features including weight loss, raised ESR, hypergammaglobulinaemia and mild anaemia. Patients present with TIAs, syncope, stroke or claudication. The diagnosis requires imaging of aortic arch, renal and other major arteries. The differential diagnosis includes syphilis and relapsing polychondritis.

Non-systemic vasculitis

- **Presentation.** Angiitis may be isolated to the central nervous system or the peripheral nervous system. There are few or no systemic features (e.g. in only 25% of primary CNS angiitis) and when present they call the diagnosis into question.
- **Differential diagnosis.** Vasculitic mimics include intravascular lymphoma, cholesterol emboli, lupus anticoagulant and bacterial endocarditis.
- **Investigations.** Biopsy is the important investigation (see above). Brain biopsy (e.g. non-dominant temporal lobe) has a morbidity of 0.5–2%. It is diagnostic in 75%, either confirming vasculitis (preferable before starting powerful immunosuppression) or revealing alternative (treatable) conditions, e.g. lymphoma, multiple sclerosis and toxoplasmosis.

Rheumatoid arthritis

This is common (prevalence 1–2%) and affects mainly women (3:1) with onset aged 35–50 years. There are several potential neurological problems.

Peripheral nerve

- **Peripheral neuropathy** affects 30% of patients; it is usually mild and managed conservatively.
- **Rheumatoid vasculitis** may also cause peripheral nerve damage. It tends to affect men with established disease or women on diagnosis. Rheumatoid vasculitis is suggested by rash, mononeuritis multiplex, or visceral involvement. The management is similar to that for vasculitis elsewhere.

Central nervous system

- **Myelopathy** has three main mechanisms:
  1. Atlanto-axial subluxation with upward migration of the odontoid process through foramen magnum (may present with occipital headache).
  2. Vertebral bony erosion or collapse.
  3. Dural thickening and fibrosis.
- **Dural rheumatoid nodules** are common and rarely thicken to become symptomatic.
- **CNS vasculitis** occasionally occurs in RA.

Medication side-effects

- **Corticosteroids** have neurological complications, e.g. myopathy.
- **Penicillamine** can cause myopathy and myasthenia gravis.

Case history outcome

The patient had Wilson's disease. He had Kayser–Fleischer rings and undetectable serum ceruloplasmin levels with abnormal LFTs. He was commenced on treatment with penicillamine and a low copper diet. His neurological problems stabilized and his LFTs normalized.

KEY POINTS

- Be aware of common general medical conditions presenting with acute neurological problems.
- Take care in sedating patients with general medical conditions: liver or respiratory patients.
- Consider haematological conditions as a cause for stroke.
- Metabolic derangement is a common cause of encephalopathy.

Further Reading

Aminoff M. Neurology and general medicine. London: Elsevier; 2001.

Functional neurology

16

Case history

A 21-year-old woman, 20 weeks pregnant, had been brought to casualty at midnight, convulsing and unconscious. Her blood sugar, arterial oxygen saturation, pulse rate, BP and ECG were normal. She had been given oxygen and intravenous diazepam. The convulsions came and went and were asynchronous in the arms and legs; at times she arched her back. Her eyes were shut; she resisted eye opening so the fundi were obscured. Her pupils reacted to light, her reflexes were present and her plantars were flexor. She withdrew her arm on gently squeezing her index finger. While talking to her, the movements lessened and she became tearful.

INTRODUCTION

Functional illness is common in every clinical speciality; 30% of neurology patients have some symptoms unexplained by organic disease. Functional neurological symptoms include motor and sensory disturbances, movement disorders and non-epileptic attacks.

CLASSIFICATION

Patients, when asked, prefer the term 'functional' to describe their non-organic symptoms. The disorders can broadly be classified as somatoform (which are common) or factitious (which are rare).

Somatoform disorder

This implies a physical problem arising from psychological factors.

- **Conversion disorder** where physical symptoms result from a painful psychic conflict.
- **Panic disorder.** Discrete panic attacks are associated with apprehension and fear. The symptoms are intermittent, of sudden onset and without obvious provoking factors.
- **Somatization disorder** is characterized by a heightened awareness of bodily sensations (that others might regard as normal), leading to numerous reported somatic symptoms. These include gynaecological, gastrointestinal and neurological problems. The prevalence of the full syndrome (women more than men) is 1 in 1000, but mild degrees are common.

Factitious disorder

The patient presents with physical symptoms (apparently 'put on') to satisfy a psychological need.

- **Münchausen syndrome**, where numerous and often dramatic symptoms are reported, intending to provoke unnecessary medical intervention. 'Münchausen by proxy' is where a child is presented with apparently serious symptoms, fabricated or induced by the parent.
- **Malingering** implies illness faked to avoid work, or to gain compensation.

PATHOPHYSIOLOGY

Functional somatoform symptoms are genuine and not intentionally feigned. Functional imaging supports this, e.g. single photon emission computed tomography shows reduced thalamic and basal ganglia blood flow contralateral to the functional sensorimotor loss. These structures modulate motor behaviour and may interfere with readiness to move; other studies have shown downstream abnormalities, e.g. inhibition of willed movements from the orbitofrontal or cingulate cortex.

DIAGNOSING FUNCTIONAL SYMPTOMS

Medical training understandably emphasizes disease diagnosis. Trainees in particular are often reluctant to diagnose functional illness, wanting to avoid overlooking serious pathology. Recent studies show that regional and tertiary centres misdiagnose 5% of functional illnesses, far fewer than Slater's 1960s report, the study that shaped many neurologists' perception of missed organic diagnoses.

History taking

Diagnostic clues to functional illness are the large number of symptoms, the numerous previous clinical consultations and (careful here) an inability to obtain a clear and consistent account of the symptoms.

- **List all the problems:** this may include many symptoms, not all neurological. When and how did they start?
- **Go through the previous medical records.** Has the patient seen numerous specialists or had many operations without finding clear pathology?
- **Previous experiences and explanations from clinicians:** these will guide your approach and explanation.
- **Identify illness beliefs;** concerns about particular diseases can be specifically addressed with the patient.
- **Illness behaviour and predicament (handicap).** How does the patient spend a typical day? Are there relevant social (job, compensation claim, caring for sick relatives) or family dynamics hindering recovery.

- **Emotional aspects.** Ask about appetite, activity and sleep (insomnia is often psychiatric or psychological, whereas excessive sleepiness often organic). Listen to the patient's speech prosody. Ask whether their problems get them down.
- **Hyperventilation.** This is a common anxiety manifestation; it may result from anxiety about neurological symptoms (and so complicate the clinical picture) and may itself provoke neurological symptoms. Ask about breathlessness, sensations of incomplete lung filling, tingling around the face and peripheries, throat and chest tightness and light-headedness.
- **Dissociation symptoms:** depersonalization (oneself is not real) or derealization (the world is not real).
- **Post-traumatic stress.** While not routine practice to ask about abuse, enquiring about childhood (e.g. age at first memory), schooling, relations with other family members, etc. may facilitate appropriate disclosure.

Examination

Accessories

Patients using accessories, e.g. cervical collar, back brace, or seemingly unnecessary crutches, sticks, or wheelchair, raise suspicion of non-organic disease. Such equipment should bear evidence of frequent use and not be used only to visit the doctor.

Motor signs

- **'Slow motion'.** Patients with functional disorders often appear to use great deliberation and effort.
- **'Giving-way'.** Collapsing weakness may be functional, but may result from pain, attention difficulty, or even some neurological illnesses (see below). The arm drop test is performed by the examiner placing an apparently flaccid upper limb above the patient's face and allowing it to 'drop'. In functional paralysis the descent of the limb is slow and jerky.
- **Variability of strength.** Functional weakness may improve with encouragement: ask the patient to look at the limb and to try very hard, encouraged in a firm voice.
- **Hoover's sign.** This demonstrates absent contralateral limb stabilization during straight leg raising: i.e. a hand beneath the left heel should detect a pressing down on attempted elevation of the right leg.
- **Gait.** 'Bizarre' gaits may accompany non-organic motor symptoms. Features include leg dragging without other hemiparetic features, odd limb posturing or a tendency to topple towards the examiner without falling.
- **Other inconsistencies.** The patient with weakness may be unable to their lift legs from couch, yet swing them around when climbing off; or unable to lift an arm on command, yet do so when dressing. However, note that higher motor disorders may show a similar disparity (see below).

Sensory signs

There are no clear signs of functional sensory loss, but the combination of factors may suggest the diagnosis.

- **Hemisensory loss** (usually left sided) is a well-recognized functional symptom closely linked to hyperventilation. Superficial reflexes over apparently numb areas, e.g. superficial abdominal or corneal reflexes, are preserved.
- **Midline sensory loss.** Consider a thalamic cause. Vibration sense should be preserved over such an area.
- **Hairline boundary.** Sensory loss either stopping or starting at the hairline clearly does not conform to either dermatomal or trigeminal distributions. Beware of leprosy, which can have this distribution.
- **Back pain.** Some patients reporting back pain may have apparently limited straight leg raising, yet be able to sit forwards with legs extended on the couch to allow low back inspection.

Visual disorders

- **Visual loss.** A discrepancy between the ability to carry out daily tasks and the results of objective tests might suggest non-organic visual loss. Preservation of optokinetic nystagmus despite complete blindness might support a functional cause.
- **Visual field abnormalities.** Tubular field defects ('tunnel' rather than 'funnel') are not consistent with the science of optics.

COMMON FUNCTIONAL NEUROLOGICAL SYNDROMES

Non-epileptic attack disorder

These can be categorized into two main groups: panic disorder and conversion disorder. In general, non-epileptic attacks from anxiety are common in patients with pre-existing epilepsy, whereas conversion disorder patients often do not have epilepsy. Most neurologists do not witness many seizures: seizures occurring in clinic are statistically more likely to be psychogenic.

Panic disorder

Panic symptoms commonly cause diagnostic confusion with complex partial seizures for three reasons:

1. **Panic symptoms resemble seizures,** e.g. epigastric sensations, light-headedness, distant feelings and even loss of consciousness from hyperventilation.
2. **Panic symptoms exacerbate epilepsy.** Hyperventilation lowers the seizure threshold and disrupted sleep pattern from anxiety may worsen epilepsy.
3. **Panic disorder may result from epilepsy.** Epilepsy is very frightening and itself provokes anxiety and sometimes panic. Since anxiety symptoms resemble seizures, this can result in a vicious cycle of apparently worsening epilepsy.

Conversion disorder

The classical patient with conversion non-epileptic attack disorder is female, with a history of apparently resistant epilepsy beginning after the age of 10 years, previous episodes of apparent status epilepticus, previous multiple hospital admissions (asthma, abdominal or chest pain), previous self harm and a history of childhood physical or sexual abuse. The diagnostic gold standard is video telemetry. Prolonged non-epileptic attacks are common: 50% of convulsive status epilepticus patients admitted to hospital are not epileptic. There may be clues in the attack semiology to non-epileptic attacks (Box 16.1).

Cognition and consciousness

- **Memory loss** reported by anxious patients is often attributable to poor concentration. Patients reporting their own memory loss often have poor concentration and anxiety rather than dementia; unconcerned patients whose carers report the problem more often have true dementia. If memory loss patients are asked to rate their memory tasks performance, patients with anxiety often report performing poorly (despite good

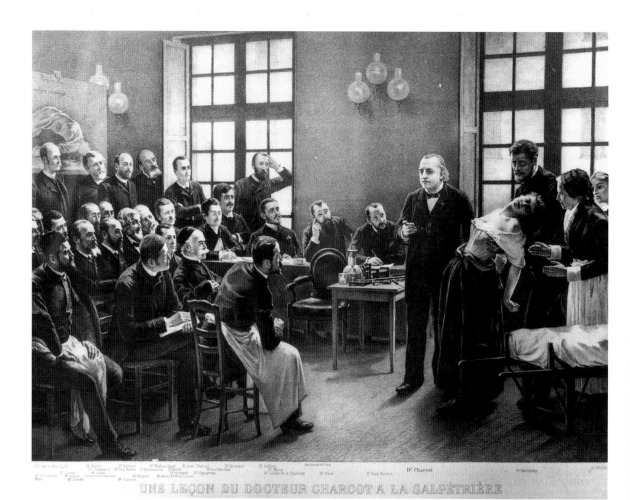

UNE LEÇON DU DOCTEUR CHARCOT A LA SALPÊTRIÈRE

Figure 16.1
Charcot demonstrating 'pseudoseizures' (with permission from the Freud Museum©, London).

> **Box 16.1: *Features distinguishing non-epileptic from epileptic attacks***
>
> - **Situation**. Non-epileptic attacks typically occur in stressful situations, e.g. in the waiting room, while shopping.
> - **Motor activity** is asynchronous, whereas in true seizures, the movements of the arms and legs are synchronous during the clonic phase. Movements come and go throughout the attack; in each component, the motor activity is unchanged, unlike a seizure, where it gradually diminishes during the clonic phase. Semi-purposeful movements may occur during pseudoseizures, e.g. pushing away, whereas automatisms of seizures are not usually purposeful.
> - **Pelvic thrusting** and opisthotonic posturing occur, but are not expected in seizures.
> - **Apnoea** and even cyanosis may accompany pseudoseizures. However, breath is held on inspiration; whereas in the tonic phase of a seizure breath is held in expiration.
> - **Eyes are closed** in typical pseudoseizures, whereas the eyes are often open in a seizure. There is resistance to eye opening. In pseudoseizures, if the eyes are forcibly opened, Bell's phenomenon occurs avoiding gaze. The pupil response is preserved, whereas in a seizure, gaze is fixed (sometimes to one side) and the pupillary light response is often absent.
> - **Biting:** In functional episodes, there may be biting of the tip of the tongue or the cheek; in a seizure the side of the tongue is bitten.
> - **Duration:** functional episodes can continue for many minutes: seizures usually last less than 2 min.
> - **Crying** afterwards is more common with functional episodes.
> - **Recovery:** patients are quickly orientated (though often report sleepiness) after a pseudoseizure, but have prolonged confusion after a seizure.

results), whereas demented patients often report performing well (despite poor results). The TOMM (test of memory malingering) may be administered; tests like this rely on patients performing worse than chance (thus suggesting deliberate underperformance).

- **Pseudocoma** can quickly be distinguished from true coma on clinical grounds. If doubt remains, then caloric testing is helpful (but cruel!): iced water into an ear induces vertigo, nystagmus and vomiting in alert patients.

Movement disorders

The unusual nature of a movement disorder does not necessarily imply that it is functional. Many dystonias, e.g. blepharospasm and writer's cramp, were originally considered entirely functional; clinicians must therefore adopt a cautious approach and an open mind. Undoubtedly, there are some functional movement disorders, especially in patients presenting with tremor or gait disorder.

Tremor

Several features suggest that a tremor is psychogenic.

- **Abrupt onset.**
- **Variable frequency.** The examining clinician may be able to change this (Fig. 16.2).
- **Variable amplitude.** This may diminish on approaching a target. Lifting a weight may change the amplitude and frequency.
- **Distractibility.** The tremor changes with distraction.
- **Entrainment.** The tremor entrains to a rhythm tapped out by the contralateral (normal) limb.

289

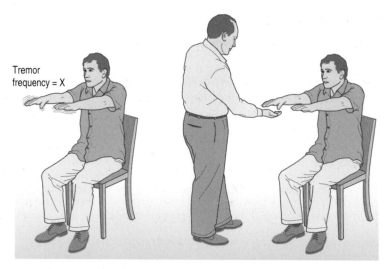

With patient sitting in chair, examiner says 'tap my hand with this rhythm', and clicks out a rhythm with foot–observes patient's free hand–and tremor frequency changes from X to that imposed by examiner

Figure 16.2
Examiner can change the frequency of the tremor. Tremor frequency (X) is measured with the patient sitting in a chair. The examiner says 'clap my hand with this rhythm' and clicks out a rhythm. Examiner observes the patient's free hand: tremor frequency change from X is that imposed by the examiner.

Dystonia

Patients with psychogenic dystonia comprise 2–3% of those attending a dystonia clinic. It is a difficult diagnosis and must be made only with caution. Important features include:

- **Occurrence at rest.** Organic dystonia generally starts on action. However, dystonia paradoxically improving with movement can occur with neuroleptic-induced dystonias.
- **Onset in the foot or leg in adults.** Whereas childhood onset dystonia can begin in the lower limbs, adult onset focal dystonia is usually in the head, neck or arm. However, foot dystonia in adults may occur in coeliac disease, corticobasal degeneration or dopa-responsive dystonia.

Speech disorder

Dysphasia. Anxious patients commonly experience difficulty saying clearly what they wish to say; although the symptom is intermittent, its distinction from mild dysphasia may be difficult.

MIMICS OF FUNCTIONAL ILLNESS

Finding non-organic signs never excludes a serious underlying disorder. It is important to consider 'functional elaboration' of an underlying disorder, where patients subconsciously 'help' the clinician by exaggerating certain signs.

Some neurological disorders may lead to an erroneous diagnosis of functional illness.

Conditions with 'give-way' weakness

- **Myasthenia gravis.** During attempted sustained effort, fewer and fewer muscle fibres contract leading to an abrupt 'give way'.
- **Demyelinating neuropathy.** It is alarming how frequently Guillain–Barré syndrome is initially diagnosed as functional. In some demyelinating neuropathies, attempted tetanic muscle contraction is disturbed by abnormal axon excitability, causing sudden 'giving' (hyperpolarization block).
- **Sensory inattention,** e.g. in right-sided parietal lesions, may lead to apparent giving way.
- **Sensory ataxia.** Patients with loss of position sense (e.g. in acute polyneuropathy) sometimes appear unable to sustain voluntary effort.
- **Pain** is an important reason for people to avoid full effort in strength testing.
- **Anxiety** superimposed upon organic symptoms may lead to giving way in a mildly weak or numb limb.

Episodic disorders

- **Paroxysmal dystonias** may present with bizarre episodic movements induced by tasks, alcohol or caffeine.
- **Episodic weakness** may be secondary to periodic paralysis, myasthenia gravis or Uthoff's phenomenon in demyelination. Some spinal cord vascular malformations may cause periods of weakness related to exercise or heavy meals.
- **Frontal lobe seizures.** There may be bizarre hypermotor features, sometimes with retained consciousness, resistance to medication and even a normal ictal EEG ('pseudo-pseudoseizures'). The clue is that they are typically brief and stereotyped and usually begin in sleep.
- **Hypoglycaemia** may cause intermittent altered consciousness and bizarre behaviour.
- **Porphyria.** Symptoms may occur in acute relapses and be associated with pain and psychiatric symptoms: this can easily be mis-labelled as functional.

Other motor problems

- **Praxis disorders.** Gait apraxia may cause profound walking difficulty, yet examination on the couch may be relatively normal. There may be disparity between parts of the examination. For example, an elderly patient who cannot walk may have strong arms and legs, intact joint position sense, no cerebellar signs and have no parkinsonian features: consider hydrocephalus or small vessel disease.
- **Axial ataxia** (usually from alcohol) may be disabling only when the patient tries to stand or walk.
- **Frontal lobe syndromes.** Frontal meningioma and frontal lobe dementia (including variant CJD) are often diagnosed late. They often present first with behaviour changes unmatched by changes on routine mental function testing.

Swallowing and speech disorders

- These are not well localized and cannot be readily tested for; they are therefore easily mislabelled as non-organic. Important causes include myopathy, neuromuscular junction

disorders, peripheral nerve disease and sometimes brain disorders. There are also mechanical causes, e.g. osteophytes, tumours at tongue base and achalasia.
- Oro-buccal dyspraxia, e.g. in frontotemporal dementia, means the patient cannot cough voluntarily but will cough if something goes down the wrong way.

Sensory symptoms

- MS (even glioma) presenting with somatic sensory symptoms may show no definite physical signs in the early stages. Naturally, the patient will be anxious; it is easy to mis-label these symptoms as functional. Careful examination may identify 2-point discrimination abnormalities, especially with lateralized symptoms.
- Unusual patchy sensory loss, for example, stopping at the hairline, may occur with leprosy.

INVESTIGATIONS

Presumed functional symptoms are often investigated to reassure patients or clinicians. It is worth outlining to the patient the type of pathology being sought and the risk of uncovering irrelevant abnormalities, e.g. incidental sinus disease or even a small meningioma that may not explain the symptoms. Some imaging 'abnormalities,' e.g. white dots on MR brain scan, incidental lumbar or cervical spondylosis, may only reinforce the patient's misplaced notion of organic disease.

In patients with non-epileptic attacks, particularly if the events continue, or if the patient or family doubt the diagnosis, a prolonged EEG, ideally capturing one of the events, gives greater certainty. Informing the patient about the results and perhaps watching a recorded event together can be useful. If possible, the investigations should be performed reasonably quickly and the results promptly discussed with the patient.

MANAGEMENT

Patients with functional symptoms form a large proportion of the outpatient workload: it is worth investing time and effort to develop helping strategies. When diagnosed and appropriately managed early, the prognosis can be excellent. But once established, many patients remain considerably disabled; 30–50% of patients with functional weakness are unchanged after 1 year.

An explanation (following any investigations) is the key to managing the patient. This should emphasize:

- There is no test to prove or disprove a functional diagnosis: the patient and clinician must each accept that there is some uncertainty, but that stress factors are a definite and treatable component of the symptoms.
- This type of symptom is common, real and disabling; they are not made-up or willed. It can be helpful to involve the family, e.g. what should they do if the patient were to have another funny turn.

- Avoid 'reassurance' without evidence: patients with symptoms will not be reassured simply by being told that there is nothing to worry about; some will worry more and seek further opinions.
- An explanation of the mechanism of symptoms is sometimes helpful. Some symptoms are akin to flushing, sweaty palms, pupil size: they happen normally and automatically, with no control over them. A computer analogy may help: the problem is with the software; the hardware is working; the system needs rebooting. Thus the symptoms have the potential to improve.
- Gentle encouragement to move an affected limb passively (or asking a partner to help). Encourage gentle regular exercise, e.g. swimming.
- Agree achievable goals, e.g. to be met before the review appointment: goals are appropriate to all rehabilitation situations and give clear purpose to a therapy.
- Physiotherapy can rebuild confidence and extend treatment goals.
- Medications occasionally help, although generally are best avoided in this situation. Consider agreeing a 2–3 months trial of antidepressants (e.g. amitriptyline or SSRI) in those where pain, mood changes or sleep disturbance predominate (the number needed to treat is 2–3).
- The patient's predicament is at least partly due to the diagnosis itself (e.g. of epilepsy) as opposed to the symptoms: the clinician should appreciate that removing a diagnosis may appear disadvantageous to the patient who risks losing credibility with family and friends, as well as the secondary gains of sickness benefits, support and attention.
- Clinical psychology or psychiatry colleagues may help, particularly with more resistant symptoms; some tertiary neuropsychiatry units specifically manage functional illness.
- Follow-up should be arranged, with neurology and/or with clinical psychology.
- Admission of patients with chronic problems to rehabilitation wards gives little lasting success.
- Written information is important, including copies of letters to the general practitioner and recommended websites. Patients must be confident that the clinician is being entirely open with them.

Case history outcome

The diagnosis was psychogenic non-epileptic attack disorder. The first management step was to obtain a more detailed history from the patient and her family. There was a history of previous similar episodes, but no previous diagnosis of epilepsy and no immediately obvious triggers to this attack. The vital signs, blood sugar and ECG were normal. The clinician explained that this was not an epileptic seizure and that anti-epileptic drugs would not help. The patient agreed to be seen by the clinical psychologist. Over a series of consultations, the patient disclosed several emotionally traumatic issues; these were appropriately addressed and the episodes settled.

KEY POINTS

- Functional illness is common; with appropriate work-up, few serious diagnoses are missed.
- Examination looks for inconsistency in symptoms and signs. Hoover's test is particularly helpful.

- Anxiety symptoms resemble neurological symptoms (tingling, blurred vision, headache) and commonly co-exist with organic neurological symptoms.
- Finding definite 'hysterical' signs (e.g. tunnel vision) does not exclude underlying organic disease: anxious patients may subconsciously exaggerate signs.
- 'Give way' weakness can be organic (myasthenia gravis, demyelinating neuropathy, pain, inattention) as well as functional.
- If you are going to investigate, do so quickly and discuss results promptly; do not opt to do more and more investigations.
- Non-organic aspects of disease are often more treatable than the underlying condition (e.g. depression in dementia or MS).
- Explanation is the key: consider using analogies; avoid reassurance and certainty, but rather share the evidence.
- Agree small but realistic goals and plan review.
- Exercise caution in diagnosing non-organic disease if the patient is >40 or the doctor is <40 years of age.

Further Reading

Stone J, Zeman A, Sharpe M. Functional weakness and sensory disturbance. J Neurol Neurosurg Psychiatry 2002; 73(3): 241–245.

Index